PRIMARY ANGIOPLASTY

PRIMARY ANGIOPLASTY

MECHANICAL INTERVENTIONS FOR ACUTE MYOCARDIAL INFARCTION

SECOND EDITION

Edited by

DAVID ANTONIUCCI

Careggi Hospital
Florence, Italy

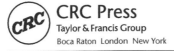

CRC Press
Taylor & Francis Group
Boca Raton London New York

CRC Press is an imprint of the
Taylor & Francis Group, an **informa** business

CRC Press
Taylor & Francis Group
6000 Broken Sound Parkway NW, Suite 300
Boca Raton, FL 33487-2742

First issued in hardback 2017

ISBN 13: 978-1-138-11465-4 (pbk)
ISBN 13: 978-1-84184-662-0 (hbk)

Library of Congress Cataloging-in-Publication Data

Primary angioplasty : mechanical interventions for acute myocardial infarction / edited by David Antoniucci. — 2nd ed.
    p. ; cm.
  Includes bibliographical references and index.
  ISBN-13: 978-1-8418-4662-0 (hardcover : alk. paper)
  ISBN-10: 1-8418-4662-7 (hardcover : alk. paper)   1. Angioplasty. 2. Myocardial infarction. I. Antoniucci, David.
  [DNLM: 1. Myocardial Infarction—surgery. 2. Angioplasty—methods.
WG 300 P9513 2009]
  RD598.5.P747 2009
  617.4′13—dc22

                                                                                                                2009000132

**Visit the Taylor & Francis Web site at
http://www.taylorandfrancis.com**

**and the CRC Press Web site at
http://www.crcpress.com**

Preface

The advances in the percutaneous mechanical treatment of acute myocardial infarction since the publication of the first edition of *Primary Angioplasty* have required an extensive revision of all chapters.

During this period several randomized trials provided a definite answer about the role of new devices and drugs for the treatment of myocardial infarction. This new edition analyzes critically the results of studies on antiembolic and thrombectomy devices, including negative studies such as the EMERALD and the AIMI trials, and studies on drug-eluting stents and new adjunctive antithrombotic treatments, such as the HORIZONS trial. Moreover, a new chapter on the impact of bleeding on outcome has been added, while the revised chapter on imaging modalities provides an updated definition of the role of echographic, scintigraphic, and MRI studies for the assessment of the efficacy of reperfusion and of complex processes such as ventricular remodeling.

To minimize fragmentations and inconsistencies and to avoid the impersonal tone of many multiauthored texts, I chose to confirm the enlistment of the same authors of the first edition and to include new authors from the same investigator group of the Careggi Hospital in Florence, Italy.

The text maintains the same structure that includes four sections: the clinical perspective, the technical perspective, the vessel perspective, and the efficacy perspective. In the new edition, we have included more than 40 exemplary cases captured in the accompanying DVD. Many of these cases contain specific features that were approached using strategies made on individual basis without the help of the indications provided by randomized trials that usually excluded very elderly patients and patients with very complex coronary anatomy from randomization.

All sections are structured as independent components and provide an updated patient- and lesion-specific approach, including "tips and tricks" learned by personal experience in thousands of patients with acute myocardial infarction.

I hope that this new edition will confirm the approval of the first edition, and will prove useful to those involved in primary percutaneous coronary interventions and aid in the care of patients with acute myocardial infarction. To the extent that it achieves this goal, credit must be given to the persons involved in its preparation.

My appreciation goes to the authors who contributed to this text and the editorial and production staff at Informa Healthcare for all their help in making this edition a reality.

David Antoniucci

Contents

Case Index (DVD)
Renato Valenti, Angela Migliorini, and Guido Parodi

1. Anterior AMI. Multilesion LAD PCI.

2. Inferior AMI and multivessel disease.

3. Inferior AMI. Direct RCA stenting complicated by distal macroembolization.

4. Anterior AMI complicated by cardiogenic shock. LM thrombotic occlusion
   and RCA ostium stenosis.

5. Inferior AMI. Primary multivessel intervention.

6. NSTEMI. LM calcific lesion and 3-vessel disease. Multivessel DES
   revascularization.

7. NSTEMI complicated by cardiogenic shock. Multivessel DES revascularization
   of LM complex anatomy trifurcation and 3-vessel disease.

8. NSTEMI complicated by heart failure. Diffuse multivessel disease. Aorto-iliac
   kinking. Multivessel DES revascularization.

9. Lateral AMI. Multivessel PCI: culprit OM branch and nonculprit LAD.

10. Anterior AMI. Three vessel simultaneous thrombosis. Multivessel PCI.

11. Inferior AMI. Large thrombus post-RCA stenosis. Thrombectomy aspiration.

12. Anterolateral AMI complicated by heart failure. Multivessel disease. Ulcerated
    plaque of LAD with macroembolization. Rheolytic thrombectomy and multivessel PCI.

Contributors

Piergiovanni Buonamici   Division of Cardiology, Careggi Hospital, Florence, Italy

Nazario Carrabba   Division of Cardiology, Careggi Hospital, Florence, Italy

Giampaolo Cerisano   Division of Cardiology, Careggi Hospital, Florence, Italy

Emilio Vincenzo Dovellini   Division of Cardiology, Careggi Hospital, Florence, Italy

Angela Migliorini   Division of Cardiology, Careggi Hospital, Florence, Italy

Guia Moschi   Division of Cardiology, Careggi Hospital, Florence, Italy

Guido Parodi   Division of Cardiology, Careggi Hospital, Florence, Italy

Giovanni Maria Santoro   Division of Cardiology, San Giovanni di Dio Hospital, Florence, Italy

Renato Valenti   Division of Cardiology, Careggi Hospital, Florence, Italy

Supplementary Resources Disclaimer

Additional resources were previously made available for this title on CD. However, as CD has become a less accessible format, all resources have been moved to a more convenient online download option.

You can find these resources available here: www.routledge.com/9781841846620

Please note: Where this title mentions the associated disc, please use the downloadable resources instead.

Section 1
The Clinical Perspective

1

Pathophysiology Basics of Acute Myocardial Infarction

GUIDO PARODI

Division of Cardiology, Careggi Hospital, Florence, Italy

THE EPICARDIAL VESSEL

Atherosclerotic plaque rupture in the coronary arteries is thought to underlie most acute coronary syndromes (ACSs), including unstable angina and acute myocardial infarction (AMI), as well as many cases of sudden cardiac death, and thus is a major cause of overall mortality and morbidity (1). This process characterizes the clinical transition from stable coronary artery disease to ACSs.

Intracoronary thrombosis, the immediate result of plaque rupture, was hypothesized to be the cause of AMI as early as 1912 by Herrick (2). However, plaque rupture and resulting intracoronary thrombosis were not universally accepted as major mechanisms underlying the ACS until the modern medical era. Large-scale randomized, controlled trials confirming the efficacy of thrombolytic therapy were not performed until over 70 years after Herrick's report.

Mortality from ACS began declining before thrombolysis became routine therapy (3), even as a result of treatments that ameliorate the effects of atherosclerotic plaque rupture (i.e., antithrombotics, antianginal therapy, and revascularization techniques). Thrombolytic therapy in the most recent large-scale randomized trials still yields high one-month mortality and recurrent cardiac event rates (4).

A novel approach in the treatment of AMI was found to be necessary despite declining overall cardiac mortality.

Atherosclerotic Plaque Morphology

Types of atherosclerotic plaques vary widely in morphology even when found in different locations in the coronary arteries of the same patients (Table 1.1).

Recent insights into the basic mechanism involved in the atherogenesis indicate that deleterious alterations of endothelial physiology, also referred to as endothelial dysfunction, represent a key early step in the development of atherosclerosis and are also involved in plaque progression and the occurrence of atherosclerotic complications (5). The initiation of atherosclerosis plaque has been correlated with the presence of a number of risk factors (e.g., hyperlipidemia, diabetes mellitus, hypertension, smoking, aging, obesity), leading to endothelial dysfunction. This endothelial dysfunction is characterized by increased permeability, reduced synthesis and release of nitric oxide, and overexpression of adhesion molecules (e.g., intracellular adhesion molecule-1, vascular cell adhesion molecule-1, and selectins) and chemoattractans

Table 1.1 Atherosclerotic Lesion Types

Plaque type	Characteristics of plaque	Clinical syndrome
I	Intimal thickening, macrophages, isolated foam cells	Asymptomatic
II, "Fatty streak"	Accumulation of intracellular lipid in infiltrating macrophages and smooth muscle cells	Asymptomatic
III	Incipient extracellular lipid and connective tissue deposition	Asymptomatic
IV, "Atheroma"	Large extracellular intimal lipid core; inflammatory cell infiltration, including macrophages, foam cells, and T cells	Usually asymptomatic; can also be associated with stable angina
Va	Atheroma with fibrous layer or layers	Stable angina
Vb	Atheroma with extensive calcification in the lipid core or elsewhere	Stable angina
Vc	Fibrosed atheroma or organized mural thrombus with minimal or absent lipid components	Stable angina
VI, "Complicated"	Disrupted type IV or V lesion with intramural hemorrhage and/or thrombosis	Acute coronary syndrome or asymptomatic lesion progression

Source: From Ref. 8.

[e.g., monocyte chemoattractant protein-1 (MCP-1), macrophage colony-stimulating factor, interleukin-1 and interleukin-6, and interferon-α and interferon-γ]. These processes facilitate the recruitment and internalization of circulating monocytes and low-density lipoprotein. The lipid material accumulated within the subendothelial space becomes oxidized and triggers an inflammatory response that induces the release of different chemotactic and proliferative growth factors. In response to these factors, smooth muscle cells and macrophages activate, migrate, and proliferate, resulting in the thickening of the arterial wall (5,6).

The earliest recognizable lesion of atherosclerosis is the intimal thickening (type I lesion), an aggregation of lipid-rich macrophages and T lymphocytes within the innermost layer of the artery wall, the intima. Early lesions mature into others with smooth muscle cell infiltration and lipid (type II, "fatty streak") and connective tissue deposition (type III) (7). The ubiquity and precocity of the atherosclerotic process are attested by the finding of fatty streak in the coronary arteries of half of the autopsy specimens from children aged 10 to 14 years. The early lesions develop within the first three decades of life in areas of localized turbulent flow within the coronary arteries (7). Their development is accelerated by conditions such as hypercholesterolemia, diabetes mellitus, hypertension, and smoking. As these early lesions grow into softer plaques with a high extracellular lipid and cholesteryl ester content and progressively thinner fibrous cap (types IV—Va, "atheroma"), they become more vulnerable to disruption (8). Ruptured plaques with overlying thrombus (type VI) are described as "complicated lesions." These lesions contain a great number of cell types, including inflammatory cells and smooth muscle cells. When they achieve a significant degree of stenosis to decrease flow without sufficient collateral circulation, these lesions result in ACSs. In the period after the plaque

rupture, thrombus over the complicated disrupted lesion organizes and the lesion calcifies (type Vb) or fibroses (type Vc) into chronic stenotic lesions (8). However, the advanced, stenotic plaques are not the only types prone to disruption. In fact, plaque disruption occurs independently of lesion size and degree of stenosis, and the relationship is complicated by vascular remodeling (3). Most AMIs actually result from disruption of lesions that are not initially flow limiting, with rapid progression to occlusion. Culprit lesions in AMI (Fig. 1.1) tend to have less calcification, which implies a certain softness of the plaque and vulnerability to shear forces and inflammatory components. Often, the complicated lesion has a central lipid core. However, the lipid composition and burden of complicated plaques can vary. Disrupted and thrombosed plaques with little lipid content have been described (3).

Atherosclerotic Plaque Growth

The coronary atherosclerotic lesion does not grow in a linear way. The gradual process by which material accumulates within the lesion is occasionally associated with the sudden increase in plaque growth that occurs with plaque rupture and resulting intracoronary thrombosis. It is by these abrupt episodes of plaque rupture that even mildly or moderately stenotic plaques can acutely progress to totally occlusive lesions (3). Thus, abrupt episodes of plaque disruption and growth account for many AMIs. However, these episodes occur against a background of gradual atheromatous plaque growth that progresses over decades. The persistence of risk factors favors the lesion growth, usually in an outward direction (positive remodeling), for many years while preserving the lumen, and the silent inflammatory process continues (9).

Several facts have been ascertained (10): (*i*) plaque progression and clinical outcome are not necessarily closely related; (*ii*) many plaques progress episodically

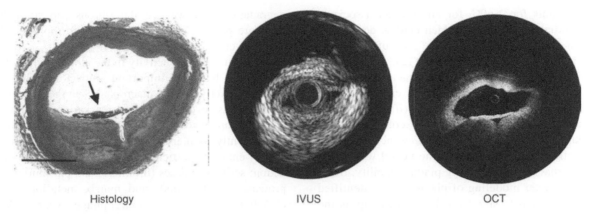

Histology   IVUS   OCT

Figure 1.1 Histology, IVUS, and OCT imaging of a plaque rupture complicated by thrombus formation. *Abbreviations*: IVUS, intravascular ultrasound; OCT, optical coherence tomography.

because of episodes of thrombosis triggered by rupture, erosion (denudation), or occasionally, by endothelial activation or inflammation; (*iii*) some thrombi remain mural rather than occlusive and produce few, if any, symptoms unless they embolize, and if lysis is incomplete and followed by reendothelialization, the result is a plaque growth; (*vi*) the hemorrhage into the plaque can result in rapid plaque growth too; (*v*) plaques within a given patient often progress unpredictably and largely independently from the others.

This frustrating unpredictability of patient outcome is probably due in part to fluctuation of risk factors and triggers (e.g., day-to-day changes in diet, blood pressure, smoking, activity, stress, pollution, infection). Nevertheless, independent plaque behavior in a given patient must be due in large measure to the marked heterogeneity of plaque histology and to differences in the physical forces to which plaques are subjected. There is growing interest in the possibility that identification and treatment of vulnerable plaques and vulnerable patients can enhance the progress made against coronary artery disease. Most vulnerable plaque detection devices in development are designed to detect thin-cap fibroatheromas. Because these devices will not detect erosion sites in advance, their sensitivity for predicting cardiac events will be limited. Specificity of a thin-cap fibroatheroma detector for predicting plaque rupture will also be limited because not all thin-cap fibroatheromas will rupture, nor will all ruptures lead to a cardiac event. Moreover, in the future it will be easy to predict the affirmation of the upcoming concept of "vulnerable blood" (a specific milieu needed for plaque rupture to cause a clinical event); thus, for secondary prevention purposes there is considerable discussion about the relative effort that should be devoted to combating the systemic versus focal manifestations of atherosclerosis (11).

The development and growth of the coronary atherosclerotic plaque can be subdivided into five phases on the basis of lesion morphology and associated clinical sequelae (12):

Phase 1: Asymptomatic development of lesions types I to III occurs in most individuals in the first few decades of life.

Phase 2: Atheroma (lesions IV and Va) develops and is usually asymptomatic or may be accompanied by stable angina pectoris.

Phase 3: Plaque disruption occurs, resulting in a nonocclusive overlying mural thrombus and in the sudden growth of a complicated lesion (type VI) and is often asymptomatic, but may be accompanied by stable angina pectoris.

Phase 4: Plaque disruption (also type VI lesion) is complicated by a large, often occlusive thrombus and is associated with AMI, unstable angina, or sudden cardiac death.

Phase 5: Phases 3 and 4 are followed by the development of chronic calcified (type Vb), or fibrotic (type Vc) lesions, which are often marked by stable angina pectoris. Severely stenotic lesions can occlude without plaque rupture from stasis in the vessel, leading to thrombus. Occlusions of a phase 5 lesion are often clinically silent, as distal myocardium is frequently supplied by collateral flow.

Atherosclerotic Plaque Rupture

Various mechanisms have been proposed as the initial cause of plaque rupture. The identification of mechanical and biological factors of plaque rupture has enhanced our understanding of the pathophysiology of AMI.

Pathological studies have established the association between plaque rupture and thrombus formation. Two primary mechanisms can trigger the development of thrombus formation: frank rupture of the atheromatous fibrous cap and superficial denudation of the endothelium.

Rupture accounts for $\geq 60\%$ for all thrombi associated with myocardial infarction or sudden cardiac death. Plaque erosion constitutes approximately 35% of the underlying mechanism of coronary thrombi (12).

Morphological and microscopic characteristics of the unstable plaque include (*i*) thin fibrous cap (<65 μm), (*ii*) eccentric, large lipid core, and (*iii*) infiltrating macrophages (13). Nevertheless, any combination of cap thickness and atheroma size may occur. Blood flow impacting on the plaque and the vessel wall stress are key external factors affecting plaque stability. Studies using computer modeling of plaques have identified circumferential tensile stress on the fibrous cap as the most important mechanical factor involved in plaque rupture (14). Most plaques rupture at sites of high calculated circumferential stress, which is often at the periphery of eccentric plaques. These studies also showed the importance of the thickness of the fibrous cap (thickness in millimeters being inversely related to the peak stress in the cap) and the stenosis rate (circumferential stresses in the plaque gradually decreased when stenosis severity increased).

Richardson et al. (15) studied the effects of mechanical stress on the fibrous cap in individuals who died of AMI. By evaluating different geometries of plaques that caused lethal coronary thrombosis, they observed increased levels of stress concentrating at the edges of the fibrous cap, at the border with the normal intima. It was also observed that in those cases with very small lipid pools, the point of maximum stress was located over the center of the plaque. This concentration of mechanical stress in the fibrous cap regions is possibly due to the inability of the soft lipid core to bear the large mechanical stresses that develop during elevation of blood pressure or repetitive dynamic stress caused by pulsatile blood pressure.

Moreover, it was observed that mechanical stress was higher in ruptured regions than that in nonruptured ones. However, it was also found that the location of plaque rupture was not always the area of greatest stress in an individual lesion. In plaque stability matter, the importance of fibrous cap thickness is crucial to be emphasized. In addition, weakening of tissue by compression of the fibrous cap such as by collapse of the artery due to the pressure gradient caused by the stenosis, or by arterial spasm, remain possible mechanisms (13).

The variable and unpredictable nature of plaque rupture despite apparent lesion similarity has focused attention on the fibrous cap as an active biological structure. When tissues are injured or inflammated, the repair process begins, and both synthetic and degradative processes greatly accelerate. The predominant component of all fibrous cap is connective tissue matrix proteins, particularly collagens types I and III, but also elastin and proteoglycans. Diminished collagen synthesis or increased degradation will weaken the fibrous cap strength and therefore produce a greater tendency to rupture at lower levels of circumferential stress (13).

Inflammatory cell activity in the atherosclerotic plaque appears to have an important impact on fibrous cap thickness. Activation of macrophages in the atheromatous plaque leads to the secretion of a variety of proteolytic enzymes capable of degrading the extracellular matrix and consequently weakening the atheroma. Three major families of enzymes participate in extracellular matrix degradation: serine proteases (urokinase and plasmin), cysteine proteases (cathepsins), and matrix metalloproteinases (MMPs). For instance, macrophages secrete MMPs, which have activity against the collagen component of the plaque and may act to weaken the fibrous cap (3). Macrophages in the atherosclerotic plaque derive from circulating monocytes, which adhere to the vessel wall in areas of turbulent flow. Monocytes are drawn into the vessel wall by chemotactic factors, such as MCP-1, which also acts to induce tissue factor expression in monocytic and smooth muscle cells. In addition to macrophages, T lymphocytes are found in abundance in the atherosclerotic plaques (13). Systemic infections (e.g., *Chlamydia pneumoniae*, *Cytomegalovirus*, and *Helicobacter pylori*) have been linked to atherosclerotic disease, although a causal relationship is far from being clarified. Infectious agents may affect endothelial function and activate monocytes and macrophages to secrete inflammatory cytokines. These cytokines, in turn, stimulate the production of reactive oxygen species and proteolytic enzymes, which may influence plaque tendency to rupture at lower levels of circumferential stress (16). Moreover, apoptotic cell death of T lymphocytes, macrophages, and smooth muscle cells in the fibrous cap may contribute to the destabilization of advanced atherosclerotic plaques. Oxidative stress and the antioxidant capacity of the arterial wall appear to play important roles in plaque rupture in addition to the progression of atherosclerotic disease (3).

Thrombosis Following Plaque Rupture

Fracture of the fibrous cap exposes intensely thrombogenic material to the blood elements within the vessel lumen. Platelets accumulate over a layer of fibrin, forming the initial "white clot," which directly overlies the disrupted plaque. Subsequently, a fibrin and erythrocyte-rich "red clot" forms over the white platelet clot, in a process strongly enhanced by blood stasis (3). Among the components of the plaque, the lipid core appears to have the highest thrombogenicity. This increased thrombogenicity largely results from factors, such as the tissue factor, apparently elaborated by cells infiltrating the plaque, and possibly by vascular smooth muscle cells and macrophages. Tissue factor, the most potent trigger of the coagulation cascade, forms a high-affinity complex with factors VII/VIIa, leading to activation of factors IX and X, thereby triggering both the intrinsic and extrinsic blood coagulation cascades (6). Tissue factor concentration is higher in the lipid core of the atheromatous plaque than in other areas of the arterial wall. In atherectomy specimens, the tissue factor staining tends to colocalize with areas of macrophage infiltration (3).

Thrombus accumulates over the disrupted plaque, leading to a spectrum of clinical possibilities. The clinical manifestation of the event may range from asymptomatic progression of the lesion to significant impairment of coronary blood flow, resulting in symptomatic myocardial ischemia. Often, many systemic factors, such as platelet and inflammation activation, coexist with local factors and increase thrombogenicity around the ruptured plaque. Acute plaque rupture may change the geometry of the atherosclerotic lesion, thereby increasing turbulence in the overlying vessel lumen. The resulting alteration in blood flow leads to stasis around the ruptured plaque and expansion of thrombus (3).

Plaque disruption and thrombus formation are not uncommon features. Any form of endothelial denudation leads to activation of the coagulation system. Microscopic foci of endothelial loss associated with platelet thrombi are present on the surface of many advanced plaques. They have no clinical implications at least on the short term, but may stimulate plaque growth through thrombin and platelet-derived growth factor (PGDF)-related stimulation of smooth muscle growth and matrix synthesis (17). Larger, but apparently clinically silent, ruptures have been observed also at autopsy in coronary arteries of 9% of persons who died of noncardiac disease, increasing to 22% in those with diabetes or hypertension. Most of these ruptures are old intra-plaque hemorrhages due to entrance of blood into the lipid core of the lesion and followed by healing of the rupture. These findings suggest that the coagulation cascade is often activated at an early stage after plaque rupture (18). Deep intimal tears, which extend into the highly thrombogenic lipid core of lesions and sometimes showing extrusion of parts of the atheroma, are often associated with massive thrombosis. They are found in most cases of acute transmural myocardial infarction, and plaque rupture frequently results in extrusion of atheromatous debris into the vessel lumen (17).

In young patients and in females, plaque erosions are common causes of coronary thrombosis underlying myocardial infarction (18). Thrombosis caused by endothelial erosion can be seen at sites of preexisting high-grade stenosis and may depend on a hyperthrombogenic state triggered by systemic factors, including elevated low-density lipoprotein, cigarette smoking, hyperglycemia, and others states associated with increased blood thrombogenicity (6).

Vasospasm Following Plaque Rupture

Vasoconstriction is frequent at the site of the ruptured plaque, and may often exacerbate the ACS. Systemic cathecholamine release, prompted or enhanced by the stress of the event, contributes to vasoconstriction. Platelet-derived factors, as well as thrombin, may stimulate vasoconstriction in the presence of a damaged coronary vessel wall. In addition, vessel spasm may derive from abnormal endothelial responses and hypercontractile vascular smooth muscle associated with atherosclerotic plaques (3). Vasoconstriction of both infarct-related artery and nonculprit vessels has been reported (19). Furthermore, the relationship between the epicardial vessel disease and the microvascular spasm in its distribution areas is not yet fully elucidated (5).

Clinical Sequelae Following Plaque Rupture

From a clinical point of view, a spectrum of acute coronary events may follow atherosclerotic plaque rupture. These events range from the asymptomatic to those resulting in ACS and sudden cardiac death. The pathophysiology underlying these clinical events involves a reduction in blood flow supporting myocardium distal to the site of acute plaque rupture. Blood flow is reduced by accumulated thrombus, as well as vasospasm over the ruptured plaque. The severity of the resulting coronary event appears to be related to the change in blood flow around the site of plaque disruption. In those cases where blood flow is essentially unaffected, plaque rupture may result only in asymptomatic progression of the atherosclerotic lesion. If blood flow is reduced, it may result in unstable angina. If complete acute vessel occlusion follows plaque rupture in the absence of sufficient collateral blood flow, AMI results (3). Of note, thrombotic component of the acute coronary occlusion can vary widely, but it is constantly present.

Role in Plaque Stabilization of Percutaneous Coronary Intervention

Although not usually classified as such, percutaneous coronary intervention is an effective method of short-term stabilization of a disrupted and/or thrombotic plaque. Even though percutaneous coronary intervention results in vessel wall injury at the site of the procedure, expansion of the lumen particularly with a properly opposed stent results in an axial redistribution of plaque away from the center of the lesion toward the reference segments, and possibly in plaque compression. Theoretically, this change in plaque geometry may seal the intimal tears and allow for intimal healing. Combined with the improvements in blood flow due to expanded lumen and reduced shear rates, the net result will be a short-term strong reduction in local thrombogenicity. In patients with AMI, stent placement, usually with the use of adjunctive platelet GP IIb/IIIa receptor inhibitors, has been efficacious in reducing subsequent adverse events (20). This result supports the evidence that beyond the complex interplay of multiple systemic and local factors, a normal flow is likely to be the strongest antithrombotic factor, as that achievable by percutaneous coronary intervention. The practical implication of the antithrombotic role of a normal flow is the need for an optimal result of the interventional procedure (21).

THE MICROCIRCULATION

In the past century, most of AMI research interest and treatment strategies focused on epicardial coronary arteries. Little attention has been paid to the coronary microcirculation. Until recently, there was limited access to the assessment of microvascular integrity and function in patients with AMI. The availability of imaging technologies has revealed that microvascular dysfunction, even after optimal recanalization of the epicardial vessel, may exist in a far greater proportion of patients than was previously thought possible and may play a key role in the outcome (22).

In AMI, the extent of myocardial salvage is critically dependent on blood flow to the risk area (23). Thus, the primary objective of reperfusion therapies should be not only to achieve rapid and sustained epicardial patency but also to restore microvascular flow and myocardial tissue perfusion. Microvascular disruption, embolization of plaque contents, thrombus or platelet aggregates in the microcirculation, and inflammatory process activation lead to mechanical obstruction and may compromise the recovery of perfusion at tissue level (24), a phenomenon known as no-reflow.

In patients with AMI successfully treated with mechanical reperfusion, microvascular dysfunction within the risk area is a powerful independent predictor of post-infarction left ventricular (LV) dilation and long-term clinical outcome (25–27). Thus, microvascular integrity and adequate tissue reperfusion, even after optimal epicardial recanalization, represent the true standard for success of reperfusion.

Understanding the pathophysiology of the microvascular dysfunction during AMI is the prerequisite for the management of this condition. The exact mechanism of microvascular dysfunction in AMI is not fully elucidated, but it is certainly multifactorial, and a variety of events contribute to it.

Endothelial Dysfunction

After prolonged coronary occlusion and the restoration of blood flow in the epicardial coronary artery, the structural damage of the microvasculature by ischemic injury may be sufficient to prevent the restoration of normal flow to the myocytes. In addition, the damage of the microvessel network prevents the recruitment of collateral flow. This phenomenon is more pronounced with long periods of coronary occlusion.

Microscopic examination of the myocardium within the no-reflow area showed that the cardiac cells are swollen and the capillary endothelium is damaged and exhibits areas of regional swelling with intraluminal protrusion that, in some cases, appeared to plug the capillary lumen. The cellular edema and the ischemic myocardial cell contracture compress the microvessel network and contribute to microvascular obstruction (22).

Different studies indicate that ischemic endothelial damage may be at least in part reversible. The final extent of endothelial damage within the infarcted territory may be completed during the coronary occlusion or may progress after reperfusion (i.e., reperfusion injury) up to 48 hours after coronary reflow (28). Studies using myocardial contrast echocardiography demonstrate that ischemic microvascular damage, as well as LV function, may recover in the late stage of AMI. This improvement may continue up to six months and is dependent on the persistence of epicardial vessel patency. These observations confirm the presence of the so-called microvascular stunning (29).

Embolization

New evidence has underscored the high frequency and clinical importance of spontaneous atherothrombotic embolization into the microvasculature. Paradoxically, embolization may be enhanced by reperfusion treatments. Plaque and vessel wall constituents, including lipid, necrotic core, matrix, endothelial cells, and old and fresh thrombi, can all embolize. Embolization sets up the potential for microvascular dysfunction (or obstruction), with loss of endothelial integrity, release of vasoactive and proinflammatory agents from platelets and lipid core, increased vascular tone, and potentiation of platelet thrombus (24).

Tanaka et al. (30) have shown that the angiographic no-reflow phenomenon after mechanical reperfusion correlates with lesion morphology, as assessed by intravascular ultrasound (IVUS). Lipid pool-like images, fissured/dissected lesions, and eccentric plaques were observed before intervention more frequently in patients with no-reflow after the restoration of epicardial flow, as compared with patients without no-reflow. Again, a large vessel is a high-risk feature for no-reflow, probably secondary to the fact that large vessels are able to contain large amounts of plaque or thrombus.

Microembolization may occur when artificial plaque rupture is induced during coronary intervention, and the lipid pool with additional thrombus formation is washed out of the atheromatous plaque into the microcirculation.

We can now begin to recognize a certain profile of patients who are most apt to show emboli at the time of a revascularization procedure. Diffuse disease, friability of the atheromatous lesion (lipid-rich), and presence of platelet thrombus would seem the most likely predisposing features once an artery is manipulated. The friability of the lesion may well link to inflammation, and many studies have underscored the clinical meaning of the elevation in C-reactive protein, interleukins, vascular adhesion molecules, and other inflammatory markers in predicting this phenomenon. On demographic characteristics, diabetes mellitus is a strong risk factor of embolization in atherosclerotic disease. This can be attributed to the extension of atherosclerotic involvement, the preexisting microvascular disease that reduces the adaptive capacity to embolization, or other metabolic factors (24).

Blood Cell Plugging

Intravascular plugging of leukocytes plays an important role in the pathophysiology of the no-reflow phenomenon. Experimental studies showed that in the canine model reperfusion leads to rapid accumulation of leukocytes in the microvasculature (22). Reperfusion with leukocytes-depleted blood may reduce myocardial no-reflow (31). Again, in the rat model the no-reflow phenomenon was prevented by rendering the rats neutropenic. Leukocytes may interfere with blood flow by mechanical plugging, and perhaps by release of oxygen-free radicals that are able to add further injury to the capillary endothelium (22).

The potential for a cardioprotective effect of adenosine in AMI appears to be, at least in part, related to the inhibition of neutrophil-related processes (32), which are the principal mediators of ischemia-reperfusion injury.

Experimental and postmortem histological studies have demonstrated a time-dependent shift in the location of the leukocytes in postischemic myocardium from intravascular (which peaks about 1 hour after reperfusion) to interstitial (which peaks > 5 hours after reperfusion) (33).

Microvascular Spasm

Previous studies have shown that intracoronary administration of calcium and sodium channel blockers, such as verapamil and nicorandil, may attenuate microvascular dysfunction after reperfusion (34,35). These data support the hypothesis that a vasoconstriction of a distal microvasculature may play a role in the progression of capillary damage, likely mediated by abnormal calcium and sodium

concentration and by the vasoactive substance released from activated platelets such as serotonin.

The vasodilator reserve is impaired in postischemic vessels, secondary to endothelial dysfunction, leading to reduced generation of nitric oxide and prostacyclin, enhanced endothelin formation, and the damage to vascular adrenergic receptors. In addition, activated neutrophils release vasoconstriction mediators. The prevalence of vasoconstriction in postischemic vessels reduces pressure gradient in the capillary bed and favors further neutrophil cell accumulation (36).

Coronary ischemia and stretch are known to reflexly increase the cardiac sympathetic nerve activity by the stimulation of cardiac ventricular and coronary receptors. After angioplasty, an α-receptor-mediated vasoconstriction has been described. So during mechanical reperfusion of AMI, an intense α-adrenergic vasoconstriction can take place in the infarct-related artery and then reduce myocardial perfusion (37).

In patients with AMI, the coronary regulatory function may be significantly impaired even in the areas of myocardium not directly supplied by the infarct-related artery. The impairment of microvascular function in remote areas may be explained by several possible mechanisms. An elevated LV diastolic pressure may affect blood flow in both infarct-related artery and in remote regions by decreasing coronary perfusion pressure. The generalized increase in neurohormonal sympathetic activity could lead to an impairment of vasodilator responsiveness in the remote regions after infarction. Vasoconstrictor substances released at the site of coronary occlusion (such as serotonin, thrombin, thromboxane A_2) can constrict the vascular smooth muscle surrounding the thrombus, but they can also constrict distal vessels, leading to further blood-flow stasis and coronary thrombosis. The vascular bed of the non-infarct-related arteries can be influenced by systemic and local neurohormonal constrictor stimuli, resulting in an increase of the ischemia extent and reducing collateral flow to the infarct-related artery (38).

Collateral Circulation

Coronary collaterals offer an important alternative source of blood supply when the original vessel fails to provide sufficient blood, and timely recruitment of collaterals may avoid transmural myocardial infarction at the time of coronary occlusion (36).

The functional coronary collateral circulation results from hypertrophic evolution of vessels with a lumen diameter of 20 to 350 μm present in normal hearts at birth. Recurrent and severe ischemia is assumed to stimulate the development of coronary collateral circulation.

In fact, myocardial ischemia, per se, can be a sufficient stimulus to induce coronary collateral development, possibly through biochemical signals, including release of angiogenic growth factor. The process is mediated mechanically through an increase of shear stresses. In the case of a hemodynamically relevant coronary stenosis a pressure gradient is created and collateral arteries are recruited. Because of the decrease in arterial pressure distal to the stenosis, blood flow is redistributed through the preexistent arterioles that now connect a high-pressure area with a low-pressure one. These modifications result in an increased flow velocity and therefore increased shear stress in the preexistent collaterals arteries, which leads to a marked activation of the endothelium, the upregulation of cell adhesion molecules, and increasing adherence of monocytes, which transform into macrophages. Subsequently, several morphological changes and vascular remodeling occur. Different growth factors and chemokines are involved in this process (39). At present, it is not clear why there are differences between individuals in their capability of developing a sufficient collateral circulation.

Previous studies have shown that recurrent episodes of angina in the 24 hours before AMI are a stimulating factor for the development of collateral channels (40). Early recruitment of collateral circulation was more frequent in patients with acute right coronary artery occlusion, suggesting a more extensive collateralization from the left coronary system to the area supplied from the right coronary artery. Recruitment of collateral flow was also favored by a longer delay from symptom onset to treatment (39). Another condition associated with the development of coronary collaterals in AMI is the presence of total chronic occlusion. Conversely, cardiogenic shock and baseline infarct artery TIMI grade flow >1 are associated with a poor recruitment of collaterals (41). Moreover, it has been documented that after the implantation of a drug-eluting stent the coronary collateral function may be impaired (42).

In patients treated with primary angioplasty for ST-segment elevation AMI within six hours from symptoms onset, the presence of collateral circulation is not an independent predictor of survival (41). Likely, transmural myocardial ischemia subsequent to infarct artery occlusion is not significantly reduced by the early recruitment of collateral vessels, whereas the early restoration of the anterograde flow in the infarct artery, provided by mechanical intervention, instantaneously overcomes the collateral flow in the area at risk. However, the development of coronary collaterals may help protect the myocardium from infarction during episodes of prolonged ischemia and may extend the limited numbers of "golden hours" from the onset of coronary occlusion to successful tissue reperfusion.

THE MYOCARDIUM

Ischemic Injury

The myocardium can tolerate brief minutes (up to 15 minutes) of severe or even total ischemia without resultant cardiomyocyte death. Although the cells suffer ischemic injury, the damage is reversible with prompt tissue reperfusion. With increasing duration and severity of ischemia, however, greater myocytes damage can develop, with a predisposition to irreversible cell damage or necrosis. Complete necrosis of all myocardial cells at risk requires at least four to six hours or longer of ischemia, depending on the presence of collateral blood flow into the ischemic zone, the persistent or intermittent artery occlusion, and the sensitivity of the myocytes (43).

Sudden occlusion of a coronary artery is followed by physiological and metabolic changes that appear within seconds of the cessation of coronary flow. Energy metabolism shifts from aerobic or mitochondrial metabolism to anaerobic glycolysis after only eight seconds (44). Simultaneously, effective contractions diminish and then cease, and the myocardium stretches rather than shortens with each systole. The membrane potential decreases and the electrocardiographic changes appear. The demand of the myocytes for energy far exceeds the supply from anaerobic glycolysis, and from reserves of high-energy phosphate, resulting in decreased tissue ATP and accumulation of ADP. Anaerobic glycolysis provides 80% of the new high-energy phosphate produced in zones of total or severe ischemia, utilizing glucose from glycogenolysis as its substrate. The lactate and its associated H^+ accumulate. After only 10 minutes of ischemia, intracellular pH decreases, and the load of intracellular osmotically active particles (lactate, inorganic phosphate, creatine, etc.) increases markedly, resulting in intracellular edema. In the absence of oxidative phosphorylation, ADP is converted to AMP, which in turn is broken down to adenosine and ultimately to inosine, hypoxantine, and xantine. Various substances, such as bradykinin, opioids, norepinephrine, and angiotensin, are released into the extracellular fluid. These agents interact with adenosine, and stimulate intracellular signaling systems (44). A variety of potential causes of irreversible myocytes injury has been described: high-energy phosphates depletion and the cessation of anaerobic glycolysis; catabolism without resynthesis of macromolecules; reduced transsarcolemmal gradients of Na^+ and K^+; calcium overload; cell swelling; activation of phospholipases and proteases; impaired mitochondrial function; activation of ATPases; catabolite accumulation (lactate, inorganic phosphate, free radicals, H^+, ammonia, fatty acid derivatives); enzyme denaturation; membrane damage; and increased intracellular osmolarity.

Reperfusion Injury

Timely reperfusion has clearly been shown to be the most effective means to prevent progression of ischemic cell necrosis after coronary artery occlusion, and it is now widely accepted that prompt reopening of the occluded vessel, by either primary angioplasty or thrombolysis, must be pursued as soon as possible in patients with AMI. However, reperfusion of the previously ischemic myocardium may not be entirely beneficial, as there is also evidence that it may carry injurious components that may in part counteract the beneficial effects of the restoration of blood flow. This phenomenon has been called "reperfusion injury" (36).

The principal mediators of reperfusion injury are oxygen radicals and neutrophils, which are redistributed by reperfusion in the previously ischemic tissue. Oxygen radicals can attack every biologically relevant molecule. One important cardiac consequence might be peroxidation of unsaturated lipids of cell membranes. This may be an important mechanism of cell damage because the activity of membrane-bound enzymes can be affected by oxidation of membrane lipids. In addition to a direct oxidative attack, oxygen radicals can also modulate various cellular activities that are important mediators in the sequence of events leading to tissue injury during reperfusion. Superoxide radical inactivates nitric oxides, whereas hydrogen peroxide can induce adherence of neutrophils to intact vessels via ICAM-1 and CD18 interaction (36).

Myocardial stunning is the best-established clinical manifestation of reperfusion injury. It is defined as "prolonged postischemic dysfunction of viable tissue salvaged by reperfusion" (44,45). This myocardium, after a prolonged but reversible dysfunction, requires a prolonged period before complete functional recovery.

Microvascular dysfunction is another manifestation of reperfusion injury. Reperfusion causes marked endothelial cell dysfunction, which results in vasoconstriction, platelet and leukocyte activation, increased oxidant production, and increased fluid and protein extravasation.

Finally, reperfusion of a severely ischemic myocardium may also result in myocyte death and necrosis (lethal reperfusion injury). A disruptive type of necrosis, termed "contraction band necrosis," has been documented and is ascribed to massive myofibril contraction after reperfusion-induced calcium reentry. This form of reperfusion injury is the most severe and is clearly irreversible (43).

The past two decades have witnessed several pharmacological interventions designed to limit reperfusion injury. Unfortunately, no agent has shown convincing efficacy. The lack of a consistent clinical benefit may be related to a variety of factors, including poor clinical trial design, inadequate pharmacokinetic/pharmacodynamic studies, and the complexity of the phenomenon (43).

Myocardial Stunning and Hibernation

There is convincing evidence that the myocardium that has been reperfused after a relatively short period of ischemia is characterized by a variety of unfavorable, but not lethal, cellular changes that, given sufficient time, will revert to normal. The most prominent of these changes is myocardial stunning, which is the prolonged contractile dysfunction that occurs despite the absence of irreversible injury and normal blood flow. Mechanical stunning is associated with a constellation of reversible derangements, including ATP depletion, collagen damage, cell swelling, increased capillary permeability, and impaired microvascular responsiveness. The duration of the dysfunction greatly exceeds the one of the antecedent ischemia, for example, after 15 minutes of ischemia in dogs, myocardial function remains depressed for 24 hours (46). It seems certain that stunning also occurs in myocardium salvaged by arterial reperfusion after periods of one to three hours, i.e., periods that result in substantial amounts of necrosis in damaged tissue (46,47).

A number of candidate underlying mechanisms for stunning have been investigated. Experimental studies have shown clearly that 50% to 70% of the stunning effect is due to a burst of O_2-derived free radicals (in particular the hydroxyl radical) liberated during the first few minutes from reperfusion. This means that much of the stunning effect is a complication of reperfusion and therefore is a form of reperfusion injury (44). O_2-derived free radicals react quickly with proteins, phospholipids, and thiols. Nevertheless, a number of O_2-derived free radical scavengers have been tested without consistent benefits in human studies of myocardial infarction.

Inotropic agents can override stunning. Administration of catecholamine, such as dobutamine, will restore contractile function to control level showing that the contractile system of the myocyte (including those allowing Ca^{2+} entry and sarcoplasmic reticulum function, the myofibrils, and the mitochondria) is sufficiently preserved to allow full contraction. The exact changes that lead to the failure of contraction in myocardial stunning are unknown. Among the possibilities are any alterations in the availability of Ca^{2+}, and the sensitivity of the contractile apparatus to calcium (44).

During an AMI a progressive wave front of cell death moves across the wall of the left ventricle from the subendocardial to the subepicardial layer. Myocardium salvaged by reperfusion is located primarily in the subepicardium and midmyocardium, and these layers display the properties of stunned myocardium. Recovery of this tissue can be observed over the course of a variable period of time (from 3 days to 6 months), although most of the improvement is likely to take place within the first 30 days after infarction (44,48). It has been documented that after successful mechanical reperfusion of AMI nearly half of the patients show poor LV functional recovery (<10% increase in ejection fraction). Moreover, early (within 30 days) and late (between 30 days and 6 months) functional recovery patterns were detected in 44% and 14% patients, respectively. In particular, 89% of the overall functional recovery was confined in the first month. However, the time course of LV functional recovery during six months (early vs. late) did not significantly affect long-term survival (48).

Hibernation is a state of persistently impaired myocardial and LV function at rest due to reduced coronary blood flow that can be partially or completely restored to normal if the myocardial oxygen supply/demand relationship is favorably altered, either by improving blood flow and/or by reducing demand (45,49). It was proposed that the functional state of contractile failure of hibernation is due to chronic stunning caused by multiple episodes of more severe ischemia. Other experimental studies, however, suggest that hibernation does occur with a chronic low-flow state (45). Whether the myocardial dysfunction is due to the downregulation of metabolism or to the chronic stunning, the treatment is clear: arterial flow must be improved.

Ischemic Preconditioning

Preconditioning is a powerful mechanism to protect the myocardium from ischemic damage. In the strictest sense, it refers to the delay of infarct development by one or more episodes of ischemia before persistent coronary occlusion. It is important to realize that the evolution to cell death is delayed but not prevented. Moreover, it appears that there is a bimodal distribution of protection, with an early phase (classic preconditioning) and a late phase (50).

The mechanisms of ischemic preconditioning appear to be complex and involve second messenger pathways. The myocardium that is preconditioned exhibits the striking metabolic changes noted during the ischemic reversible injury, including a smaller adenine nucleotide pool (ATP + ADP + AMP), a creatine phosphate overshoot, an excess of intracellular glucose and lactate, and stunning. It has been postulated that preconditioned tissue dies slowly because of the reduction in energy demand (45). The results of some experimental studies provide strong evidence that adenosine is involved in preconditioning with the potassium channels involved in mediating the effect of adenosine. Strong data exist that the beneficial effect of adenosine on preconditioning may be mediated via the A1 receptor (45).

Several clinical studies suggest that brief episodes of ischemia (angina) occurring before an AMI may have protective effects by ischemic preconditioning. Pre-infarction angina can reduce myocardial infarct size, and arrhythmias, resulting in improved LV function,

prevention of LV remodeling, and increase in survival (45,51). However, not all pre-infarction angina studies have showed its protective effect (52), and there is still debate as to whether pre-infarction angina has any benefit in elderly patients.

Ventricular Remodeling

The acute loss of myocardium results in an abrupt increase in loading conditions that induces a remodeling process involving the infarcted border zone and remote noninfarcted myocardium. Myocyte necrosis and the resultant increase in load trigger a cascade of biochemical intracellular signaling processes that initiate and subsequently modulate reparative changes, which include dilation, hypertrophy, and collagen synthesis. This balance is determined by the size, transmurality, and location of the infarct, patency of the infarct-related artery, residual myocardial viability, microvascular integrity in the area at risk, LV diastolic function, extracellular matrix activity, and neurohormonal activation (Fig. 1.2) (27,53–55). Remodeling encompasses cellular changes including myocyte hypertrophy, necrosis, apoptosis and fibrosis, and increased fibrillar collagen and fibroblast proliferation. As the heart remodels, its geometry changes; it becomes less elliptical and more spherical; ventricular mass and volumes increase, all of which may adversely affect cardiac function (53). Post-infarction remodeling has been arbitrarily categorized into an early phase (within 72 hours) and a late phase (beyond 72 hours). The early phase involves expansion of the infarct zone, which may result in early ventricular rupture or aneurysm formation. Late remodeling involves the LV globally and is associated with chambers dilation, distortion of ventricular shape, and mural hypertrophy. The failure to normalize increased wall stresses results in progressive ventricular dilation, recruitment of border zone myocardium into the scar, and deterioration of contractile function (52). LV remodeling after AMI is an important predictor of

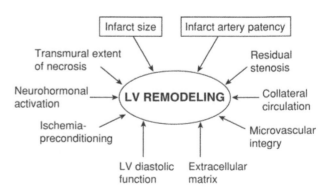

Figure 1.2 Factors influencing LV remodeling after acute myocardial infarction. *Abbreviation*: LV, left ventricular.

hospitalization for heart failure and mortality. The remodeling process is heterogeneous, but the specific pattern of LV dilation (early, late, and progressive) does not affect independently clinical outcome (55). Interestingly, particular subgroups of patients, such as diabetics or hypertensives, are at higher risk of post-infarction heart failure because their LV is unable to appropriately dilate and remodel (56,57).

Infarct Expansion

Infarct expansion results from the degradation of the intermyocytes collagen struts by serine proteases and the activation of MMPs released from neutrophils. Infarct expansion occurs early from myocyte injury and results in wall thinning, ventricular dilation, and elevation of diastolic and systolic wall stresses. Infarct expansion causes the deformation of the border zone and remote myocardium, which alters the Frank–Starling relations and augments shortening. Perturbation in circulatory hemodynamics triggers the sympathetic adrenergic system, which stimulates catecholamine synthesis, activates the renin-angiotensin-aldosterone system, and stimulates the production of atrial and brain natriuretic peptides. Augmented shortening and increased heart rate from sympathetic stimulation result in hyperkinesis of the noninfarcted myocardium and temporary circulatory compensation. In addition, the natriuretic peptides reduce intravascular volume and systemic vascular resistance, normalize ventricular filling, and improve pump function (53,58).

REFERENCES

1. Maseri A, Fuster V. Is there a vulnerable plaque? Circulation 2003; 107:2068–2071.
2. Herrick JB. Clinical features of sudden obstruction of the coronary arteries. J Am Med Assoc 1912; 59:2015–2020.
3. Gutstein DE, Fuster V. Pathophysiology and clinical significance of atherosclerotic plaque rupture. Cardiovasc Res 1999; 41:323–333.
4. Keeley EC, Boura JA, Grines CL. Primary angioplasty versus intravenous thrombolytic therapy for acute myocardial infarction: a quantitative review of randomized trials. Lancet 2003; 361:13–20.
5. Lerman A, Holmes DR, Herrmann J, et al. Microcirculatory dysfunction in ST-elevation myocardial infarction: cause, consequence, or both? Eur Heart J 2007; 28:788–797.
6. Corti R, Fuster V. New understanding, diagnosis, and prognosis of atherothrombosis and the role of imaging. Am J Cardiol 2003; 91(suppl 3A):17A–26A.
7. Ross R. The pathogenesis of atherosclerosis: a perspective for the 1990s. Nature 1993; 362:801–809.
8. Stary HC, Chandler AB, Dinsmore RE, et al. A definition of advanced types of atherosclerotic lesions and a histologic classification of atherosclerosis: a report from the Committee on Atherosclerosis. American Heart Association. Circulation 1995; 92:1355–1374.
9. Libby P. Vascular biology of atherosclerosis: overview and state of the art. Am J Cardiol 2003; 91(suppl 3A):3A–6A.
10. Casscells W, Naghavi M, Willerson JT. Vulnerable atherosclerotic plaque. A multifocal disease. Circulation 2003; 107:2072–2075.
11. Waxman S, Ishibashi F, Muller JE. Detection and treatment of vulnerable plaques and vulnerable patients: novel approaches to prevention of coronary events. Circulation 2006; 114:2390–2411.
12. Fuster V, Lewis A. Mechanisms leading to myocardial infarction: insights from studies of vascular biology. Circulation 1994; 90:2126–2146.
13. Arroyo LH, Lee RT. Mechanisms of plaque rupture: mechanical and biologic interactions. Cardiovasc Res 1999; 41:369–375.
14. Cheng GC, Loree HM, Kamm RD, et al. Distribution of circumferential stress in ruptured and stable atherosclerotic lesions: a structural analysis with histopathologic correlation. Circulation 1993; 87:1179–1187.
15. Richardson PD, Davies MJ, Born GVR. Influence of plaque configuration and stress distribution on fissuring of coronary atherosclerotic plaques. Lancet 1989; 2:941–944.
16. Ross R. Atherosclerosis: an inflammatory disease. N Engl J Med 1999; 340:115–126.
17. Rentrop KP. Thrombi in acute coronary syndromes. Revisited and revised. Circulation 2000; 101:1619–1626.
18. van der Wal AC, Becker AE. Atherosclerotic plaque rupture. Pathologic basis of plaque stability and instability. Cardiovasc Res 1999; 41:334–344.
19. Hanratty CG, Koyama Y, Rasmussen HH, et al. Exaggeration of nonculprit stenosis severity during acute myocardial infarction: implications for immediate multivessel revascularization. J Am Coll Cardiol 2002; 40:911–916.
20. Ambrose JA, Martinez EE. A new paradigm for plaque stabilization. Circulation 2002; 105:2000–2004.
21. Parodi G, Valenti R, Carrabba N, et al. Long-term prognostic implications of nonoptimal primary angioplasty for acute myocardial infarction. Catheter Cardiovasc Interv 2006; 68:50–55.
22. Rezkalla SH, Kloner RA. No-reflow phenomenon. Circulation 2002; 105:656–662.
23. Reiner JS, Lundergan CF, Fung A, et al. Evolution of early TIMI 2 flow after thrombolysis for acute myocardial infarction. GUSTO-1 Angiographic Investigators. Circulation 1996; 94:2441–2446.
24. Topol EJ, Yadav JS. Recognition of the importance of embolization in atherosclerotic vascular disease. Circulation 2001; 101:570–580.
25. Ito H, Maruyama A, Iwakura K, et al. Clinical implications of the "no-reflow" phenomenon. A predictor of complications and left ventricular remodeling in reperfused anterior wall myocardial infarction. Circulation 1996; 93:223–228.
26. Wu KC, Zerhouni EA, Judd RM, et al. Prognostic significance of microvascular obstruction by magnetic resonance imaging in patients with acute myocardial infarction. Circulation 1998; 97:765–772.

27. Bolognese L, Carrabba N, Parodi G, et al. Impact of microvascular dysfunction on left ventricular remodeling and long-term clinical outcome after primary coronary angioplasty for acute myocardial infarction. Circulation 2004; 109:1121–1126.

28. Rochitte CE, Lima JC, Bluemke DA, et al. Magnitude and time course of microvascular obstruction and tissue injury after acute myocardial infarction. Circulation 1998; 98:1006–1014.

29. Agati L. Microvascular integrity after reperfusion therapy. Am Heart J 1999; 138(suppl 2):S76–S78.

30. Tanaka A, Kawarabayashi T, Nishibori Y, et al. No-reflow phenomenon and lesion morphology in patients with acute myocardial infarction. Circulation 2002; 105:2148–2152.

31. Byrne JG, Appleyard RF, Lee CC, et al. Controlled reperfusion of the regionally ischemic myocardium with leukocytes-depleted blood reduces stunning, the no-reflow phenomenon, and infarct size. J Thorac Cardiovasc Surg 1992; 103:66–72.

32. Marzilli M, Orsini E, Marraccini P, et al. Beneficial effects of intracoronary adenosine as an adjunct to primary angioplasty in acute myocardial infarction. Circulation 2000; 101:2154–2159.

33. Christiansen JP, Leong-Poi H, Klibarov AL, et al. Noninvasive imaging of myocardial reperfusion injury using leukocyte-targeted contrast echocardiography. Circulation 2002; 105:1764–1767.

34. Taniyama Y, Ito H, Iwakura K, et al. Beneficial effect of verapamil on microvascular and myocardial salvage in patients with acute myocardial infarction. J Am Coll Cardiol 1997; 30:1193–1199.

35. Ito H, Taniyama Y, Iwakura K, et al. Intravenous nicorandil can preserve microvascular integrity and myocardial viability in patients with reperfused anterior myocardial infarction. J Am Coll Cardiol 1999; 33:654–660.

36. Ambrosio G, Tritto I. Reperfusion injury: Experimental evidence and clinical implications. Am Heart J 1999; 138 (suppl 2):S69–S75.

37. Gregorini L, Marco J, Kozàcova M, et al. α-Adrenergic blockade improves recovery of myocardial perfusion and function after coronary stenting in patients with acute myocardial infarction. Circulation 1999; 99:482–490.

38. Uren NG, Crake T, Lefroy DC, et al. Reduced coronary vasodilator function in infarcted and normal myocardium after myocardial infarction. N Engl J Med 1994; 331: 222–227.

39. Koerselman J, van der Graaf Y, de Jaegere PPT, et al. Coronary Collaterals. An important and underexposed aspect of coronary artery disease. Circulation 2003; 107:2507–2511.

40. Rentrop KP, Cohen M, Blancke H, et al. Changes in collateral channel filling immediately after controlled coronary artery occlusion by an angioplasty balloon in human subjects. J Am Coll Cardiol 1985; 5:587–592.

41. Antoniucci D, Valenti R, Moschi G, et al. Relation between preintervention angiographic evidence of coronary collateral circulation and clinical and angiographic outcomes after primary angioplasty or stenting for acute myocardial infarction. Am J Cardiol 2002; 89:121–125.

42. Meier P, Zbinden R, Togni M, et al. Coronary collateral function long after drug-eluting stent implantation. J Am Coll Cardiol 2007; 49:15–20.

43. Verma S, Fedak PWM, Weisel RD et al. Fundamentals of reperfusion injury for the clinical cardiologist. Circulation 2002; 105:2332–2336.

44. Kloner RA, Jennings RB. Consequences of brief ischemia: stunning, preconditioning, and their clinical implications. Part I. Circulation 2001; 104:2981–2989.

45. Kloner RA, Jennings RB. Consequences of brief ischemia: stunning, preconditioning, and their clinical implications. Part II. Circulation 2001; 104:3158–3167.

46. Braunwald E, Kloner RA. The stunned myocardium: prolonged, postischemic ventricular dysfunction. Circulation 1982; 66:1146–1149.

47. Ferrari R, Pepi P, Ferrari F, et al. Metabolic derangement in ischemic heart disease and its therapeutic control. Am J Cardiol 1998; 82(suppl 5A):K2–K13.

48. Parodi G, Memisha G, Carrabba N, et al. Prevalence, predictors, time course, and long-term clinical implications of left ventricular functional recovery after mechanical reperfusion for acute myocardial infarction. Am J Cardiol 2007; 100:1718–1722.

49. Rahimtoola SH. The hibernating myocardium. Am Heart J 1989; 117:211–221.

50. Ferrari R, Ceconi C, Curello S, et al. Ischemic preconditioning, myocardial stunning, and hibernation: basic aspects. Am Heart J 1999; 138(suppl 2):S61–S68.

51. Iglesias-Garriz I, Fernàndez-Vasquez F, Perez A, et al. Preinfarction angina limits myocardial infarct size in non-diabetic patients treated with primary coronary angioplasty. Chest 2005; 127:1116–1121.

52. Zahn R, Schiele R, Schneider S, et al. Effect of preinfarction angina pectoris on outcome of patients with acute myocardial infarction treated with primary angioplasty (Results from the Myocardial Infarction Registry). Am J Cardiol 2001; 87:1–6.

53. St John Sutton MG, Sharpe N. Left ventricular remodeling after myocardial infarction. Pathophysiology and therapy. Circulation 2000; 101:2981–2988.

54. Cohn JN, Ferrari R, Sharpe N. Cardiac remodelling. Concepts and clinical implications: a consensus paper from an International forum on cardiac remodeling. J Am Coll Cardiol 2000; 35:569–582.

55. Bolognese L, Neskovic N, Parodi G, et al. Left ventricular remodeling after primary coronary angioplasty: patterns of left ventricular dilation and long-term prognostic implications. Circulation 2002; 106:2351–2357.

56. Carrabba N, Valenti R, Parodi G, et al. Left ventricular remodeling and heart failure in diabetic patients treated with primary angioplasty for acute myocardial infarction. Circulation 2004; 110:1974–1979.

57. Parodi G, Carrabba N, Santoro GM, et al. Heart failure and left ventricular remodeling after reperfused acute myocardial infarction in patients with hypertension. Hypertension 2006; 47:706–710.

58. Mukherjee R, Brinsa TA, Dowdy KB, et al. Myocardial infarct expansion and matrix metalloproteinase inhibition. Circulation 2003; 107:618–625.

2

Major Subgroups at Presentation

ANGELA MIGLIORINI, GIAMPAOLO CERISANO, PIERGIOVANNI BUONAMICI, AND GUIA MOSCHI

Division of Cardiology, Careggi Hospital, Florence, Italy

ELECTROCARDIOGRAPHY

The electrocardiogram (ECG) remains a crucial tool in the timely identification of acute myocardial infarction (AMI) and in the early selection of patients who will benefit from reperfusion therapies. A detailed analysis of patterns of ST-segment elevation may influence decisions regarding the use of percutaneous coronary interventions (PCIs) that are, according to the recommendation of the Task Force of the European Society of Cardiology, "the preferred therapeutic option when it can be performed within 90 minutes after the first medical contact" (1).

The specificity of the ECG in AMI is limited by large individual variations in coronary anatomy as well as by the presence of preexisting coronary artery disease, particularly in patients with a previous myocardial infarction, chronic occlusion, collateral circulation, or previous coronary bypass surgery. The ECG is also limited by its inadequate presentation of the posterior, lateral, and apical walls of the left ventricle (2). The optimum ECG variables for the detection of AMI are ST-segment elevation $\geq$ 1 mm in at least 1 lead, either inferior (II, III, aVF) or lateral (V5, V6, I, aVL), and ST-segment elevation $\geq$ 2 mm in at least 1 anterior lead (V1–V4). Such a model has 56% sensitivity and 94% specificity. Changing the degree of ST-segment elevation greatly modifies both sensitivity and specificity (3).

Left Anterior Descending Coronary Artery Occlusion

The earliest signs of AMI are subtle and include increased T-wave amplitude over the affected area. T waves become more prominent, symmetrical, and pointed ("hyper-acute"). These changes in T waves are usually present for only 5 to 30 minutes after the onset of the infarction, and are followed by ST-segment changes. In practice, ST-segment elevation is often the earliest recognized sign of AMI (4).

After occlusion of the left anterior descending coronary artery (LAD), ST-segment elevation $\geq$ 1 mm is most frequently observed in V2 (sensitivity, 91–99%) and then, in decreasing order of frequency, in V3, V4, V5, aVL, V1, and V6. The maximum ST-segment elevation is recorded in V2 or V3 (3).

Powerful predictors of proximal LAD occlusion include ST elevation in leads I and aVL, and ST depression in inferior leads. ST-segment elevation in leads I and aVL often coexists with inferior ST-segment depression (3).

The electrical activity of the anterolateral wall of the left ventricle (supplied by both the first diagonal and the first obtuse marginal branches) is well captured by the leads aVL and I. During an acute anterior infarction, a culprit lesion at the level of the first diagonal can be suspected when precordial ST elevation is associated with

ST-segment elevation in aVL (highly specific) and when ST-segment elevation is present in both leads I and aVL (highly sensitive combination also for diagonal occlusion). Occlusion of the first diagonal may produce unique ECG changes characterized by ST-segment elevation in the noncontiguous leads aVL and V2, plus ST depression in leads III and aVF or in V4. When ST-segment elevation in leads I and aVL is accompanied by ST depression in lead V2, the culprit lesion is usually the first marginal branch of the left circumflex artery (LCX) (3).

Moreover, four ECG signs were recently found to be specific for occlusions at the level of the first septal perforator; these include ST-segment elevation in aVR, disappearance of preexisting septal Q waves in lateral leads, ST-segment depression in V5, and right bundle branch block (3,5).

Distal LAD occlusions usually have ST-segment elevation ≤ 3.2 mm in V2 and slight to moderate ST-segment elevation in V3. Other common findings are new Q waves in V4–V6 and augmented R-wave amplitude in V2. This pattern of acute right septal conduction delay results from an ischemic disruption of the right septal activation vectors, and may be indistinguishable from the changes observed in recent or old posterior infarction (3).

The significance of ST-segment elevation in lead V1 deserves a specific comment. Lead V1 captures electrical phenomena from the right septal area, which is supplied by the septal branches of the LAD. In some patients, the septum is additionally protected by blood supply from a conal branch of right coronary artery (RCA). This explains why approximately two-thirds of patients with anterior AMI have no ST-segment elevation in V1. The presence of ST-segment elevation in V1 correlates strongly with ST elevation in V3R and predicts the less common anatomic scenario in which a small conal branch of the RCA does not reach the interventricular septum. RCA occlusion is found in 7% of the patients, with ST-segment elevation in leads V1 through V4, who undergo coronary angiography (3).

Right Coronary Artery or Circumflex Occlusion

The typical ECG pattern of inferior infarction consists of ST-segment elevation in leads II, III, and aVF. The occlusion is in the RCA in 80% to 90% of the cases, and in the LCX in the remaining patients. Higher ST elevation in lead III than in lead II strongly suggests RCA disease. Because the only lead that faces the superior part of the left ventricle and directly opposes the inferior wall is aVL, ST depression in lead aVL is almost always determined by RCA occlusion. Injury in leads II, III, and aVF without ST depression in aVL indicates proximal LCX occlusion (2).

The arteries that supply the posterolateral region of the left ventricle are the obtuse marginal branch of the LCX, the posterolateral, and the LAD branches. Thus, ST-segment changes in leads V5–V6 indicate posterolateral ischemia triggered by either RCA or LCX occlusion. When ST elevation is significant (>2 mm), it is probably a sign of a large ischemic burden related to a very large artery (3). Precordial ST depression accompanying inferior injury is more likely to develop from LCX than RCA occlusion. The degree of ST depression in V3 compared with the degree of ST elevation in lead III ("V3/III ratio") is highest (1.2) when the occlusion is in the LCX and lowest (<0.5) when it is in the proximal RCA. Occlusions of the mid-RCA produce V3/III intermediate ratios. The absence of ST depression in leads V1–V2 rules out LCX occlusion, with a predictive value of >90% (6). ST-segment elevation in leads I–aVL or V5–V6 is frequently accompanied by ST depression in lead aVR. This sign is independent of ST depression in V1, and indicates a larger infarct size. However, lead aVR is frequently ignored in clinical practice, despite the demonstration of high predictive value of ST-segment changes by this lead (3).

The vascular beds of LCX have broad anatomic variability and may supply a rather small ventricle area. This is why the standard 12-lead ECG shows ST-segment elevation in less than half of the cases of LCX occlusion. When present, ST elevation is more often seen in leads II, III, and aVF, followed by leads V5, V6, and aVL. One-third of patients with chest pain secondary to LCX occlusion have isolated ST depression in the ECG; ST depression in leads V1–V2 is a sensitive sign. Another third of patients will not have any changes in the 12-lead ECG (3).

Special Electrocardiographic Injury Patterns

Anterior Plus Inferior Injury

The combination of anterior and inferior ST-segment elevation in the ECG may give the impression of a critical mass of myocardial injury. However, it often results from distal occlusion of a long LAD, which "wraps around" the apex and results in wall motion abnormalities circumscribed to the apex. Another possible cause can be an acute occlusion of the RCA that was supplying the collateral circulation for a chronically occluded LAD.

When injury in leads II, III, and aVF is accompanied by ST elevation in V1 but ST depression in V2, right ventricular, rather than apical, infarction is likely (3,7).

Left Main Disease

The ECG of patients with chest pain secondary to occlusion or subocclusion of the left main coronary artery frequently shows a combination of ST-segment elevation in aVR and

ST depression in leads I, II, and V4–V6. A sum of ST changes >18 mm is 90% sensitive for left main disease (3).

Diffuse ST-segment depression, as the marker of large subendocardial infarction, often signals left main trunk or triple vessel disease. On the other hand, diffuse precordial (and often inferior or lateral) ST depression with peak in leads V4–V6 may be caused by subendocardial ischemia from a subtotal obstruction of the LAD (3).

ST-Segment Depression

Many patients with acute chest pain have "reciprocal" ST-segment depression (ST depression concomitant with ST elevation in a lead group different from the one showing ST elevation). The mechanism underlying this ST depression is usually mirroring a phenomenon of electrical reflection of the transmural injury onto the opposite ventricular wall.

Another possible mechanism for ST depression is regional subendocardial ischemia or infarction. In patients with prolonged chest pain and predominant ST depression in any lead except aVR, ST depression of ≥4 mm is 97% specific (and 20% sensitive) for AMI (3).

The presence of ST-segment depression in the antero-lateral leads in the admission ECG of anterior AMI patients with reciprocal changes in inferior leads is associated with the presence of multivessel disease. While, among patients with inferior wall AMI, left precordial ST-segment depression predicts a high prevalence of multivessel disease (3).

Patients with isolated ST-segment depression AMI are likely to be older, with a high prevalence of previous myocardial infarction, triple vessel or left main trunk disease (8) (DVD: Case 7).

Right Ventricular Infarction

Transmural injury of the right ventricle translates into ST-segment elevation ≥1 mm in precordial leads. ST elevation in V1 is highly specific for proximal RCA occlusion. In 7% of patients, ST elevation extends to lead V5, suggesting anterior infarction. However, this ST elevation decreases toward V4, whereas in anterior injury the ST segment is more elevated in V2–V3, than in V1. Right ventricular infarction is usually concurrent with infarcts of the inferior wall. Fifty-four percent of patients with inferior injury have ST elevation in lead V4R (sensitivity for right ventricle infarction of 93%). Isolated right ventricular infarction is rare and occurs mainly in patients with right ventricular hypertrophy (2,3).

Left Bundle Branch Block

Spontaneous or pacing-induced left bundle branch block (LBBB) can obscure the electrocardiographic diagnosis of AMI. An indicator of AMI in the presence of LBBB is ST deviation in the same (concordant) direction as the major QRS vector. Concordant ST changes in the presences of LBBB include ST-segment depression of at least 1 mm in lead V1, V2, or V3 or in lead II, III, or aVF and elevation of at least 1 mm in lead V5. Extremely discordant ST deviation (>5 mm) is also suggestive of myocardial infarction in the presence of LBBB (9).

The left bundle branch usually receives blood from the LAD and the RCA. When a new LBBB occurs in the context of an AMI, the infarct is usually anterior and large and mortality extremely high (10).

Nonspecific ECG

Fifteen percent to eighteen percent of patients with AMI do not show changes in the initial ECG, and an additional 25% show nonspecific changes (3). Although nondiagnostic ECG in patients with chest pain is often associated with lesion in branch vessels, the probability of detecting AMI increases by recording serial ECG. However, because reperfusion therapies are more effective when administered early, it is ideal to maximize the information provided by the admission ECG. On the other hand, patients presenting with normal or nonspecific ECGs have a favorable prognosis, mainly due to smaller amount of myocardium at risk (11).

ECHOCARDIOGRAPHY

In patients with reperfused AMI, two main questions need to be promptly answered: (*i*) Has myocardium been optimally reperfused, and how much myocardium has the potential to further recover during follow-up? (*ii*) Is monitoring of left ventricular (LV) function/geometry able to identify early predictors of unfavorable remodeling?

Beyond its traditional diagnostic role (Table 2.1), echocardiography has become an important and powerful tool

Table 2.1 Echocardiography in Patients with Acute Myocardial Infarction: Key Points

Traditional role of echocardiogram
- Diagnosis of AMI in patients with a nondiagnostic ECG
- Risk stratification through the assessment of LV function
- Diagnosis of mechanical complications of AMI

Emergent role of echocardiogram
- Evaluation of effectiveness of reperfusion therapy
- Evaluation of functional recovery of post-ischemic myocardium (myocardial viability)
- Early risk stratification for LV remodeling
- Evaluation of intravenous MCE imaging for determining optimal AMI treatment strategies

Abbreviations: AMI, acute myocardial infarction; ECG, electrocardiogram; LV, left ventricular; MCE, myocardial contrast echocardiographic.

because it has the potential to adequately address these two main issues and to participate in therapeutic process.

This chapter focuses on emergent aspects of echo-evaluation of post-infarction LV remodeling in the setting of AMI treated by means of primary PCI.

Early Echocardiographic Monitoring of Post-Infarction LV Remodeling

Beyond infarct size (12,13), infarct-related artery (IRA) patency is thought to be one of the most important factors driving the LV remodeling process (14–16). However, LV dilation also occurs after successful PCI, despite the persistence of the IRA patency and the absence of significant residual stenosis, and still retains its poor prognostic significance (17). Multiple factors may contribute to LV remodeling, including the infarct location (18), the adequacy of reperfusion (19), the abrupt alteration of loading conditions (18), and the activation of circulating neurohormones and local autocrine tropic factors (20). Echo-Doppler provides simple and reliable information on most of the old (infarct location) and emerging (myocardial viability and diastolic function) risk factors that might strongly influence LV remodeling after primary PCI.

Myocardial Infarct Location

In one study on 285 consecutive patients (21), the incidence of a six-month LV remodeling progressively increased (10%, 23%, and 51%, respectively; $p < 0.001$) from the lowest to the highest tertile of infarct size, as assessed by the peak of MB-creatine-kinase. However, LV dilation was similar in anterior and non-anterior myocardial infarct in the group with medium and large infarct size, respectively, while it was significantly higher in patients with anterior infarct location and small infarct size (Fig. 2.1). Thus, patients successfully treated with primary PCI and relatively small infarcts should not be considered at low risk for LV

remodeling if infarct location is anterior. This fact helps to explain and clarify why in the work of Stone et al. (22) mortality is significantly increased in patients with anterior infarction compared with non-anterior infarction despite adjustment for infarct size, but this difference is evident only in the lowest quartile of infarct size as assessed by peak CK release.

Microvascular Dysfunction and Myocardial Viability

In patients with AMI, the absence of microvascular perfusion assessed by myocardial contrast echocardiography (MCE) with intracoronary injection early after mechanical recanalization may be found in up to 30% of the patients despite a thrombolysis in myocardial infarction (TIMI) grade 3 flow in the epicardial vessel (no-reflow phenomenon) (23,24). The no-reflow phenomenon predicts lack of recovery of resting LV systolic function, and a poor prognosis. In a study based on 100 patients with AMI treated by PCI the incidence of no-reflow was 18% (23). In patients with no-reflow, LV volumes progressively increased and at six months were larger than those of patients with MCE reflow (end-diastolic LV volume: 171 ± 61 mL vs. 115 ± 30 mL; $p < 0.0001$). By stepwise multiple regression analysis, microvascular dysfunction in the infarct-risk area resulted in the most important independent predictor of late LV dilation ($p = 0.0001$). These findings confirm experimental results (25) and expand the previous observations by Ito et al. (19), who found that microvascular integrity in the infarct zone—a sensitive marker of myocardial viability—prevents LV remodeling in reperfused patients.

Although MCE enhancement generally indicates normal perfusion and viable myocardium, contractile performance failed to improve in more than 50% of the segments that manifested normal opacification early after reperfusion (26,27), and an additional assessment

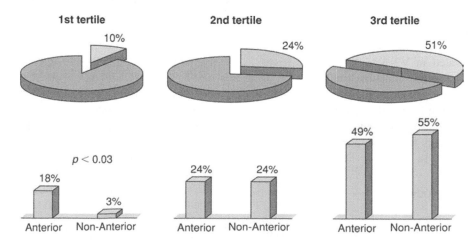

Figure 2.1   Incidence of LV remodeling according to infarct size and location. *Abbreviation*: LV, left ventricular.

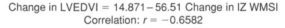

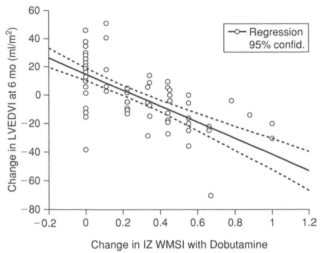

Figure 2.2 Relation between infarct zone viability expressed as changes in IZ WMSI at peak dobutamine and changes in LVEDVI at six months ($r = -0.66$; $p < 0.00001$). *Abbreviations*: IZ WMSI, infarct zone wall motion score index; LVEDVI, left ventricular end-diastolic volume index. *Source*: From Ref. 30.

of the contractile reserve with dobutamine stress may be necessary to establish viability and to evaluate the risk of LV remodeling (28,29). Consistently, the absence of residual infarct zone viability, as assessed by low-dose dobutamine echocardiography at day 3 after primary PCI, has discriminated patients who had progressive LV dilation from those who maintained normal LV geometry, despite a patent IRA and the absence of residual IRA stenosis in both groups (Fig. 2.2) (30). These data were confirmed by Nijland et al. (31). The future of echocardiographic assessment of myocardial post-reperfusion viability is focused on the intravenous MCE imaging (32). This technique permits a more reliable analysis of microvascular integrity in acute phase of myocardial infarction, as well as after microvascular convalescent stage is reached (33,34).

The recent AMICI (Acute Myocardial Infarction Contrast Imaging) trial (35) studied myocardial perfusion by using MCE in 110 consecutive patients who underwent successful primary or rescue PCI within six hours of ST-elevation AMI onset. MCE was performed within one day of PCI, and echo reperfusion was compared with TIMI flow grade, myocardial blush grade, peak CK, ST-segment resolution, and echocardiographic wall motion score. The end point was LV remodeling, which occurred in 25% of patients and was defined as a 20% increase in LV end-diastolic volume at the six-month follow-up echocardiography. At multivariate analysis, only the endocardial length of the myocardial perfusion

defect on MCE and a TIMI flow grade <3 predicted LV remodeling. Furthermore, in the subset of patients with a TIMI flow grade 3, only the endocardial length of MCE perfusion defect predicted LV remodeling.

In AMI patients treated by primary coronary stenting, the extent of late recovery of resting systolic function correlates with the extent of perfusion by intravenous MCE at three to five days after IRA recanalization. Furthermore, the presence of MCE patchy effect in the regions with persistent severe abnormalities of resting wall thickening identifies areas with contractile reserve (36), which may be beneficial for preventing adverse LV remodeling independently of recovery of resting function.

Currently available contrast agents are not yet approved for myocardial perfusion, thus their use is limited to clinical investigations. A future approval for their use in the clinical arena for assessing myocardial perfusion during AMI will allow to choose the optimal treatment strategies for individual patients.

Diastolic Function

In the early stages of coronary occlusion, there are marked alterations in diastolic behavior, with impaired ventricular relaxation and greatly elevated myocardial stiffness (36). These changes in ventricular chamber properties may be followed by the increase in end-diastolic filling pressure, which reflects elevated ventricular chamber stiffness within the ischemic zone (37). Doppler echocardiography of transmitral flow has emerged as a powerful noninvasive tool to assess the characteristics of LV filling, producing insights into diastolic function and its effect on filling pressure (38). Among the different Doppler variables, the deceleration time (DT) of the early filling wave has been found to have a strong negative correlation with chamber stiffness (39,40). Moreover, a shortening of DT, indicative of a restrictive filling pattern (RFP), has been found to affect early LV remodeling (41) and to predict an adverse outcome of patients with LV systolic dysfunction after AMI (42–44). In particular, an RFP, as expressed by a short DT (<130 milliseconds) at day 3 after primary PCI, was the most powerful predictor of LV remodeling even after controlling for infarct size, and the degree of LV dilation was related to the severity of impairment of LV filling (Fig. 2.3) (41). Furthermore, in a subgroup of patients with AMI and LV dysfunction, a short DT at day 3 after primary PCI resulted as a more powerful predictor of early LV dilation than brain natriuretic peptide levels (42). Although the prognostic value RFP may arise partly because it reflects a large infarct (43), the mechanisms linking the RFP to LV remodeling over and above the effects of infarct size, systolic dysfunction, and early patency of IRA are unclear (41,44). LV pressure overload will cause myocyte stretch, increased wall stress, decreased

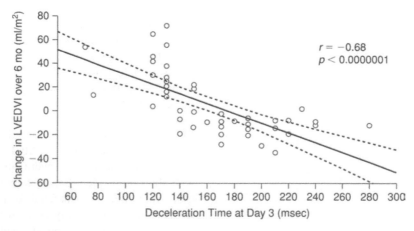

Figure 2.3 Relation between deceleration time and changes of LVEDVI at six months. *Abbreviation*: LVEDVI, left ventricular end-diastolic volume index. *Source*: From Ref. 41.

subendocardial perfusion, and reduced energy production. These variables in turn are associated with neurohormonal activation and ventricular remodeling. Although the remodeling process will initially restore stroke volume and systemic hemodynamics, continuing dilation will have a detrimental effect on long-term LV function and survival. These findings may provide the critical linkage between RFP and worse prognosis after AMI (44–47). Consistently, several studies have suggested that an RFP, irrespective of the method for its assessment, is an independent predictor of poor outcome post-AMI (44–47). However, the conclusions of these studies are limited by the small sample sizes and the low overall event rates. This fact has precluded a definite conclusion on the independent importance of an RFP, especially when overall LV systolic function is preserved. More recently, the Meta-analysis Research Group in Echocardiography (MeRGE) study on 3396 AMI patients has confirmed the important individual prognostic power of an RFP (as assessed by a Doppler pattern of mitral inflow) (48). In this meta-analysis RFP was associated with all-cause mortality (HR, 2.67; 95% CI 2.23–3.20; $p < 0.001$) and remained an independent predictor in multivariate analysis (HR, 2.35; 95% CI 1.94–2.83; $p < 0.0001$) with age, gender, and LV ejection fraction (LVEF). The overall prevalence of RFP was 20%, and it was higher (36%) in the quartile of patients with lower LVEF (<39%), and lower (9%) in patients with higher LVEF (>53%; $p < 0.0001$). RFP remained significant within each quartile of LVEF, and no interaction was found for RFP and LVEF ($p = 0.42$). RFP also predicted mortality in patients with above and below a median end-systolic volume index, and in different Killip classes.

A major unresolved question is how to optimally manage patients with abnormal LV filling. To date, no interventional trial has been undertaken with hard end points in which patient selection has been based on abnormalities in LV filling. In a study on 104 consecutive

patients with a first anterior AMI successfully treated with primary PCI, among patients without RFP, two-year cumulative mortality rate was only 3%, and the occurrence of death, AMI, and congestive heart failure

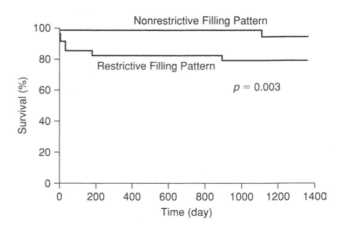

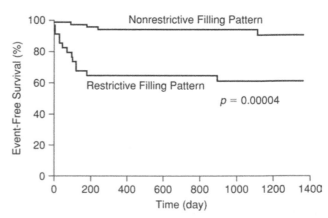

Figure 2.4 Cumulative survival rates for cardiac mortality (*top graph*) and for all major cardiac events (death, hospital admission for heart failure or myocardial infarction) (*bottom graph*). *Source*: From Ref. 44.

occurred in only 6%. On the other hand, one-third of patients had evidence of RFP, and among these patients, the two-year mortality rate was 24% and the adverse event rate was 39% (Fig. 2.4) (44). Although patients with restrictive filling appeared sicker compared with those without RFP, echocardiographic diastolic dysfunction remained an independent predictor of mortality (44). Although LV volumes increased at six months among patients with RFP, compared with patients with normal LV filling, they remained unchanged from 6 to 24 months, as did LVEF and diastolic and systolic eccentricity indexes (Fig. 2.5) (44). It is reasonable to speculate that mechanical reperfusion and persistent late patency may have blunted the remodeling process or at least attenuated its effects on LV shape and geometry, and therefore may have exerted a positive influence on the progression of heart failure and prognosis.

Mitral Regurgitation

Ischemic mitral regurgitation (MR) should be distinguished from MR due to structural leaflet disease (degenerative or rheumatic disease or mitral valve prolapse) and casually associated with coronary artery disease.

The mitral valve has a complex anatomy contributing actively to the process of systolic valvular closing. This mechanism consists of a combination of interactions of the ventricle, annulus, and papillary muscles. Any alteration in one or more of these structures may contribute to the regurgitation. Papillary muscle dysfunction and dilatation or loss of contraction of the mitral annulus, the two mechanisms historically cited to cause MR (49), do not adequately explain ischemic MR and have been challenged. Extensive evidence has shown that ischemic MR results from LV distortion, which displaces the papillary muscles and tethers the mitral leaflet apically, resulting in systolic tenting of mitral valve leaflets away from the annulus with incomplete closure of the valve (50–54).

The frequency of post–myocardial infarction MR reported in the literature differs greatly owing to baseline differences in study populations or to the technique used to detect MR. Post–myocardial infarction MR remains frequent, up to 74% (55–57), despite modern management of myocardial infarction, including a high rate of reperfusion

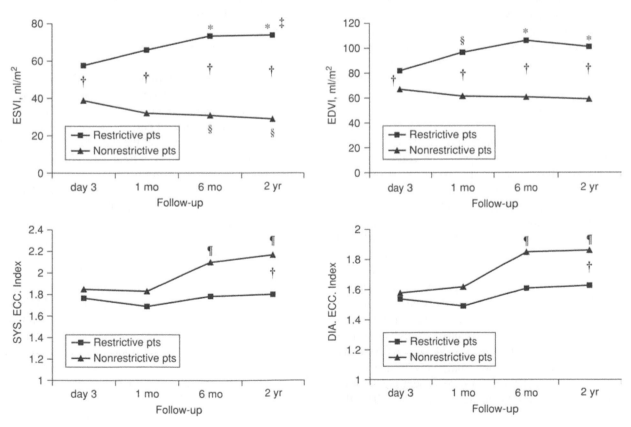

Figure 2.5 Time course of LV end-systolic (*top left graph*) and end-diastolic (*top right graph*) volume indexes (ESVI and EDVI, respectively) in the restrictive and nonrestrictive filling groups. Time course of LV systolic (SYS.) (*bottom left graph*) and diastolic (DIA.) (*bottom right graph*) eccentricity (ECC.) indexes in the restrictive and nonrestrictive filling groups. Analysis of variance: * $p < 0.0005$ vs. baseline within groups; † $p < 0.001$ between groups; ‡ $p < 0.05$ vs. 1 month within groups; § $p < 0.05$ vs. baseline within groups; ¶ $p < 0.005$ vs. baseline and 1 month within groups. *Abbreviation*: LV, left ventricular. *Source*: From Ref. 44.

and nearly systematic use of antiremodeling therapies (58,59). Color Doppler echocardiography is the most sensitive technique and allows qualitative evaluation of the mitral valve apparatus to best define the etiology of MR and quantitative analysis by measuring the effective regurgitant orifice area and the regurgitant volume (60).

Patients with MR after myocardial infarction are usually older (56,61–64) and more likely to be women (61,65–67) to have a history of previous infarction (56), a more diffuse coronary disease, and larger infarctions compared with patients without MR (68). Reports on the association between MR and the location of the infarction are conflicting; while one study reported an association with inferior infarction (69), other studies reported a higher prevalence of MR in anterior myocardial infarction or no difference in infarct location (61,65).

Published studies differ greatly in design, inclusion criteria, duration of follow-up, and technique of MR assessment. However, they consistently indicate that MR after myocardial infarction carries an adverse prognosis with increased risk of death and heart failure independently of previously known indicators of risk after myocardial infarction (61,63,65,70–72), electrocardiographic pattern (with or without ST elevation) (65,72), and rate and modality of reperfusion (61,65,71). The only report to advice caution in the interpretation of MR after myocardial infarction is the recent study of Hillis et al., which suggests that increased mortality in patients with MR is primarily determined by other related factors, such as increased age and poorer LV systolic function (62).

The predictive value of MR could greatly vary according to the timing of echocardiography, because the early days or weeks after MI are characterized by recovery of stunned or hibernating myocardium and significant changes in LV function and geometry, which may significantly affect the degree of MR (73). LV remodeling could be the link between post-myocardial infarction functional MR and poor prognosis after AMI. In patients successfully treated with primary PCI, early high-degree MR was associated with a higher prevalence of six-month LV remodeling (66% vs. 22%, $p < 0.0001$) and of two-year heart failure (39% vs. 12%, $p < 0.0002$) (65); in this study a significant correlation was found between effective regurgitant orifice area of MR and LV dilation ($r = 0.54$, $p = 0.0004$). By stepwise multivariate regression analysis, effective regurgitant orifice area of MR was an independent predictor of LV remodeling ($p = 0.001$) and heart failure ($p < 0.0001$).

ANGIOGRAPHY

In the setting of AMI, coronary angiography procedure should not be the one that is routinely performed for elective diagnostic purpose. Time factor is crucial. Therefore, the diagnostic examination must be ductile, intervention oriented, and time and contrast medium containment guided. The radiographic views must be just the sufficient number to detect the IRA and to plan the PCI and proper device selection. Only in the event of uncertain identification of infarct-related artery or angiographic findings not consistent with clinical and electrocardiographic features it is wise to take time to achieve an accurate diagnosis. These can be reached even by using more, nonstandard radiographic views, and in some cases completing the examination with left ventricle and/or ascending aorta angiography.

The Coronary Artery Disease

During AMI, the most common finding at emergency coronary angiography is a cutoff sign at the point of acutely occluded coronary vessel, associated with a variable amount of thrombotic burden. Younger patients are more likely to have lower plaque burden and higher thrombotic burden than older subjects. On the other hand, older patients present more frequently diffuse and multivessel coronary artery disease with a higher total plaque burden. The presence of coronary thrombus is revealed by the feature of a convex margin that stains with contrast and persists for several cardiac cycles. Definite intraluminal globular filling defect can be visualized if the vessel is not totally occluded. The sites of acute coronary artery occlusion are analogous of those found in patients with chronic stable angina pectoris, representing different stages of the same disease. Therefore, an acute coronary occlusion is frequent to involve a bifurcation site or a coronary bend.

Atherosclerotic aneurysmal dilatation of the IRA is an uncommon angiographic finding (about 2% of all cases) (74), and it is frequently associated with high-burden thrombus formation. Three patterns of coronary dilatation have been described: the ectasia type (diffuse dilatation of ≥50% more of the length of the IRA), the fusiform type (defined as a spindle-shaped dilatation), and the saccular type (defined as a localized spherical-shaped dilatation). There are incidences of 70%, 20%, and 10%, respectively, of ectasia, fusiform, and saccular types. The right coronary artery is the one more frequently involved in the aneurysmal dilatation (>50% of cases), followed by the LAD and LCXs. Aneurysmal dilatation may involve multiple coronary sites (74) (cases 21 and 38).

In a series of more than 1000 consecutive, unselected patients treated by the Florence group for ST-segment elevation AMI from 1995 to 1999, the culprit lesion was located in the LAD, RCA, LCX, left main trunk, and bypass grafts in 51%, 36%, 12%, 1%, and 1% of the cases, respectively (75).

Multivessel coronary artery disease is present in about half of the patients (75,76).

Significant exaggeration of nonculprit lesion stenoses severity may occur at angiography if a focal increase in vascular tone develops in the acute phase. This phenomenon may affect multivessel revascularization decision-making (77). The incidence of associated chronic coronary occlusion is 12% (75,78). Angiographic evidence of collateral flow [Rentrop (79) grade >1] to the IRA was present in about 23% of patients with AMI admitted within six hours from symptoms onset (78).

Inability to identify the IRA occasionally occurs, and generally, in AMI without ST-segment elevation. Angiographic results must always fit with clinical and electrocardiographic findings to correctly identify the infarct-related vessel.

The TIMI Flow Grade of the Infarct Artery

Coronary blood flow in the IRA can be graded using the classification developed by the TIMI group (80). At baseline coronary angiography, the most common finding is a 0 to 1 TIMI grade flow (about 70–80% of patients) (76).

In a previously published series of AMI patients treated by primary angioplasty, TIMI grade 3 flow has been found in about 10% to 20% of patients at the time of initial angiography, possibly owing to endogenous fibrinolysis or pretreatment with aspirin, heparin, and ADP antagonists (81,82). In the 2507 patients enrolled in the four PAMI trials (81), a spontaneously open IRA at the baseline angiography favorably affected the outcome. In patients with TIMI grade flow 3 at baseline angiography, the in-hospital mortality rate was 0.5% versus 2.4% of patients with TIMI grade flow 0 to 2 ($p = 0.02$).

Early reperfusion before definitive angioplasty is associated with improved survival by enhancing myocardial salvage and reducing complications related to LV failure. Theoretically, the procedural success rate of angioplasty may be improved by lytic-mediated thrombus-burden reduction (resulting in less distal microembolization) and a patent infarct vessel before angioplasty, facilitating road mapping and proper device selection.

ELDERLY

The Bias Selection of Elderly Patients for Percutaneous Intervention for Acute Myocardial Infarction and the Effectiveness of a Routine Aggressive Reperfusive Strategy

Age is a strong predictor of cardiogenic shock (CS) and death in patients with AMI, and elderly patients comprise the fastest growing segment of Western country populations. It should be highlighted that many patients with AMI admitted to community hospitals currently do not receive any emergency reperfusive treatment because of late presentation for fibrinolysis (>6 hours from symptom onset) or contraindication for high risk of bleeding and stroke. Elderly is frequently associated with comorbidities that contraindicate fibrinolytic therapy, and many elderly patients are currently excluded from fibrinolytic treatment. This high-risk subset of patients may have a strong benefit from primary mechanical intervention, while the benefit of fibrinolysis may be mild or absent for the decreased efficacy in reperfusion and the high risk of stroke. The reperfusive option in elderly patients has to be considered as a first-line problem considering that in Western countries elderly patients represent one-third of all patients admitted with a diagnosis of ST-segment elevation AMI. Despite this trend, few data exist about the benefit of an early mechanical reperfusive treatment in elderly patients with AMI. Moreover, a number of survey studies have shown that there is a bias selection of patients referred for emergency mechanical revascularization favoring younger patients (83–88). The National Registry of Myocardial Infarction investigators have shown that in the past decade the proportion of ideal patients not receiving acute reperfusion therapy decreased by one-half (20.6% in 1994–1997, and 11.6% in 2000–2004, $p < 0.001$) (89). However, use of reperfusive therapy remained lower in patients 75 years or older. Elderly patients who were ideal for reperfusive treatment had a nearly 40% lower probability to receive reperfusion compared with patients younger than 55 years (adjusted OR for receiving acute reperfusion therapy 0.63, 95% CI 0.58–0.68).

Furthermore, elderly patients are poorly represented or excluded in previous randomized trials on primary PCI. This selection bias makes it very difficult to get a correct analysis of the impact of an emergency percutaneous revascularization strategy in elderly patients.

In the CADILLAC (Controlled Abciximab and Device Investigation to Lower Late Angiographic Complications) trial, which compared coronary angioplasty and provisional infarct artery stenting with routine infarct artery stenting with or without abciximab, the median age of the enrolled population was only 59 years, and more than 20% of eligible patients with AMI were excluded from randomization (76). Patients consented but not randomized were older (median age 61.9 vs. 59.0 years, $p = 0.002$) and had a higher in-hospital mortality compared with randomized patients (4.0% vs. 1.6%, $p = 0.001$) (90). Again, the median age of 59 years is not consistent with those of large survey studies representative of the "real world" of AMI that showed a higher mean age of patients due to the higher percentage of elderly patients. The National Registry of Myocardial Infarction showed a mean age of

61.8 ± 13.3 years of the 66,883 patients with AMI recruited in the 2000 to 2003 period (89). This selection bias is evident also in extremely high-risk setting, such as CS due to predominant ventricular failure, where mechanical reperfusion may be considered as the only effective therapeutic option. In the SHOCK (SHould we emergently revascularize Occluded Coronaries for cardiogenic shock) trial, patients selected for randomization were younger than nonrandomized patients (mean age of randomized patients 65.8 ± 10.4 years; mean age of nonrandomized patients 68.5 ± 12.1 years, $p < 0.001$) and the incidence of patients 75 years and older in the SHOCK registry cohort was twofold higher than that in the randomized trial cohort (32.4%) (88,91). The bias selection is present also in single high-volume center experiences. Laster et al. reported the results of coronary angioplasty in 55 octogenarians that represented only 4.4% of the overall treated population (92). The Mayo Clinic experience of primary PCI for AMI in octogenarians treated between 1979 and 1997 includes only 127 patients, less than 8% of the overall treated population (93). In the National Cardiovascular Network, a registry based on 109,708 patients who underwent PCI, only 418 octogenarian patients had PCI for AMI, and the mortality rate in this subset of very elderly patients was 11% (94). This percentage is inferior to those reported by survey studies, where octogenarians represent at least 10% of the overall population of patients with AMI (95), suggesting that many elderly patients are excluded from reperfusive treatment also in centers with a program- of primary PCI for AMI.

Sakai et al. reported the results of PCI in a series of 1063 patients with AMI. Of these, 261 were 75 years and older (24%). The in-hospital mortality rate was 8.4% in elderly patients, and 3.7% in patients younger than 75 years ($p < 0.01$) (96). It is important to highlight that in this experience, a substantial minority of death in the elderly was noncardiac (noncardiac mortality rate was 2.3% in the elderly and 0.6% in the younger patient group, $p < 0.005$), suggesting an increased incidence in the elderly of comorbidities and competing illness that may have a significant impact on outcome despite successful coronary revascularization.

In Florence, from 1995, all patients with AMI are considered eligible for primary PCI without any restriction based on age or clinical status on presentation. It is likely that the use of routine PCI for all patients with AMI minimizes any bias selection favoring younger patients for an aggressive revascularization strategy and allows a correct assessment of the feasibility, safety, and efficacy of current PCI techniques in elderly patients.

Overall, from starting of the program of primary PCI in 1995, 3035 consecutive patients underwent primary PCI. The median age was 65 ± 13 years (range 23–99 years), 24% of patients were older than 75 years, and 12% were octogenarians or older. These age characteristics are consistent with those of large survey studies and confirm that this population may be considered representative of the "real world" of AMI. The overall six-month mortality was 7.1%, and by Cox analysis, age was strongly related to the risk of death (HR 1.05, 95% CI 1.04–1.07, $p < 0.001$). The other variables independently related to the risk of death were CS, anterior AMI, previous myocardial infarction, and primary PCI failure. When patients are categorized on the basis of ages 75 years and older and younger than 75 years, it is evident that elderly patients beyond this age category have a worse baseline clinical profile, with a greater incidence seen in women and those with hypertension, CS, previous myocardial infarction, and multivessel disease. Despite this higher baseline risk profile, the procedural success rate in the elderly group was slightly lower than in the younger patient group (94% and 98%, respectively; $p < 0.001$), and coronary stenting was accomplished in the large majority of patients (87% in both groups; $p = 0.795$). However, despite the high procedural success rate, the mortality rate in elderly patients was more than threefold higher than the one of younger patients (15% vs. 5%; $p < 0.001$). After adjusting for differences in baseline characteristics, age remained a strong predictor of death (HR 1.07, 95% CI 1.03–1.1, $p < 0.001$).

Elderly and Cardiogenic Shock

Routine emergency revascularization strategy in elderly patients with AMI complicated by CS due to predominant ventricular failure is a matter of debate. The SHOCK trial did not show any benefit of an emergency revascularization strategy compared with an initial medical stabilization strategy that included intra-aortic balloon counterpulsation and fibrinolytic treatment in elderly patients (91). The overall one-month mortality rate did not differ significantly between the emergency revascularization group and the medical therapy group (46.7% and 56.0%, respectively, $p = 0.11$). A positive interaction between emergency revascularization and subgroup variables was found only for patients younger than 75 years. In patients 75 years or older, emergency revascularization was associated with increase in the relative risk of death despite the randomized population having a lower risk profile than patients enrolled in the registry (88). Patients 75 years or older and randomized to emergency revascularization had a one-month mortality rate of 75%, while patients younger than 75 years had mortality rate of 41.4%. The results of this study, i.e., the only concluded randomized trial comparing an emergency revascularization strategy with an initial medical stabilization strategy in patients with CS, have been considered for the

ACC/AHA guideline Task Force that recommended an emergency revascularization strategy in patients with CS only for those younger than 75 years (97). However, as suggested by the SHOCK investigators, the small number of elderly patients enrolled in the trial (only 56 patients!) may explain the lack of a benefit of an emergency revascularization strategy in elderly patients, as well as the worse baseline risk profile of patients randomized to emergency revascularization compared with patients randomized to initial medical stabilization (98).

However, to explain the negative results of emergency revascularization in elderly as shown by the SHOCK trial, major limitations in logistic and procedural outcome should be highlighted along with the differences in baseline risk profile between patients randomized to emergency revascularization or initial medical stabilization. Explanations for the lack of benefit of emergency revascularization in elderly patients may lie within the very long delay from CS diagnosis to randomization, time to treatment being a strong determinant of survival in patients with CS, and the nonuse of stents in the majority of patients, which results in a very low procedural success rate (77%) (91). In the SHOCK trial population, the median time from myocardial infarction onset to the diagnosis of CS was only five hours, and this delay is similar to the one of the SHOCK registry population (88), but the abnormally long time from CS diagnosis to randomization (>4 hours) resulted in a median time to treatment of 11 hours, while only a minority of patients (25%; 38 of 152 patients randomized to the emergency revascularization arm) received the reperfusive treatment within six hours of the diagnosis. The subgroup analysis in the SHOCK trial suggests an inverse relation between time to treatment and survival, but this interaction was not significant due to the small number of patients who underwent revascularization within six hours after infarction (91). Another major criticism raised from the results of the SHOCK trial is based on the very low procedural success rate, due, at least in part, to the nonuse of stents in the large majority of patients. This criticism is supported by the different mortality rate according to the successful or unsuccessful procedure. Among patients assigned to revascularization, successful PCI was associated with a one-month mortality rate of 38%, while unsuccessful PCI was associated with a one-month mortality rate of 79% ($p = 0.003$) (91).

As suggested by the negative results of the SHOCK trial in the elderly, the effectiveness of a routine PCI strategy in elderly patients with AMI complicated by CS due to predominant ventricular failure are strongly dependent by the logistic model used and the quality of the revascularization procedures.

The impact of these two variables on patient outcome seems to be confirmed by the Florence experience (99).

Of 280 patients with CS due to predominant ventricular failure, the elderly group (age $\geq$ 75 years, mean age 81 ± 5 years) included 104 patients (37%), while the remaining 176 patients were younger than 75 years (mean age 62 ± 9 years). The large majority of patients (92% of the elderly group, and 90% of the younger patient group) were admitted within six hours from symptom onset. Overall, there were 13 primary PCI failures (4.6%), 8 in the elderly group (8%) and 5 in the younger patient group (3%, $p = 0.062$). IRA stenting was accomplished in most patients of both groups (80% in each group). The six-month mortality rate was 56% in the elderly group and 26% in the younger patient group ($p < 0.001$). There were no differences in reinfarction rate between groups. The large majority of deaths in both groups occurred during hospitalization, and refractory CS or congestive heart failure accounted for most deaths. After multivariate analysis, the variables related to mortality were age (HR 1.07, 95% CI 1.02–1.12, $p = 0.005$) and primary PCI failure (HR 4.01, 95% CI 1.53–10.51, $p = 0.005$).

The most relevant demographic characteristic of this CS population is the high incidence (37%) of elderly patients. This incidence is superior to those of previous survey studies of patients undergoing primary PCI, and to the one of the SHOCK trial (91). In the SHOCK trial the incidence of patients 75 years or older was only 16% (24 patients of 152 randomized to emergency revascularization). This discrepancy may be explained by a referral bias for PCI that excluded from an emergency revascularization treatment older and sicker patients. Thus, one may infer that the Florence policy of routine primary PCI in all patients with AMI without any restriction based on age resulted in a representative sample of the population of elderly patients with AMI complicated by CS.

Another unique feature of this series is that the large majority of the patients had reperfusive treatment within six hours from AMI symptom onset. The short time to treatment, as revealed in this series of patients, may be explained, in part, by the logistic model used that included in the Florence metropolitan area a network of mobile coronary care units, allowing the diagnosis of AMI at home and simultaneously alerting the invasive cardiology team; the effective assistance during transportation (intubation, inotropic, and antiarrhythmic treatment) from home directly to the catheterization laboratory; and a zero door-to-balloon time, which make it possible for a large number of patients with CS on presentation to reach the catheterization laboratory within six hours from AMI onset (100).

The procedural success rate was higher compared with the SHOCK trial, and similar in elderly and younger patient groups. This figure may be explained by the use of stents in the majority of patients, since it has be shown that infarct artery stenting is strongly associated with higher acute procedural success and lower incidence of target vessel failure after a successful PCI (101–106).

The six-month mortality rate was more than twofold higher in the elderly patients compared with the one of younger patients, and multivariate analysis confirmed age as a strong predictor of mortality, in spite of a successful mechanical revascularization. Consistent with the results of previous studies, the other variable independently related to the risk of death was primary PCI failure (107–109). The six-month mortality rate of 56% for patients 75 years or older compares favorably with those of previous studies. This favorable outcome may be explained in part by the high procedural success rate, and in part by the short time from CS onset and revascularization.

Several studies have shown that procedural success is strongly associated with survival (107–109). Time to treatment is another variable that is strongly related with survival in high-risk AMI patients, mainly in patients with CS (100,110–112). However, the comparison of the outcome of the Florence series of patients with that of other studies should be done cautiously due to the inherent biases that have contributed to treatment approaches. In the SHOCK registry, only 62% of patients with CS due to predominant ventricular failure underwent coronary angiography, and only 35.4% of the women and 31% of the men had PCI (113).

The apparent benefit of emergency PCI in elderly with AMI complicated by CS, as revealed in the Florence experience, strongly supports the use of a routine emergency PCI strategy in elderly with AMI complicated by CS. Age, itself, remains an important outcome predictor among elderly patients, but the higher mortality in them should not discourage the emergency revascularization strategy since many data suggest that the magnitude of the benefit of a treatment is directly related to the risk of death. As a consequence, the measured benefit of emergency PCI in elderly patients could be considered superior to the one in younger patients despite a twofold higher mortality rate in the elderly compared with younger patients. In support of this hypothesis are the data from randomized trials comparing primary PCI with fibrinolysis that showed a stronger benefit of percutaneous mechanical revascularization with increasing age in patients with AMI without CS on admission (114,115).

A critical appraisal to the results of the SHOCK trial, as well as the results of the published registries, resulted in a revision of the ACC/AHA guidelines for the treatment of CS complicating AMI, and emergent PCI should be viewed as applicable to all patients including those 75 years or older (116).

Technical Issues

There are no technical aspects of AMI PCI that are specific to the elderly. However, several technical aspects are more frequently encountered with increasing age, and most are subsequent to the increased diffusion of the atherosclerotic process in the coronary system as well as in the other vascular districts. The inability to identify the infarct artery is more frequent in patients with non-ST-segment elevation on the presentation ECG. In these patients baseline coronary angiography frequently reveals diffuse disease and multiple coronary occlusions that make the correct recognition of the target vessel difficult (DVD: Case 29). On the contrary, the inability to identify the infarct artery in ST-segment elevation AMI may be considered a remote possibility. The electrocardiographic location of AMI and the staining contrast medium at level of acute coronary occlusion due to the thrombotic component of the occlusion make the identification of the infarct artery easy in nearly all cases.

Anatomic coronary characteristics that are more frequently associated with increasing age are diffuse calcification and tortuosity of coronary arteries (case 6 and 22). Both these characteristics suggest the use of very trackable and high support coronary wires, as well as guiding catheters with high backup (Voda, Amplatz left, and Hockey Stick may be considered the first choice guiding catheters). Predilation before coronary stenting should be considered mandatory in patients with diffusely calcified and tortuous vessel to decrease the risk of coronary stenting failure.

The femoral access may be difficult or even impossible in patients with diffuse atherosclerosis and tortuosity of the iliac-femoral axes. The use of hydrophilic wires and long shafts under fluoroscopic guidance may solve the access problem. Extremely tortuous aorto-iliac trees may prevent the advancement of the guiding catheter over a long shaft: the more direct solution to this problem is the use of guiding catheters smaller than the size of the shaft (typically a 6F guiding catheter on an 8F shaft) and of a 0.63 wire for the guiding catheter (DVD: Case 8). The radial or brachial access is alternative to the femoral access. However, it should be highlighted that in nearly all patients with a tortuous aorto-iliac axis, the tortuosity will be a problem even by using the alternative brachial approach.

For patients who need intra-aortic balloon counterpulsation, the balloon assistance should be stopped as soon as possible because of the increased risk in elderly patients of device-related fatal complications (e.g., retroperitoneal hematoma and visceral embolism).

It should be remembered that in elderly patients a substantial minority of in-hospital deaths are due to noncardiac cause (96), and great attention deserves the correct use of heparin and contrast medium to decrease the risk of hemorrhagic complications and renal insufficiency.

No specific contraindication exists to the use of abciximab in elderly patients, and the safety profile of the drug in elderly is similar to the one in younger patients (117).

WOMEN

Epidemiology

Cardiovascular diseases are the leading cause of death in women in the Western countries. In the United States, in 2000, 41% of deaths in women were due to coronary artery disease (118). Moreover, all survey studies show that the mortality rate of women with AMI is higher than men, regardless of the treatment received (85,119–126). A statistical survey analysis in the United States revealed a one-year mortality of 38% of women after AMI (127).

A unique feature of the risk of death of women with AMI is the so-called age paradox. The odds of in-hospital death for AMI increase with decrease in age for women versus men (119,128,129). This means that the younger the patient, the higher the risk of death for women relative to men. Data from the second National Registry of Myocardial Infarction show that the mortality rate in women is higher than in men for all age groups younger than 80 years, and that this difference reaches a peak in age groups younger than 50 years. In patients younger than 50 years, the mortality rate for women is more than twofold that of men (6.3% vs. 3.0%). It has been suggested that younger women (younger than 65 or 70 years) may represent a distinct high-risk group (128). The higher risk was only partially accounted for differences in coexisting conditions, clinical characteristics, and early management. However, in this large database of 384,878 patients, an analysis by type of treatment was not performed; thus, it is unknown if an interaction between sex and age also exists in patients who undergo primary PCI. The age paradox is evident also among the survivors in the acute phase of AMI. A study based on a sample of 1935 patients surviving the acute phase of myocardial infarction showed that for patients younger than 50 years, women had a lower long-term survival compared with men, while for those 70 years or older, men had a poorer long-term survival compared with women (130).

Another unique feature associated with the higher mortality rate in women is the impact of diabetes mellitus (DM). DM is a stronger risk factor for women compared with men. Barnett-Connor et al. in a study based on a follow-up of 14 years have shown that the adjusted risk of DM for death was higher in women than in men (3.32 vs. 1.89, respectively) (131). It has been suggested that DM in women could be considered a coronary heart disease equivalent due to its high detrimental effect on the course of atherosclerotic cardiovascular disease in this sex (132).

Despite these impressive epidemiological data, several studies have shown a referral selection bias for reperfusive therapy for AMI, pharmacological or mechanical, favoring men (85,89,122,123,133,134), and making the analysis of the benefit of primary PCI in women complex and difficult. Few data exist on the impact of female gender on outcome of patients with AMI undergoing primary PCI, and the complex interplay of selection bias owing to primary PCI eligibility, the higher risk of procedural complications in women than in men, and the differences in baseline risk factors have not been evaluated completely.

In a series of 670 patients, Vacek et al. reported a long-term mortality of 7% in women and 9% in men (135). In the Primary Angioplasty in Myocardial Infarction (PAMI) and PAMI-2 trial cohorts, in-hospital mortality was considered similar in women and in men, and PAMI investigators suggested that primary coronary angioplasty may offset the effects of high-risk demographic characteristics of women (136). This hypothesis was not confirmed by the outcome analysis of the Stent-PAMI patient cohort (137). In the Stent-PAMI trial, 900 patients with AMI were randomized to primary coronary angioplasty or primary stenting. At six months, women had a higher rate of mortality (7.9% vs. 2.0%, $p = 0.0002$) and reinfarction (6.4% vs. 2.7%, $p = 0.01$) than men, whereas the late target vessel revascularization rates were similar (13.8% vs. 10.5%, $p = 0.20$). Moreover, primary infarct artery stenting improved the prognosis of men but not of women.

In the CADILLAC trial a more complete analysis that also included body surface area provided different results from the PAMI studies (138). In this study that included 2082 patients with AMI randomized to angioplasty or stenting, with and without abciximab, women accounted for 27% of the entire population. In comparison with men, women were older, had lower body surface area, and a higher incidence of DM, hypertension, hyperlipidemia, and a longer delay to treatment. The unadjusted one-year mortality was higher in women compared with men (7.6% vs. 3.0%, $p < 0.001$), as well as target vessel revascularization rate (16.7% vs. 12.1%, $p = 0.006$), major adverse event rate (23.9% vs. 15.3% $p < 0.001$), and moderate-severe bleeding rate (7.2% vs. 2.8%, $p < 0.001$). Female gender was an independent predictor of one-year major adverse events (HR 1.64, 95% CI 1.24–2.17, $p = 0.0006$), but not of death (HR 1.11, 95% CI 0.53–2.36, $p = 0.78$), while body surface area was independently related to mortality (HR 0.13, 95% CI 0.02–0.77, $p = 0.03$). Compared with balloon angioplasty, infarct artery stenting resulted in a strong reduction of major adverse events (28.1–19.1%, $p = 0.01$) and target vessel revascularization (20.4–10.8%, $p = 0.002$).

The stringent eligibility criteria for enrolment used in the PAMI randomized studies and CADILLAC study may, in part, explain the conflicting results from the analysis of the patient cohorts. The randomization criteria used resulted in the exclusion from enrollment of many patients at higher risk of death, such as patients in Killip class III or IV, or elderly patients who were represented in very small numbers in these studies.

The performance of routine PCI in all patients with AMI may help to minimize bias and generalize results. As a consequence, the analysis of registry studies, based on unselected consecutive patient series, may help to correctly assess the impact of gender on outcome of patients undergoing primary PCI, since in these studies, any bias selection process was avoided.

These conditions were satisfied in a series of 1019 patients (789 men and 230 women) reported by the Florence investigators (75). The high incidence of very elderly patients and CS is the most relevant demographic characteristics of this population. The mean age of women was 70.3 ± 11.6 years, and 39% of female patients were younger than 75 years versus 13% of male patients (p < 0.001). In the female group there was a greater incidence of diabetes (20% vs. 13%, $p = 0.007$), hypertension (40% vs. 32%, $p = 0.017$), and CS (19% vs. 11%, $p = 0.003$). There were no differences in onset of symptoms to treatment time. The only differences in baseline angiographic characteristics were smaller infarct arteries in women than in men, as defined by the reference vessel diameter, and a lower incidence of collateral Rentrop grade 2 to 3 flow supplying the infarct area in women. The six-month mortality rate was twofold higher in women than in men (12% vs. 7%, $p = 0.028$). After multivariate analysis, female gender did not emerge as an independent predictor of mortality, and the higher mortality in women could be explained only by older age, and by the greater incidence of CS. In this series of patients there were no differences between women and men in admission and treatment delay times, suggesting that the outcome was not influenced by a longer delay in women, as reported from previous studies (119,121,133). Similar results were reported by two other observational studies. Cariou et al. in a series of 400 consecutive unselected patients who underwent primary or rescue angioplasty showed a higher in-hospital mortality in women than in men (19% vs. 7%, respectively), but female gender was not an independent predictor of death (134). Brodie in a series of 1490 patients treated with primary PCI, reported a mortality rate higher in women than in men (11.6% and 6.9%, respectively) (139). Again, when the mortality rate was adjusted for differences in baseline variables, female gender was not a significant predictor of death (139).

The age paradox was not revealed in these studies, and this fact may be due to the relatively small number of patients in these single-center databases, associated with the large predominance of elderly women, or very elderly women, that accounted for the large majority of deaths.

Efficacy of Primary Infarct Artery Stenting in Women

In the Florence patient series, primary stenting rate was similar in men and women despite smaller infarct arteries in women. Primary stenting was an independent predictor of better event-free survival at six months, mainly for a reduction in repeat target vessel revascularization, and the benefit of stenting was similar in men and women. The six-month angiographic follow-up showed a lower restenosis rate both in men and women with stented infarct arteries than in patients who underwent coronary angioplasty alone. In the Stent-PAMI trial, the prognosis of women was not improved by infarct artery stenting: the need for late target vessel revascularization was similar in women with stented infarct arteries and conventional coronary angioplasty alone (12% vs. 15.5%, $p = 0.47$) (137). The variability in results probably reflects differences in populations studied because of the eligibility criteria used for randomization. Moreover, the Stent-PAMI trial design did not prevent the crossover of a substantial percentage of patients from the angioplasty arm to stenting (15%) (104), and the crossover was more frequent for women than men (19.4% vs. 13.4%, respectively), resulting in a reduction in the measured benefit of stenting by the intention-to-treat analysis (unpublished data). The same investigators reported opposite results in the CADILLAC trial patient cohort. In this trial, the benefit of infarct artery stenting extended to women, with a significant reduction in the number of 12-month adverse cardiac events in stented women compared with angioplasty alone (OR 0.53; 95% CI 0.35–0.821, $p = 0.003$) (76).

Women and Cardiogenic Shock

A number of survey studies have shown that the bias selection of women with AMI referred for emergency mechanical revascularization works also in the subset of women with CS due to predominant ventricular failure (83,85–87,109) (case 35).

The confounding effect of bias selection favoring men on gender-related outcome is evident in the survey study on CS from California (87). In this registry, CS complicating AMI was identified in 1122 patients. Of these, only 259 (23%) had emergency mechanical revascularization. The early revascularized patients were less often women compared with the nonrevascularized patients, the incidence of women being 39% in the revascularized patient group and 48% in the nonrevascularized patient group ($p = 0.008$). Early revascularization was associated with a better survival (OR 0.2, $p < 0.0001$), while female gender was associated with an increased risk of death (OR 1.4, $p = 0.01$). The low incidence of revascularized patients among the women group may explain the worse prognosis of women.

The SHOCK registry showed similar in-hospital mortality in 115 women and 176 men who underwent PCI (49.6% and 43.8%, respectively, $p = 0.339$), suggesting that emergency mechanical revascularization may provide similar benefit in men and women (140). However, it should be highlighted in the inherent biases that have contributed to emergency revascularization treatment approaches in the SHOCK registry. Only 62% of patients with CS underwent coronary angiography, and only 35.4% of the women and 31% of the men had PCI (140).

On the contrary, the randomized SHOCK trial could not demonstrate a benefit of emergency mechanical revascularization in women (91). In the SHOCK trial, 302 patients, 205 men and 97 women, with AMI complicated by CS due to predominant LV failure were randomly assigned to an emergency revascularization strategy or an initial medical stabilization. The overall one-month mortality rate did not differ significantly between the emergency revascularization group and the medical therapy group (46.7% and 56%, respectively, $p = 0.11$). A positive interaction between emergency revascularization and subgroup variables was found only for those younger than 75 years. However, the relative risk analysis clearly suggested a benefit only for men and for patients with a short delay from AMI onset to randomization. In women, emergency revascularization was associated with increase in the relative risk of death despite that the randomized population had a lower risk profile than patients enrolled in the registry. The last figure confirmed also an adjunctive bias in selection of patients for randomization. The small sample size of the study may explain the lack of an early benefit of an emergency revascularization strategy in women. Alternative explanations may lie within the very long delay from shock diagnosis to randomization, being time to treatment a strong determinant of survival in patients with CS (100), and the nonuse of stents in the majority of patients, which resulted in a very low procedural success rate (77%) (91,141).

Again, registry studies based on unselected treated patient cohorts may help to minimize the confounding effects of bias selection, and to correctly assess gender-related differences in outcome of patients with AMI complicated by CS undergoing routine PCI.

Gender-related differences in procedural, angiographic, and clinical outcomes in 208 consecutive patients with AMI complicated by CS were assessed by the Florence investigators (142). Of 208 patients with CS, 65 were women and 143 men. Women were older than men (74 ± 10 years vs. 66 ± 12 years, $p < 0.001$) and had a greater incidence of a history of hypertension (43% vs. 29%, $p = 0.041$). Despite women having smaller infarct arteries, the procedural success rate was similar in women and men. This figure may be explained by the use of stents in the majority of patients, since it has been shown that stenting is a strong determinant of procedural success (106). The six-month mortality rate was 42% in women and 31% in

men ($p = 0.157$). There were no differences between groups in reinfarction rate and target vessel revascularization rate. Multivariate analysis showed age as the only variable independently related to the six-month mortality, while female gender was not related to the risk of death (142). The most relevant demographic characteristic of this large series of patients is the high incidence of very elderly patients in the women group. The mean age of 74 ± 10 years in the women group is higher compared with the female population of the SHOCK registry (71 ± 11 years) that included 322 women (140), as well as with the entire randomized population of the SHOCK trial (66 ± 10 years) (91). Another important figure that may explain the consistency with the results of the SHOCK registry, and the negative results of the SHOCK trial, is that the large majority of Florence patient series had the reperfusive treatment within six hours from AMI symptom onset, similar to the SHOCK registry population; in the registry, the median time from myocardial infarction onset to the diagnosis of CS was 6.2 hours (140). On the contrary, in the SHOCK trial population the median time from myocardial infarction onset to the diagnosis of CS was only five hours, but the abnormally long time from CS diagnosis to randomization (>4 hours) resulted in a median time to treatment of 11 hours (91).

Spontaneous Coronary Artery Dissection

Spontaneous coronary artery dissection is a rare cause of AMI, and in the majority of cases occurs in women, frequently in the postpartum period (143,144). However, AMI complicating spontaneous coronary artery dissection may occur also in postmenopausal women, and in men. Despite the low incidence, the correct recognition and treatment of this condition may be difficult and challenging (DVD: Cases 18, 24, 26, 28, and 40). The recognition is easy when baseline angiography clearly shows non-occlusive dissection, or the occlusion occurs distally to a dissected coronary artery segment, or the dissection process involves more than one coronary artery (exceptionally all 3 coronary arteries may be involved in the dissection process) (145,146). The recognition by angiography is difficult or even impossible when the occlusion complicates the dissection at the same level of the beginning of the dissection, or the dissection planes are distal and long and result in a diffuse and uniform reduction of the vessel lumen due to the thrombosis of the dissecting hematoma in the false lumen, which prevents contrast medium penetration. The right diagnosis may be indirectly suggested by clinical data, such as gender, postpartum period, and the absence of angiographic evidence of coronary atherosclerosis, or directly, by ultraselective angiography, using a dual lumen catheter or an over-the-wire catheter, or by intravascular ultrasound interrogation after placement of a coronary wire in the true lumen of the vessel.

The goal of PCI is the reestablishment of a brisk flow with the minimal aggressiveness to avoid the extension of the dissection, or coronary perforation or rupture. A global "soft" interventional approach includes careful manipulation of the guiding catheter and the coronary wire and the use of long balloons at low pressure. If conventional angioplasty, even with long inflation times, is unsuccessful, stenting remains the only effective therapeutic option. For long dissections involving major branches, typically in the dissections of the left coronary system, spot stenting should be considered the first stenting technique, since a short stent may be effective in reestablishment of a good flow, avoiding the complication related to long or multiple stent implantation, such as loss of major branches, and proximal or distal extension of dissection. Stent placement should be accomplished with the minimal inflation pressure sufficient to expand the stent, since high inflation pressure may be complicated by extension of the dissection. The indication in the use of IIb-IIIa inhibitors should be matched with the risk of coronary perforation or rupture, and these drugs should be administered only after the correct placement of the coronary wire in the true lumen of the vessel. Residual nonocclusive dissection, even long, should not be treated, since a normal flow may be spontaneously maintained, and also because it contributes to the spontaneous healing of the dissection.

The Tako-Tsubo Cardiomyopathy (Ballooning Ventricle)

Tako-tsubo cardiomyopathy (TTC) or stress or ballooning ventricle cardiomyopathy is a recently described clinical condition that may mimic ST-elevation AMI, being characterized by chest pain, ischemic ECG changes, transient wall motion abnormalities mainly in the mid-apical segments and limited release of cardiac injury markers, in the absence of obstructive epicardial coronary artery disease (147–149). In the large majority of cases, a stressful event triggers the syndrome. Female sex, low peak CK-MB value, and the presence of antecedent stressful event are predictors of TTC in patients with suspected anterior AMI. However, there is still no reliable way to distinguish TTC associated with ST-segment elevation on the presenting ECG from ST-segment elevation AMI due to coronary artery disease. Therefore, most patients with TTC undergo urgent coronary angiography (DVD: Cases 23 and 37). Whether the identification of specific characteristics in the future will allow the detection of TTC noninvasively is unknown.

It is now believed that TTC is not so rare as initially thought. The 2% incidence in the overall AMI population

rises to 12% when the attention is focused on women with suspected anterior AMI (150). Thus, it seems to be mandatory to consider TTC in the differential diagnosis in women with chest pain and ST-segment elevation in the precordial leads.

The syndrome generally has a favorable outcome, and the LV dysfunction due to catecholamine-induced myocardial stunning recovers within days or few weeks (147–151). However, in the acute phase some complications may occur and may require left ventricle support treatment (151).

EDITOR'S COMMENT

Women with AMI have a worse clinical and angiographic profile compared with men. Women have more frequently diffuse coronary artery disease and smaller vessels compared with men. The worse baseline profile is associated with a higher mortality compared with men. However, the benefit of early PCI for AMI is similar in women and men, and any potential referral bias in the use of PCI based on gender differences should be avoided.

DIABETICS

DM independently predicts mortality after thrombolytic therapy for AMI (152,153). DM appears to confer a three- to fourfold increase in risk of death after AMI (154,155). The impact of primary PCI on outcome of DM patients with AMI is not well defined, and the results of previous randomized trials comparing PCI with fibrinolysis may not be considered fully representative of the subset of DM patients with AMI.

In the Global Utilization of Streptokinase and Tissue plasminogen activator for Occluded coronary arteries (GUSTO)-IIb study 1138 patients (177 DM patients and 961 non-DM patients) with AMI were randomized to receive either primary angioplasty or accelerated alteplase (156). Of 472 patients randomized to PCI, 81 (17%) had DM. At one-month follow-up there was no significant difference in mortality between DM patients and non-DM patients (8.1% and 5.2%, respectively, $p = 0.252$). This lack of influence of diabetic status may be explained by the low overall risk of the enrolled population. Nearly all GUSTO-IIb patients (99%) were in Killip class I or II, and only two patients were in Killip class IV. Moreover, only a minority of DM patients (27%) required insulin. The relatively low-risk profile of the entire GUSTO-IIb population may explain, in part, also the lack of interaction between diabetic status and reperfusion strategy, PCI, or fibrinolysis. Consistent with the results of the subanalysis of the GUSTO-IIb trial, a combined analysis of GUSTO-IIb trial and RAPPORT (ReoPro and Primary PTCA Organization and Randomized Trial) trial cohorts showed that the presence of DM does not independently predict death or reinfarction at 30 days (157). In the Stent-PAMI trial, 893 patients with AMI were randomized to infarct artery stenting or conventional angioplasty (158). Of 893 patients, 135 (15%) had DM. There were no differences in one-year mortality between DM patients and non-DM patients, and among DM patients, between non-insulin-dependent and insulin-dependent patients. Again, as in GUSTO-IIb study, the lack of influence of diabetes status on mortality may be explained by the low-risk enrolled population: the mean age of DM patients was 64 years, most of them were non-insulin dependent (112 patients; 83%), and patients with CS or high-risk coronary anatomy were excluded from the enrolment. Another possible explanation for the lack of influence of diabetic status on mortality, as revealed by these studies, may be related also to the small number of DM patients, since the incidence of DM in these cohorts of patients is inferior to those reported by U.S. epidemiological studies.

An observational study based on a sample of 1071 patients with AMI treated by PCI showed that DM patients receiving PCI for AMI had a more than twofold higher mortality rate at six months compared with non-DM patients (159). At six months, the mortality rate was 15% in DM group and 7% in the non-DM group ($p < 0.001$). DM was present in 168 (15.7%) patients, and 86 had DM requiring insulin (51% of DM patients). DM patients were older, more frequently women, and had a greater incidence of CS, multivessel disease, chronic occlusion, smaller infarct arteries, and were less frequently smokers. Among DM patients, those requiring insulin had a greater incidence of CS (27% vs. 13%, $p = 0.032$).

The difference in mortality between DM and non-DM patients was mainly due to the subgroup of patients requiring insulin, who reached a six-month mortality rate of 26%, which was higher than non-requiring insulin DM patients (8%, $p < 0.001$). The majority of deaths in both groups occurred during hospitalization and were due to refractory CS or congestive heart failure. The more frequent cause of death after discharge was congestive heart failure. By Cox analysis, DM was not independently related to the six-month mortality. When adjusting for insulin/non-insulin treatment, only DM requiring insulin was independently related to the risk of death (HR 2.28, 95% CI 1.38–3.76, $p = 0.001$), while non-requiring insulin DM was not related to the risk of death.

The categorization of DM patients, based on insulin/non-insulin treatment, also provided an explanation for the higher mortality of requiring insulin patients after adjustment for the worse baseline risk profile. In insulin-treated DM patients the effectiveness of PCI in achieving myocardial reperfusion was lower than the other patients. The no-flow phenomenon was revealed more frequently in DM patients requiring insulin than in non-requiring insulin DM patients (13% vs. 2%, $p = 0.012$). Again, early ST-segment elevation resolution rate was higher in non-DM patients than in those with DM (76% vs. 65%, $p = 0.002$), and among DM patients, early ST-segment resolution was more frequent in non-requiring insulin DM patients (78% vs. 52%, $p = 0.005$). Both figures, the no-reflow phenomenon and early ST-segment elevation resolution, which are strong markers of the efficacy of reperfusion (160–162), suggest a less effective reperfusion and myocardial salvage in patients requiring insulin, despite a successful mechanical restoration of the epicardial flow. Thus, the link between DM requiring insulin and increased mortality might be the lack of an effective myocardial reperfusion at microcirculatory level in many patients with a patent infarct artery. The reasons for a less effective reperfusion despite a successful procedure are not yet defined. One may hypothesize the contribution of several negative factors, such as an already damaged coronary microvessel network (163), increased risk of atherothrombotic peripheral embolism, decreased cell viability due to the metabolic disorder of the diabetic status, and decreased myocardial resistance to ischemia due to the poor collateral flow (164). The results of this study, based on a series of DM patients, larger than previous PCI studies, are consistent with those from major fibrinolytic trials. In the GUSTO-I trial, based on a population of more than 40,000 patients with AMI, the one-year mortality rate was 14.5% among the 5944 patients with DM and 8.9% in non-DM patients, with the highest mortality rate being observed in DM patients who were treated with insulin (152). In the FTT (Fibrinolytic Therapy Trialists') collaborative pooled analysis of data from large fibrinolytic trials, patients with DM had an almost twofold higher rate of mortality at 30 days than non-DM patients (13.6% vs. 8.7%, $p < 0.05$) (153).

The CADILLAC trial investigators have shown in a cohort of 1301 patients enrolled in the myocardial blush grade substudy that DM patients (232 of the 1301 patients) are more likely to have abnormal myocardial reperfusion (myocardial blush grade 0–1 56% in DM patients vs. 47.1% in non-DM patients, $p = 0.001$) and that DM was an independent predictor of absent myocardial reperfusion as assessed by myocardial blush grade and ST-segment resolution (HR 2.94, 95% CI 1.64–5.37, $p = 0.005$) (165).

The EMERALD (Enhanced Myocardial Efficacy and Removal by Aspiration of Liberated Debris) trial investigators have confirmed a decreased effectiveness of mechanical myocardial reperfusion in DM patients (166). This trial, based on a cohort of 501 patients with

AMI randomized to conventional PCI or PCI supported by an antiembolic device, included 62 diabetics. Compared with non-DM patients, DM patients had more frequently angiographic evidence of no reperfusion (post-PCI blush grade 0–1 34% vs. 16%, $p = 0.002$), lower rate of complete ST-segment elevation resolution (45% vs. 65%, $p = 0.005$), larger infarct size as assessed by sestamibi scintigraphy (median infarct size 20% vs. 11%, $p = 0.005$). As a consequence of the decreased myocardial reperfusion, DM patients had a higher incidence of heart congestive failure (12% vs. 4%, $p = 0.016$) and six-month death (10% vs. 1%, $p < 0.0001$).

Heart congestive failure is not invariably related to a higher propensity of DM patients for LV remodeling and depressed systolic function, since diastolic dysfunction also may play a role in the developing of heart congestive failure (167).

The impact of abciximab treatment on the reperfusion of the microvessel network in DM patients with AMI treated with infarct artery stenting is not defined, and it is unknown if the strong benefit revealed in AMI populations by observational (117,168) and randomized controlled studies is maintained in DM patients (169–171). Again, it is unknown if the increased benefit of abciximab in elective PCI DM patients (more than 50% reduction in target vessel revascularization rate at six-month follow-up) is preserved also in AMI DM patients (172).

All studies show that also in the subset of AMI, DM patients have a higher restenosis rate compared with non-DM patients, and although coronary stenting may improve the angiographic outcome, DM patients continue to fare worse than non-DM patients. In the Stent-PAMI trial, infarct artery stenting compared to angioplasty provided a benefit in terms of clinical events related to restenosis or reocclusion only in non-DM patients or non-insulin-dependent DM patients (158). In the CADILLAC trial, DM patients accounted for 16.6% of the entire population, and stenting compared to conventional angioplasty provided the same benefit in DM patients and in non-DM patients, with a decrease in the incidence of the composite end point of death, reinfarction, target vessel revascularization and disabling stroke (76). The differences in the rate of the primary end point was driven by the lower rates of target vessel revascularization in the stenting group than in the angioplasty group, suggesting a benefit of infarct artery stenting on target vessel failure rate also in DM patients.

An increased angiographic restenosis rate in DM patients was reported also by the Florence investigators, with the higher restenosis rate in DM requiring insulin patient subset, confirming that DM is a strong predictor of in-stent restenosis also in the setting of AMI in addition to its established role in the development of in-stent restenosis following elective PCI (159,173).

CARDIOGENIC SHOCK

Patients with CS account for a large proportion of deaths from AMI. The incidence of CS complicating AMI ranges from 5% to 15% (83,174–177). Population-based estimates of temporal trends in CS suggest that this incidence remains relatively stable over time (177). The same studies show in-hospital mortality over 70%, and a significant progressive improvement in the in-hospital survival, particularly during the 1990s. This improvement is coincident with the increased use of myocardial revascularization techniques during the same period (178).

Most of the observational studies have shown that percutaneous myocardial revascularization in CS may have a strong impact on survival, with survival contingent both on the successful establishment of coronary reperfusion, and on the duration of shock. Nevertheless, reported one-month survival rates are very different, ranging from 40% to 74% (83,106,107,109,179–185). These differences may be explained mainly by the differences in the success rates of mechanical reperfusion, and in the duration of CS. In addition, the definition of shock itself has varied, and this fact may have resulted in different outcomes.

Despite the very encouraging results with primary or rescue coronary angioplasty in many observational studies, the efficacy of emergency mechanical revascularization has been questioned. It has been postulated that the difference in survival between an aggressive mechanical reperfusion strategy and conventional therapy might reflect only a selection bias resulting in the exclusion of the most critically ill and unstable patients from reperfusive treatments because a poor outcome is expected (83). The selection bias for revascularization is evident from the data of the National Registry of Myocardial Infarction 2. In this U.S. registry 23,180 patients with CS could be identified. More than 60% did not have any reperfusive treatment, while 24% had thrombolytic treatment, 15% primary coronary angioplasty or coronary surgery, and 1% had rescue coronary angioplasty. The overall mortality rate was 70%. The mortality rate was 78% without reperfusive treatment, 67% with fibrinolytic treatment, and 42% with primary mechanical coronary intervention (186).

The Problem of the Assessment of the Efficacy of Percutaneous Interventions in Cardiogenic Shock

The SHOCK registry (83). Between 1992 and 1993, an international registry of patients with CS was compiled. The aim of the registry was to examine the current spectrum of CS and the apparent impact of early revascularization on survival in patients with predominant LV failure. Data of 251 patients with CS complicating AMI from 19 participating centers were prospectively registered. After the exclusion of patients with ventricular septal rupture or severe MR, 214 patients with primary LV failure were evaluated. The overall in-hospital mortality was 66%. The mortality rates were similar for 184 patients with electrocardiographic findings suggestive of transmural myocardial infarction and for 30 patients with subendocardial infarction (64% and 77%, respectively; $p = 0.215$). Only 120 patients (56%) underwent cardiac catheterization. Patients who were not taken to the catheterization laboratory were older (mean age 70 $\pm$ 12 years vs. 64 $\pm$ 11 years, $p < 0.001$), and had a greater incidence of subendocardial infarction (23% vs. 7%, $p < 0.01$). The mortality rate for patients who did not undergo cardiac catheterization was higher than that of patients who underwent invasive assessment (85% vs. 51%, $p < 0.01$). Among patients who underwent cardiac catheterization, the in-hospital mortality rates were similar for patients who had early revascularization (median time from shock diagnosis to revascularization 3 hours) and for patients who did not have any revascularization procedure (51% and 58%, respectively). Paradoxically, the mortality rates were apparently lower for patients who underwent late revascularization (median time from diagnosis 2 days—25% mortality), or very late revascularization (median time from diagnosis 1.3 weeks—0 mortality). SHOCK registry investigators concluded that the potential benefit of an early revascularization strategy remained to be determined in a randomized clinical trial. Although biased case selection for treatment may have confounded data of the registry, it was evident that some data were not commented in a proper perspective. First, among patients who underwent cardiac catheterization, the overall mortality in revascularized patients (43%) was lower than that in patients who did not have any revascularization procedure (58%). Second, the small number of patients makes it difficult to conclude the proper time of a revascularization strategy: only 17 patients underwent late or very late revascularization with a mortality rate of 18% compared with the mortality rate of 51% of patients who underwent early revascularization. Furthermore, it is likely that most patients who underwent early revascularization were highly unstable, suggesting that the comparison with patients who had late revascularization procedures is incorrect. Finally, the success rate of coronary angioplasty in the small number of patients who underwent the procedure (48 patients) was relatively low (procedural success rate = 69%) and may be explained, in part, by the nonuse of stents in this population.

Randomized Trials

The SHOCK trial (91). After the results of the SHOCK registry, in 1993 the SHOCK investigators began a randomized trial with a sample size of 302 patients with CS caused by predominant LV failure, where an immediate coronary revascularization strategy (coronary angioplasty or surgery) was compared with a more conservative approach that included fibrinolytic treatment and aortic balloon pumping (initial medical stabilization arm). The enrollment ended in 1998, six years after the start of the study. The primary end point of the study was a 20% reduction in 30-day mortality in the emergency revascularization arm as compared with the initial medical stabilization arm. The results of this trial were negative since the reduction in 30-day mortality was inferior to 20% (46.7% vs. 56.0%; difference between the groups, 9.3%; 95% CI for the difference, 20.5–1.9%; $p = 0.11$). The 30-day mortality rate was 45.3% among the 75 patients who underwent coronary angioplasty, and 42.1% among those who underwent coronary surgery. A positive interaction between early revascularization strategy and 30-day mortality was found for men younger than 75 years, time from myocardial infarction onset to randomization < six hours, and a history of prior myocardial infarction. A negative interaction between early reperfusion strategy and 30-day mortality was found for women, and patients older than 75 years. At six months, the overall mortality from all causes was lower in the emergency revascularization group than in the initial medical stabilization group (50.3% vs. 63.1%, $p = 0.027$). Despite the fact that there was no significant overall benefit of early revascularization at 30 days, and that no reasons were given for the lower six-month mortality in revascularized patients, the SHOCK investigators recommended that early revascularization should be strongly considered for patients with AMI complicated by CS, particularly for patients younger than 75 years.

A correct interpretation of data from this trial is difficult. The primary end point of the study, a 20% reduction of mortality in the emergency revascularization arm was not reached because mortality was higher than expected in the emergency revascularization arm and lower than expected in the initial medical stabilization arm. The reasons for the very high mortality rate in the early revascularization group, significantly higher than the 25% to 30% rate reported by single high-volume centers, and the 35% rate by the GUSTO investigators (184), may have several explanations. First, the success rate of coronary angioplasty remained very low until the last two years of enrollment, only 58% of patients achieving a TIMI grade 3 flow after the procedure. This poor result may be explained, in part, by the limited use of stents in the first four years of enrollment (no stent in 1993–1994, and only 14% in 1995–1996), while in 1997 and 1998 with the use of stents in 76% of treated cases, a TIMI grade 3 flow was achieved in 68% of patients. As expected, successful angioplasty resulted in decreased mortality (38%) compared with the mortality rate in patients with an unsuccessful procedure (79%). Second, the delay from CS to treatment was abnormally long: the median time from myocardial infarction onset to shock diagnosis was five hours, while the median time from myocardial infarction onset to randomization was 11 hours; the delay from randomization to treatment was 0.9 hour for coronary angioplasty and 2.7 hours for coronary surgery. Therefore, patients who underwent coronary angioplasty had treatment after a median time of 12 hours after myocardial infarction onset, and of 7 hours after shock diagnosis. This delay in treatment may partially explain the relatively poor outcome of the patients of the SHOCK trial. Among patients randomized to emergency revascularization, only 25% were randomized < six hours, and subgroup analysis suggested a positive interaction between revascularization and 30-day mortality in this subgroup of patients. This figure is consistent with the results of previous studies showing that the benefit of revascularization in shock patients is time dependent. Thus, one may infer that a higher coronary angioplasty success rate achievable with stent-supported angioplasty, as well as a shorter delay from diagnosis of shock to treatment, could have been associated with a better outcome.

The lower-than-expected 30-day mortality in the initial medical stabilization arm may be the result of the benefit of intra-aortic counterpulsation that has been showed by several investigators (187–190). Intra-aortic balloon pumping was recommended for all patients randomized to the initial medical stabilization arm, and this treatment was administered in 86% of patients.

The SMASH (Swiss Multicenter trial of Angioplasty for Shock) trial (191). The aim of this trial was to compare a strategy of emergency coronary angiography, immediately followed by percutaneous or surgical revascularization, with an initial medical management in patients with AMI complicated by CS due to predominant LV failure. The study had to be terminated prematurely due to major difficulties with patient recruitment. As a consequence, only 55 patients could be randomized, and it was not demonstrated that emergency mechanical revascularization may improve survival. At one month, the mortality rate in 32 patients randomized to emergency revascularization was 69%, while it was 78% in 23 patients randomized to an initial conservative strategy (RR = 0.88, 95% CI 0.6–1.2). The very small number of randomized patients prevents any conclusion about the efficacy of an early invasive strategy in patients with CS.

While the SMASH investigators stopped the study prematurely due to the insufficient patient enrollment, SHOCK investigators persevered in the face of low recruitment rate, which resulted in the enrollment of only 302 patients over a very long period. Major difficulties in the randomization of patients with CS in both trials suggest that it is not possible to rule out the hypothesis of a bias, which had a significant impact on the results. On the other hand, if the period of recruitment is very long, the results may be negatively affected by the nonuse of new techniques and devices in a significant number of the patients enrolled. Thus, neither of the randomized trials could evaluate the efficacy of an early revascularization strategy in patients with CS properly.

Observational Studies

The GUSTO-I trial (192). This trial of 41,021 patients with AMI included a prospective plan for examining the incidence, temporal profile, and clinical implications of shock. This key study includes the largest database of patients with CS complicating AMI. CS occurred in 2972 patients (7.2%): the majority of these patients (2657 patients; 89%) developed CS after hospital admission, frequently in the setting of recurrent ischemia or reinfarction, and only 315 of them (11%) had CS on admission. CS accounted for the majority of the deaths (58%) in the entire trial. The one-month overall mortality rate in patients with CS on admission was 57%, and 55% in patients who developed shock during the hospital stay. Coronary angioplasty was performed in only a minority of patients, 48 patients with shock on arrival, and 519 who developed shock, and it was associated with significantly improved outcome. The one-month mortality after coronary angioplasty was 43% in patients with shock on arrival compared with 61% of the patients who did not undergo the procedure ($p = 0.028$), and 32% in patients who developed shock compared with 61% of nontreated patients ($p < 0.001$). Patient selection criteria could have had a major impact in the outcomes observed. The preponderance of shock developing during the hospital stay could have been a consequence of having excluded from enrolment the patients presenting with shock, while another bias selection could have occurred in the use of angiography and coronary angioplasty, since angioplasty was performed in only 19% of patients with CS. To make a correct assessment of the impact of an aggressive strategy on mortality in patients with shock, the GUSTO investigators conducted a subsequent analysis in

2200 of 2972 patients (192). To avoid a bias in favor of an aggressive strategy, patients who died within one hour of the onset of shock were excluded, as were patients with incomplete data. This analysis showed a significant reduction in one-month mortality in patients who underwent an aggressive strategy compared with patients who were treated conservatively (38% vs. 61%, $p = 0.0001$). In the subset of 175 patients who underwent coronary angioplasty, the procedure success rate was 85%. The overall mortality rate was 42%, and 35% in patients with a successful coronary angioplasty procedure. When adjusted for differences in baseline characteristics between patients who underwent an aggressive strategy and patients who were treated conservatively, the benefit of an aggressive strategy was independently related to the reduction of one-month mortality (OR 0.43; 95% CI 0.34–0.54; $p = 0.0001$).

The Florence Registry

To correctly assess the efficacy of percutaneous mechanical revascularization in cardiogenic shock due to predominant ventricular failure, any bias selection process should be avoided. Routine coronary angioplasty should be performed in all patients with AMI. As a result of the application of a routine primary PCI strategy, treated patient populations are not biased, and the efficacy and the impact on survival of early percutaneous interventions in these populations could be correctly assessed. The Florence experience in PCI for CS complicating AMI seems to meet the criterion of a really routine treatment of all patients with CS due to predominant ventricular failure (90). Between 1995 and 2004, 2314 patients with AMI underwent primary PCI, and 280 patients (12%) had CS due to predominant ventricular failure. CS was defined as systolic blood pressure < 90 mmHg (without inotropic or intra-aortic balloon support) that was thought to be secondary to cardiac dysfunction and associated with end organ hypoperfusion such as cold or diaphoretic extremities or altered mental status or anuria. The diagnosis of CS was confirmed at cardiac catheterization by the measurement of systolic blood pressure <90 mmHg and LV filling pressure ≥20 mmHg. The high incidence of CS in this population may be easily explained: (*i*) Only a minority of treated patients (20%) with AMI are referred from community hospitals, and these patients are generally at high risk and with contraindication to fibrinolytic treatment, and include a high percentage of CS patients; (*ii*) in Florence there is a network of mobile coronary care units allowing the diagnosis of AMI at home, and simultaneously alerting the invasive cardiology team; and (*iii*) the effective assistance during transportation (e.g., inotropic agents, effective arrhythmia treatment, and intubation), the bypass of admission in the emergency room, and the subsequent zero door-to-balloon time allow a large number of patients with CS on presentation to reach the catheterization laboratory alive. This series includes a high percentage of very elderly patients (37% of patients were ≥ 75 years). The incidence of women, previous myocardial infarction, current anterior myocardial infarction, multivessel disease, and chronic occlusion is higher compared with nonshock patients. This population includes predominantly early CS: the mean time from myocardial infarction symptom onset to reperfusion was 4.2 hours. The coronary angioplasty success rate was 95%. The one-month overall mortality rate was 30.7%. At one year, the survival rate was $43 \pm 5\%$ in patients 75 years and older, and $74 \pm 3\%$ in younger patients. In this series, the only independent predictors of mortality were age (OR 1.07; 95% CI 1.02–1.12, $p = 0.005$) and primary PCI failure (OR 4.01, 95% CI 1.53–10.51, $p = 0.005$). These results were obtained in a single high-volume center using a unique logistic model that resulted in an improved outcome of patients with early CS. The effectiveness of this model should be addressed in a large multicenter outcome trial, since the favorable results reported here cannot necessarily be extrapolated to other logistic scenarios.

The German ALKK Registry (193)

This registry collected data from 80 centers in Germany regarding 9422 primary PCI for AMI. Of these, 1333 (14.2%) were performed in patients with CS. The in-hospital mortality was 46.1%. The study confirmed that primary PCI failure is a strong predictor of mortality: the mortality rates were 78.2%, 66.1%, and 37.4% in patients with TIMI grade flow 0 to 1, TIMI grade flow 2, and TIMI grade flow 3, respectively. The other variables related to in-hospital mortality were left main disease, older age, three-vessel disease, and longer time interval between symptom onset and PCI.

Despite the limitations of randomized and outcome trials, and variability of the results, available data show that emergency percutaneous mechanical revascularization may have a strong impact on survival in patients with CS. It should be underscored that the benefit of percutaneous revascularization in patients with AMI complicated CS is strongly related to the time delay from diagnosis to intervention (100,194). This critical determinant is particularly relevant in the presence of CS (100,195), since an abnormal delay increases the risk of evolution into an irreversible condition despite a successful procedure and patent infarct artery.

The Role of Coronary Stenting

Two observational studies involving more than 100 patients with CS show that infarct artery stenting is highly feasible in this setting, and suggest an initial and long-term benefit of primary infarct artery stenting compared with coronary angioplasty alone (106,196). The postulated mechanism of the benefit of coronary stenting in AMI is the correction of any residual dissection after angioplasty of an already disrupted plaque, and the restoration of a normal flow to decrease the risk of early occlusive thrombosis, and late restenosis or reocclusion of the infarct artery. Differently from patients without CS, where clinical events related to restenosis or reocclusion are recurrent angina or nonfatal reinfarction, in patients with CS due to predominant ventricular failure and successfully treated with percutaneous revascularization, acute or subacute target vessel failure due to restenosis or reocclusion may be more likely a catastrophic event. In a U.S. registry that included 483 patients with CS complicating AMI, the nonuse of stents was independently related to mortality (OR 2.55, 95% CI 1.63–3.96, $p < 0.01$) (197). Moreover, coronary stenting allows a rapid and effective multivessel revascularization in patients with CS and multivessel disease. Thus, it is likely that patients with CS may derive the greatest benefit from infarct artery stenting.

The Role of Mechanical Circulatory Support

Intra-aortic balloon pumping and other mechanical support devices should be considered a first-line therapy for patients with CS undergoing emergency PCI (see chap. 5).

Specific Conditions
Right Ventricular Infarction and Cardiogenic Shock

Isolated right ventricular infarction is a rare occurrence, but this condition may be associated with a severe low-output state and shock that may be unresponsive to fluid administration, inotropic agents, and intra-aortic balloon pumping (198). On the contrary, involvement of the right ventricle in inferior myocardial infarction is relatively frequent and associated with a poor prognosis (case 19). Percutaneous recanalization of the occluded coronary artery has a strong impact on mortality in patients with right ventricular infarction. A key study using direct angioplasty showed that restoration of normal flow in right ventricular branches resulted in dramatic recovery of right ventricular function and a mortality rate of only 2%, whereas unsuccessful reperfusion of the right ventricle was associated with persistent hemodynamic compromise and a mortality rate of 58% (199). In cases of right ventricular infarction complicated by CS and maintained LV function, the mortality rate is inferior to the one of CS complicating left ventricle failure; however, also in these relatively favorable cases the in-hospital

mortality is very high. Brodie et al. in a series of 189 patients with CS complicating AMI identified 30 patients with right ventricular infarction and maintained LV function: the late mortality rate in this subset of patients with CS was 23% (200).

Left Main Disease and Cardiogenic Shock

Disappointing results of emergency percutaneous interventions in left main disease complicated by shock were reported in two case series including, 6 and 16 patients, respectively (201,202). This scenario has dramatically changed with the improvement in interventional techniques, stent design, and antiplatelet therapy, and currently, a percutaneous revascularization approach in patients with cardiogenic shock complicating left main disease may be considered the preferred revascularization strategy. The ULTIMA (Unprotected Left Main Trunk Intervention Multi-center Assessment) registry, a prospective, multicenter, international registry of interventions of unprotected left main disease collected clinical and procedural data of 40 patients who underwent an emergency percutaneous left main intervention for AMI (203). The angiographic success rate was 88%. In-hospital mortality was 55%, and 18% of patients required in-hospital coronary surgery. There was a trend toward a lower rate of in-hospital death in patients with stented left main compared with patients who underwent coronary angioplasty alone (35% vs. 70%, $p = 0.10$). The one-year survival rates were 53% and 35% for the stented left main patients and the patients with angioplasty alone, respectively. Similar results were reported in another single-center series of 22 patients (204). Available data suggest that primary stenting may provide a superior outcome to conventional angioplasty in the subset of patients with left main disease.

Cardiogenic Shock Without ST-Segment Elevation

From an interventional viewpoint, the procedural scenario of patients with CS complicating AMI without ST-segment elevation may be quite different from the one in patients with ST-segment elevation.

The GUSTO investigators analyzed the clinical and angiographic characteristics of patients with acute ischemic syndromes with and without ST-segment elevation (205). Of the 12,073 patients enrolled in the GUSTO-IIb trial, 373 patients developed CS, 200 without ST-segment elevation, and 173 with ST-segment elevation. Patients without ST-segment elevation were older, had DM and three-vessel disease more frequently, but had less TIMI grade 0 flow at angiography. Shock development occurred considerably later in patients without ST-segment elevation (median time 76.2 hours after study entry vs. 9.6 hours in patients with ST-segment elevation), and more frequently in the setting of recurrent ischemia or recurrent infarction. Only a minority of patients without ST-segment elevation underwent mechanical revascularization (21 patients underwent coronary angioplasty, and 51 coronary surgery). Multivariate analysis showed a strong trend toward reduced mortality with percutaneous intervention (HR 0.68, 95% CI 0.45–1.00, $p = 0.052$), while coronary surgery was independently associated with increased mortality (HR 2.03, 95% CI 1.42–2.92, $p < 0.001$).

In interventional practice, patients with CS without ST-segment elevation are technically challenging because of the presence of more extensive coronary disease, more vascular comorbidities, and the frequent inability to identify the infarct artery (In the GUSTO-IIb cohort the IRA location was unknown in 24% of patients without ST-segment elevation, while the infarct artery could be identified in all patients with ST-segment elevation.) (205). On the other hand, the more progressive development of shock in this subset of patients provides a larger time window for intervention.

In AMI without ST-segment elevation complicated by CS, the only exception to the routine scenario of an elderly patient with diffuse multivessel disease and challenging coronary anatomy is the patient with a proximal occlusion of a dominant circumflex artery and a poor electrocardiographic expression. This "favorable" exception is not easily encountered and has a better prognosis compared with the other patients with CS without ST-segment elevation.

Multivessel Disease

Multivessel revascularization can be staged if the infarct artery recanalization and the adjunctive use of mechanical support result in the quick regression of the shock status, or stabilization of a diastolic blood pressure that prevents ischemia in the territories other than the infarct area. Otherwise, prompt revascularization of the arteries other than the infarct artery should be performed during the same procedure (DVD: Case 36).

EDITOR'S COMMENT

Successful early percutaneous mechanical revascularization in patients with AMI complicated by CS favorably affects the otherwise poor outcome in this patient group. Among the variables related to mortality, primary PCI failure and delay to treatment are the only modifiable ones. Since survival is linked to reperfusion status and completeness of revascularization, high performance criteria, including routine coronary stenting, intra-aortic balloon pumping, optimal adjunctive therapy, and a short delay from diagnosis to intervention, should be considered mandatory.

REFERENCES

1. The Task Force on the management of acute myocardial infarction of the European Society of Cardiology. Management of acute myocardial infarction in patients presenting with ST-segment elevation Eur Heart J 2003; 24:28–66.
2. Zimetbaum PJ, Josephson ME. Use of the electrocardiogram in acute myocardial infarction. N Engl J Med 2003; 348:933–940.
3. Sgarbossa EB, Birnbaum Y, Parrillo JE. Electrocardiographic diagnosis of acute myocardial infarction: current concepts for the clinician. Am Heart J 2001; 141:507–517.
4. Morris F, Brady WJ. ABC of clinical electrocardiography. Acute myocardial infarction—Part I. BMJ 2002; 324:831–834.
5. Engelen DJ, Gorgels AP, Cheriex EC, et al. Value of the electrocardiogram in localizing the occlusion site in the left anterior descending coronary artery in acute myocardial infarction. J Am Coll Cardiol 1999; 34:389–395.
6. Kosuge M, Kimura K, Ishikawa T, et al. New electrocardiographic criteria for predicting the site of coronary artery occlusion in inferior wall acute myocardial infarction. Am J Cardiol 1998; 82:1318–1322.
7. Yip HK, Chen MC, Wu CJ, et al. Acute myocardial infarction with simultaneous ST-segment elevation in the precordial and inferior leads: evaluation of anatomic lesions and clinical implications. Chest 2003; 123:1170–1180.
8. Barrabes JA, Figueras J, Moure C, et al. Prognostic significance of ST segment depression in lateral leads I, aVL, V5 and V6 on the admission electrocardiogram in patients with a first acute myocardial infarction without ST segment elevation. J Am Coll Cardiol 2000; 35:1813–1819.
9. Sgarbossa EB, Pinski SL, Barbagelata A, et al. Electrocardiographic diagnosis of acute myocardial infarction in the presence of left bundle branch block. N Engl J Med 1996; 334:481–487.
10. Edhouse J, Brady WJ, Morris F. ABC of clinical electrocardiography. Acute myocardial infarction—Part II. BMJ 2002; 324:863–866.
11. Welch RD, Zalenski RJ, Frederick PD, et al. Prognostic value of a normal or nonspecific initial electrocardiogram in acute myocardial infarction. JAMA 2002; 286:1977–1984.
12. Fletcher PJ, Pfeffer JM, Pfeffer MA, et al. Left ventricular diastolic pressure-volume relations in rats with healed myocardial infarction. Circ Res 1981; 49:618–626.
13. Chareonthaitawee P, Chriastian TF, Hirose K, et al. Relation of initial infarct size to extent of left ventricular remodeling in the year after acute myocardial infarction. J Am Coll Cardiol 1995; 25:567–573.
14. Jeremy RW, Hackworthy RA, Bautovich G, et al. Infarct artery perfusion and change in left ventricular remodeling in the month after acute myocardial infarction. J Am Coll Cardiol 1987; 9:989–995.
15. Hochman JS, Choo H. Limitation of myocardial infarct expansion by reperfusion independent of myocardial salvage. Circulation 1987; 75:299–306.

16. Horie H, Takahashi M, Minai K, et al. Long-term beneficial effect of late reperfusion for acute anterior myocardial infarction with percutaneous transluminal coronary angioplasty. Circulation 1998; 98:2377–2382.

17. Bolognese L, Neskovic AN, Parodi G, et al. Left ventricular remodeling following primary coronary angioplasty: pattern of left ventricular dilation and long-term prognostic implication. Circulation 2002; 106:2351–2357.

18. Gaudron P, Eilles C, Kugler I, et al. Progressive left ventricular dysfunction and remodeling after myocardial infarction: potential mechanism and early predictors. Circulation 1993; 87:755–763.

19. Ito H, Maruyama A, Iwakura K. Clinical implications of the "no reflow" phenomenon: a predictor of complications and left ventricular remodeling in reperfused anterior wall myocardial infarction. Circulation 1996; 93:223–228.

20. Colucci WS. Molecular and cellular mechanism of myocardial failure. Am J Cardiol 1997; 80(suppl 11A):15L–25L.

21. Cerisano G, Bolognese L, Sciagrà R, et al. Interactive effects of infarct location and extension on post infarction left ventricular remodeling. Eur Heart J 2000; 21(abs suppl):589.

22. Stone PH, Raabe DS, Jaffe AS, et al. Prognostic significance of location and type of myocardial infarction: independent adverse outcome associated with anterior location. J Am Coll Cardiol 1988; 11:453–463.

23. Bolognese L, Parodi G, Carrabba N, et al. Impact of microvascular dysfunction on left ventricular remodeling and long-term outcome after reperfused acute myocardial infarction. Circulation 2002; 106(abs suppl):II–598.

24. Ito H, Tomooka T, Sakai N, et al. Lack of myocardial perfusion immediately after successful thrombolysis: a predictor of poor recovery of left ventricular function in anterior myocardial infarction. Circulation 1992; 85:1699–1705.

25. Alhaddad IA, Kloner RA, Hakim I, et al. Benefits of the late coronary artery reperfusion on infarct expansion progressively diminish over time: relation to viable islet of myocytes within the scar. Am Heart J 1996; 131:451–456.

26. Iliceto S, Galiuto L, Marchese A, et al. Analysis of microvascular integrity, contractile reserve, and myocardial viability after acute myocardial infarction by dobutamine echocardiography and myocardial contrast echocardiography. Am J Cardiol 1996; 77:441–445.

27. Bolognese L, Antoniucci D, Rovai D, et al. Myocardial contrast echocardiography versus dobutamine echocardiography for predicting functional recovery after acute myocardial infarction treated with primary coronary angioplasty. J Am Coll Cardiol 1966; 28:1677–1683.

28. Hochman JS, Bulkley BH. Expansion of acute myocardial infarction: an experimental study. Circulation 1982; 65:1446–1450.

29. Pirolo JS, Hutchins GM, Moore GW. Infarct expansion: pathologic analysis of 204 patients with a single myocardial infarct. J Am Coll Cardiol 1986; 7:349–354.

30. Bolognese L, Cerisano G, Buonamici P, et al. Influence of infarct zone viability on left ventricular remodeling after acute myocardial infarction. Circulation 1997; 96:3353–3359.

31. Nijland F, Kamp O, Verhost PMJ, et al. Myocardial viability: impact on left ventricular dilation after acute myocardial infarction. Heart 2002; 87:17–22.

32. Grayburn PA, Erickson JM, Escobar J, et al. Peripheral intravenous myocardial contrast echocardiography using a 2% dodecafluoropentane emulsion: identification of myocardial risk area and infarct size in the canine model of ischemia. J Am Coll Cardiol 1995; 26:1340–1347.

33. Sakuyama T, Hayashi Y, Sumii K, et al. Prediction of short-and intermediate-term prognoses of patients with acute myocardial infarction using myocardial contrast echocardiography one day after recanalization. J Am Coll Cardiol 1998; 32:890–897.

34. Balcells E, Powers ER, Lepper W, et al. Detection of myocardial viability by contrast echocardiography in acute infarction predicts recovery of resting function and contractile reserve. J Am Coll Cardiol 2003; 41:827–833.

35. Galiuto L, Garramone B, Scarà A, et al. The extent of microvascular damage during myocardial contrast echocardiography is superior to other known indexes of postinfarct reperfusion in predicting left ventricular remodeling: results of the multicenter AMICI study J Am Coll Cardiol 2008; 51:552–559.

36. Bonow, RO. Regional left ventricular nonuniformity: effects on left ventricular diastolic function in ischemic heart disease, hypertrophic cardiomyopathy, and the normal heart. Circulation 1990; 81(suppl III):III54–III65.

37. Wijns W, Serruys PW, Slager CJ, et al. Effect of coronary occlusion during percutaneous transluminal angioplasty in humans on left ventricular chamber stiffness and regional diastolic pressure-radius relations. J Am Coll Cardiol 1986; 7:455–463.

38. Cerisano G, Bolognese L. Echo-Doppler evaluation of left ventricular diastolic dysfunction during acute myocardial infarction: methodological, clinical and prognostic implications. Ital Heart J 2001; 2:13–20.

39. Little WC, Ohno M, Kitzman DW, et al. Determination of left ventricular chamber stiffness from the time for deceleration of early left ventricular filling. Circulation 1995; 92:1933–1936.

40. Garcia MJ, Firstenberg MS, Greenberg NL, et al. Estimation of left ventricular operating stiffness from Doppler early filling deceleration time in humans. Am J Physiol Heart Circ Physiol 2001; 280:H554–H561.

41. Cerisano G, Bolognese L, Carrabba N, et al. Doppler-derived mitral deceleration time. An early strong predictor of left ventricular remodeling after reperfused anterior myocardial infarction. Circulation 1999; 99:230–236.

42. Cerisano G, Bolognese L, Pucci PD, et al. Plasma BNP versus clinical, echo and angiographic variables for predicting early left ventricular remodeling and death after reperfused acute myocardial infarction and left ventricular dysfunction. Am J Cardiol 2005; 95:930–934.

43. Popovic AD, Neskovic AN, Marinkovic J, et al. Serial assessment of left ventricular chamber stiffness after acute myocardial infarction. Am J Cardiol 1996; 77:361–364.

44. Cerisano G, Bolognese L, Buonamici P, et al. Prognostic implications of restrictive left ventricular filling in reperfused anterior acute myocardial infarction. J Am Coll Cardiol 2001; 37:793–799.

45. Nijland F, Kamp O, Karreman AJP, et al. Prognostic implications of restrictive left ventricular filling in acute myocardial infarction: a serial Doppler echocardiographic study. J Am Coll Cardiol 1997; 30:1618–1624.

46. Poulsen SH, Jensen SE, Egstrup K. Longitudinal changes and prognostic implications of left ventricular diastolic function in first acute myocardial infarction. Am Heart J 1999; 137:910–918.

47. Otasevic P, Neskovic AN, Popovic Z, et al. Short early filling deceleration time on day 1 after acute myocardial infarction is associated with short and long term left ventricular remodeling. Heart 2001; 85:527–532.

48. Møller JE, Whalley GE, Dini FL, et al. Meta-Analysis Research Group in Echocardiography (MeRGE) AMI Collaborators. Independent prognostic importance of a restrictive left ventricular filling pattern after myocardial infarction: an individual patient meta-analysis: meta-analysis research group in echocardiography acute myocardial infarction. Circulation 2008; 117:2591–2598.

49. Kisanuki A, Otssuji Y, Kuroiwa R, et al. Two-dimensional echocardiographic assessment of papillary muscle contractility in patients with prior myocardial infarction. J Am Coll Cardiol 1993; 21:932–938.

50. Sabbah HN, Kono T, Rosman H, et al. Left ventricular shape: a factor in the etiology of functional mitral regurgitation in heart failure. Am Heart J 1992; 123: 961–966.

51. Otsuji Y, Handschumacher MD, Schwammenthal E, et al. Insights from three-dimensional echocardiography into the mechanism of functional mitral regurgitation: direct in vivo demonstration of altered leaflet tethering geometry. Circulation 1997; 96:1999–2008.

52. He S, Fontaine AA, Schwammenthal E, et al. An integrated mechanism for functional mitral regurgitation: leaflet restriction vs coapting force-in vitro studies. Circulation 1997; 96:1826–1834.

53. Yiu SF, Enriques-Sarano M, Tribouilloy C, et al. Determinants of the degree of functional mitral regurgitation in patients with systolic left ventricular dysfunction. Circulation 2000; 102:1400–1406.

54. Messas E, Guerrero JL, Handschumacher MD, et al. Paradoxic decrease in ischemic mitral regurgitation with papillary muscle dysfunction. Circulation 2001; 104: 1952–1957.

55. Alam M, Thorstrand C, Rosenhamer G. Mitral regurgitation following first-time acute myocardial infarction: early and late findings by Doppler echocardiography. Clin Cardiol 1993; 16:30–34.

56. Feinberg MS, Schwammenthal E, Shlizerman L, et al. Prognostic significance of mild mitral regurgitation by color Doppler echocardiography in acute myocardial infarction. Am J Cardiol 2000; 86:903–907.

57. Golia G, Anselmi M, Rossi A, et al. Relationship between mitral regurgitation and myocardial viability after acute myocardial infarction: their impact on prognosis. Int J Cardiol 2001; 78:81–90.

58. Pierard LA. Functional mitral regurgitation in acute coronary syndrome: what determines its prognostic impact? Eur Heart J 2006; 27:2615–2616.

59. Bursi F, Enriquez-Sarano M, Jacobsen SJ, et al. Mitral regurgitation after myocardial infarction: a review. Am J Med 2006; 119:103–112.

60. Oh JK, Seward JB, Tajik AJ. Valvular heart disease. The echo manual. Philadelphia: Lippincott William & Wilkins, 1999:125.

61. Pellizzon GG, Grines CL, Cox DA, et al. Importance of mitral regurgitation in patients undergoing percutaneous coronary intervention for acute myocardial infarction (CADILLAC trial). J. Am Coll Cardiol 2004; 43:1368–1374.

62. Hillis GS, Møller JE, Pellikka PA, et al. Prognostic significance of echocardiographically defined mitral regurgitation early after acute myocardial infarction. Am Heart J 2005; 150:1268–1275.

63. Grigioni F, Enriquez-Sarano M, Zehr KJ, et al. Ischemic mitral regurgitation. Long-term outcome and prognostic implications with quantitative Doppler assessment. Circulation 2001; 103:1759–1764.

64. Koellig TM, Aaronson KD, Cody RJ, et al. Prognostic significance of mitral regurgitation and tricuspid regurgitation in patients with left ventricular systolic dysfunction. Am Heart J 2002; 144:524–529.

65. Carrabba N, Parodi G, Valenti R, et al. Clinical implications of early mitral regurgitation in patients with reperfused acute myocardial infarction. J Card Fail 2008; 14:48–54.

66. Singh JP, Evans JC, Levy D, et al. Prevalence and clinical determinants of mitral, tricuspid, and aortic regurgitation (the Framingham Heart Study). Am J Cardiol 1999; 83:897–902.

67. Tcheng JE, Jackman JD Jr., Nelson CL, et al. Outcome of patients sustaining acute ischaemic mitral regurgitation during myocardial infarction. Ann Intern Med 1992; 117:18–24.

68. Birnbaum Y, Chamoun AJ, Conti VR, et al. Mitral regurgitation following acute myocardial infarction. Coron Artery Dis 2002; 13:337–344.

69. Kumanohoso T, Otsuji Y, Yoshifuku S, et al. Mechanism of higher incidence of ischemic mitral regurgitation in patients with inferior myocardial infarction: quantitative analysis of left ventricular and mitral valve geometry in 103 patients with prior myocardial infarction. J Thorac Cardiovasc Surg 2003; 125:135–143.

70. Lamas GA, Mitchell GF, Flaker GC, et al. Clinical significance of mitral regurgitation after myocardial infarction. Circulation 1997; 96:827–833.

71. Amigoni M, Meris A, Thune JJ, et al. Mitral regurgitation in myocardial infarction complicated by heart failure, left ventricular dysfunction, or both: prognostic significance and relation to ventricular size and function. Eur Heart J 2007; 28:326–333.

72. Perez de Isla L, Zamorano J, Quezada M, et al. Prognostic significance after a first non-ST-segment elevation acute coronary syndrome. Eur Heart J 2006; 27:2655–2660.

73. Ennezat PV, Darchis J, Lamblin N, et al. Left ventricular remodeling is associated with the severity of mitral regurgitation after inaugural anterior myocardial infarction-optimal

timing for echocardiographic imaging. Am Heart J 2008; 159:959–965.

74. Yip HK, Chen MC, Wu CJ, et al. Clinical features and outcome of coronary artery aneurysm patients with acute myocardial infarction undergoing a primary percutaneous coronary intervention. Cardiology 2002; 98:132–140.

75. Antoniucci D, Valenti R, Moschi G, et al. Sex-based differences in clinical and angiographic outcomes after primary angioplasty or stenting for acute myocardial infarction. Am J Cardiol 2001; 87:289–293.

76. Stone WG, Grines CL, Cox DA, et al. The Controlled Abciximab and Device Investigation to Lower Late Angioplasty Complications (CADILLAC) Investigators. Comparison of angioplasty with stenting, with or without abciximab, in acute myocardial infarction. N Engl J Med 2002; 346:957–966.

77. Hanratty CG, Koyama Y, Rasmussen HH, et al. Exaggeration of nonculprit stenosis severity during acute myocardial infarction: implications for immediate multivessel revascularization. J Am Coll Cardiol 2002; 40:911–916.

78. Antoniucci D, Valenti R, Moschi G, et al. Relation between preintervention angiographic evidence of coronary collateral circulation and clinical and angiographic outcomes after primary angioplasty or stenting for acute myocardial infarction. Am J Cardiol 2002; 89:121–125.

79. Rentrop KP, Cohen M, Blancke H, et al. Changes in collateral channel filling immediately after controlled coronary artery occlusion by an angioplasty balloon in human subjects. J Am Coll Cardiol 1985; 5:587–592.

80. Sheehan FH, Braunwald E, Canner P, et al. The effect of intravenous thrombolytic therapy on left ventricular function. A report on tissue-type plasminogen activator and streptokinase from the Thrombolysis In Myocardial Infarction (TIMI) Phase I Trial. Circulation 1987; 72: 817–829.

81. Stone GW, Cox D, Garcia E, et al. Normal flow (TIMI-3) before mechanical reperfusion therapy is an independent determinant of survival in acute myocardial infarction. Analysis from the primary angioplasty in myocardial infarction trials. Circulation 2001; 104:636–641.

82. Zijlstra F, Ernst N, de Boer MJ, et al. Influence of prehospital administration of aspirin and heparin on initial patency of the infarct-related artery in patients with acute ST elevation myocardial infarction. J Am Coll Cardiol 2002; 39:1733–1737.

83. Hochman JS, Boland J, Sleeper LA, et al. Current spectrum of cardiogenic shock and effect of early revascularization on mortality. Results of an international registry. Circulation 1995; 91:873–881.

84. Lee KL, Woodlief LH, Topol EJ, et al. Predictors of 30-day mortality in the era of reperfusion for acute myocardial infarction. Results from a trial of 41,021 patients. Circulation 1995; 91:1659–1668.

85. Barron HV, Bowlby LJ, Breen T, et al. Use of reperfusion therapy for acute myocardial infarction in the United States: data from the National Registry of Myocardial Infarction 2. Circulation 1998; 97:1150–1156.

86. Oka RK, Fortmann SP, Varady AN. Differences in treatment of acute myocardial infarction by sex, age, and other factors (the Stanford Five-City Project). Am J Cardiol 1996; 78:861–865.

87. Edep ME, Brown DL. Effect of early revascularization on mortality from cardiogenic shock complicating acute myocardial infarction in California. Am J Cardiol 2000; 85:1185–1188.

88. Carnendran L, Abboud R, Sleeper LA, et al. Trend in cardiogenic shock: report from the SHOCK study. Eur Heart J 2001; 22:472–478.

89. Nallamothu BK, Blaney ME, Morris SM, et al. Acute reperfusion therapy in ST-elevation myocardial infarction from 1994–2003. Am J Med 2007; 120:693–699.

90. Halkin A, Stone GW, Grines CL, et al. Outcomes of patients consented but not randomized in a trial of primary percutaneous intervention in acute myocardial infarction (the CADILLAC registry). Am J Cardiol 2005; 96:1649–1655.

91. Hochman JS, Sleeper LA, Webb JG, et al. Early revascularization in acute myocardial infarction complicated by cardiogenic shock. N Engl J Med 1999; 341:625–634.

92. Laster SB, Rutherford B, Giorgi LV, et al. Results of direct percutaneous trasluminal coronary angioplasty in octogenarians. Am J Cardiol 1996; 77:10–13.

93. Singh M, Mathew V, Garrat KN, et al. Effect of age on the outcome of angioplasty for acute myocardial infarction among patients treated at the Mayo Clinic. Am J Med 2000; 108:187–192.

94. Batchelor WB, Anstrom KJ, Muhlbier LH, et al. Contemporary outcome trends in the elderly undergoing percutaneous coronary intervention: results in 7,472 octogenarians. J Am Coll Cardiol 2000; 36:723–730.

95. Gurwitz JH, Gore JM, Goldberg RJ, et al. Recent age-related trends in the use of thrombolytic therapy in patients who have had acute myocardial infarction. Ann Intern Med 1996; 124:283–291.

96. Sakai K, Nakagawa Y, Kimura T, et al. Comparison of results of coronary angioplasty for acute myocardial infarction in patients ≥ 75 years of age versus patients < 75 years of age. Am J Cardiol 2002; 89:797–800.

97. American College of Cardiology/American Heart Association Task Force on Practice Guidelines (committee on Management of Acute Myocardial Infarction). 1999 Update: ACC/AHA guidelines for the management of patients with acute myocardial infarction J Am Coll Cardiol 1999; 34:891–911.

98. Dzavik V, Sleeper LA, Picard MH, et al. Outcome of patients aged ≥ 75 years in the Should we emergently revascularize Occluded Coronaries in cardiogenic shock (SHOCK) trial: do elderly patients with acute myocardial infarction complicated by cardiogenic shock respond differently to emergency revascularization? Am Heart J 2005; 16:209–215.

99. Migliorini A, Moschi G, Valenti R, et al. Routine percutaneous coronary intervention in elderly patients with cardiogenic shock complicating acute myocardial infarction. Am Heart J 2006; 152:903–908.

100. Antoniucci D, Valenti R, Migliorini A, et al. Relation of time to treatment and mortality in patients with acute myocardial infarction undergoing primary coronary angioplasty. Am J Cardiol 2002; 89:1248–1252.

101. Rodriguez A, Bernardi V, Fernandez M, et al. In-hospital and late results of coronary stents versus conventional balloon angioplasty in acute myocardial infarction (GRAMI trial). Am J Cardiol 1998; 81:1286–1291.

102. Antoniucci D, Santoro GM, Bolognese L, et al. A clinical trial comparing primary stenting of the infarct-related artery with optimal primary angioplasty for acute myocardial infarction. J Am Coll Cardiol 1998; 31:1234–1239.

103. Suryapranata H, van't Hof AWJ, Hoorntje JCA, et al. Randomized comparison of coronary stenting with balloon angioplasty in selected patients with acute myocardial infarction. Circulation 1998; 97:2502–2505.

104. Grines CL, Cox DA, Stone GW, et al. Coronary angioplasty with or without stent implantation for acute myocardial infarction. N Engl J Med 1999; 341:1949–1956.

105. Saito S, Hosokawa G, Tanaka S, et al. Primary stent implantation is superior to balloon angioplasty in acute myocardial infarction: final results of the Primary Angioplasty versus Stent Implantation in Acute Myocardial Infarction (PASTA) trial. Catheter Cardiovasc Interv 1999; 48:262–268.

106. Antoniucci D, Valenti R, Santoro GM, et al. Systematic direct angioplasty and stent-supported angioplasty therapy for cardiogenic shock complicating acute myocardial infarction: in-hospital and long-term survival. J Am Coll Cardiol 1998; 31:294–300.

107. Gacioch GM, Ellis SG, Lee L, et al. Cardiogenic shock complicating acute myocardial infarction: the use of coronary angioplasty and the integration of the new support devices into patient management. J Am Coll Cardiol 1992; 19:647–653.

108. Lee L, Erbel R, Brown TM, et al. Multicenter registry of angioplasty therapy of cardiogenic shock: initial and long-term survival. J Am Coll Cardiol 1991; 17:599–603.

109. Perez-Castellano N, Garcia E, Serrano JA, et al. Efficacy of invasive strategy for the management of acute myocardial infarction complicated by cardiogenic shock. Am J Cardiol 1999; 83:989–993.

110. White HD. Cardiogenic shock: a more aggressive approach is now warranted. Eur Heart J 2000; 21:1897–1901.

111. Hollenberg SM, Kavinsky CJ, Parrillo JE. Cardiogenic shock. Ann Intern Med 1999; 131:47–59.

112. Hasdai D, Topol EJ, Califf RM, et al. Cardiogenic shock complicating acute coronary syndromes. Lancet 2000; 356:749–756.

113. Hochman JS, Buller CE, Sleeper LA, et al. Cardiogenic shock complicating acute myocardial infarction. Etiologies, management and outcome: a report from the SHOCK Trial Registry. J Am Coll Cardiol 2000; 36:1063–1070.

114. O'Neill WW, de Boer MJ, Gibbons RJ, et al. Lessons from the pooled outcome of the PAMI, Zwolle and Mayo clinic randomized trials of primary angioplasty versus thrombolytic therapy of acute myocardial infarction. J Invasive Cardiol 1998; 10:4A–10A.

115. de Boer M-J, Ottervanger J-P, van't Hof AWJ, et al. Reperfusion therapy in elderly patients with acute myocardial infarction. J Am Coll Cardiol 2002; 39:1723–1728.

116. Antman EM, Hand M, Armstrong PW, et al. 2007 focused update of the ACC/AHA 2004 guidelines for the management of patients with ST elevation myocardial infarction: a report of the American College of Cardiology/American Heart Association Task Force on Practice Guidelines: developed in collaboration With the Canadian Cardiovascular Society endorsed by the American Academy of Family Physicians: 2007 Writing Group to Review New Evidence and Update the ACC/AHA 2004 Guidelines for the Management of Patients With ST-Elevation Myocardial Infarction, Writing on Behalf of the 2004 Writing Committee. Circulation 2008; 117:296–329.

117. Antoniucci D, Valenti R, Migliorini A, et al. Abciximab therapy improves one-month survival rate in unselected patients with acute myocardial infarction undergoing routine infarct artery stent implantation. Am Heart J 2002; 144:315–322.

118. Heart Disease and Stroke Statistics—2003 Update. A report from the American Heart Association Statistics Committee and Stroke Statistics Subcommittee. American Heart Association 2003.

119. Vaccarino V, Krumholz HM, Berkman LF, et al. Sex differences in mortality after myocardial infarction: is there evidence for an increased risk for women? Circulation 1995; 91:1886–1891.

120. Malacrida R, Genoni M, Maggioni AP et al. A comparison of the early outcome of acute myocardial infarction in women and men N Engl J Med 1998; 338:8–14.

121. Weaver DW, White HD, Wilcox RG et al. Comparisons of characteristics and outcomes among women and men with acute myocardial infarction treated with thrombolytic therapy JAMA 1996; 275:777–782.

122. Woodfield SL, Lundergan CF, Reiner JS et al. Gender and acute myocardial infarction: is there a different response to thrombolysis? J Am Coll Cardiol 1997; 29:35–42.

123. Demirovic J, Blackburn H, McGovern PG, et al. Sex differences in early mortality after acute myocardial infarction (the Minnesota Heart Survey). Am J Cardiol 1995; 75:1096–1101.

124. Hochman JS, Tamis JE, Thomson TD, et al. Sex, clinical presentation, and outcome in patients with acute coronary syndromes. N Engl J Med 1999; 341:226–232.

125. Maynard C, Litwin PE, Martin JS, et al. Gender differences in the treatment and outcome of acute myocardial infarction: results from the Myocardial Infarction Triage and Intervention Registry. Arch Intern Med 1992; 152:972–976.

126. Lincoff AM, Califf RM, Ellis SG, et al. Thrombolytic therapy for women with myocardial infarction: is there a gender gap? J Am Coll Cardiol 1993; 22:1780–1787.

127. Heart and Stroke Facts: Statistical Update. A report from the American Heart Association Statistics Committee and Stroke Statistics Subcommittee. American Heart Association 2002.

128. Vaccarino V, Parsons L, Every NR, et al. Sex-based differences in early mortality after myocardial infarction. N Engl J Med 1999; 341:217–225.

129. Vaccarino V, Abramson JL, Valedor E, et al. Sex differences in-hospital mortality after coronary bypass surgery: evidence for higher mortality in younger women. Circulation 2002; 105:1176–1183.

130. Mukamal KJ, Muller JE, Maclure M, et al. Evaluation of sex-related differences in survival after hospitalization for acute myocardial infarction. Am J Cardiol 2001; 88:768–771.

131. Barret-Connor EL, Cohn BA, Wingard DL, et al. Why is diabetes mellitus a stronger risk factor for fatal ischemic heart disease in women than in men? The RANCHO BERNARDO Study. JAMA 1991; 265:627–631.

132. Grundy SM. United States cholesterol guidelines 2001: expanded scope of intensive low- density lipoprotein-lowering therapy. Am J Cardiol 2001; 88(suppl 7B):23J–27J.

133. Steingart RM, Packer M, Hamm P, et al. Sex differences in the management of coronary artery disease. N Engl J Med 1991; 325:226–230.

134. Cariou A, Himbert D, Golmard JL, et al. Sex-related differences in eligibility for reperfusion therapy and in-hospital outcome after acute myocardial infarction. Eur Heart J 1997; 18:1583–1589.

135. Vacek JL, Rosamond TL, Kramer PH, et al. Sex-related differences in patients undergoing direct angioplasty for acute myocardial infarction. Am Heart J 1993; 126:521–525.

136. Stone GW, Grines CL, Browne KF, et al. Comparison of in-hospital outcome in men versus women treated by either thrombolytic therapy or primary coronary angioplasty for acute myocardial infarction. Am J Cardiol 1995; 75:987–992.

137. Stone GW, Marcovitz P, Lansky AJ, et al. Differential effect of stenting and angioplasty in women versus men undergoing a primary mechanical reperfusion strategy in acute myocardial infarction—the PAMI stent randomized trial. J Am Coll Cardiol 1999; 33(2 suppl A):357A.

138. Lansky AJ, Pietras C, Costa RA, et al. Gender differences in outcomes after primary angioplasty versus primary stenting with and without abciximab for acute myocardial infarction: results of the Controlled Abciximab and Device Investigation to Lower Late Angiographic Complications (CADILLAC) trial. Circulation 2005; 111:1611–1618.

139. Brodie BR. Why is mortality rate after percutaneous transluminal coronary angioplasty higher in women? Am Heart J 1999; 137:582–584.

140. Wong SC, Sleeper LA, Monrad ES, et al. Absence of gender differences in clinical outcomes in patients with cardiogenic shock complicating acute myocardial infarction. A report from the SHOCK Trial Registry. J Am Coll Cardiol 2001; 38:1395–1401.

141. Antoniucci D. Stenting and other new developments in interventional therapy for cardiogenic shock. In: Hollenberg SM, Bates ER, eds. Cardiogenic Shock. Armonk, NY: Futura Publishing Company, 2002:145–158.

142. Antoniucci D, Migliorini A, Moschi G, et al. Does gender affect the clinical outcome of patients with acute myocardial infarction complicated by cardiogenic shock who undergo percutaneous coronary intervention? Catheter Cardiovasc Interv 2003; 59:423–428.

143. De Maio SJ, Kinsella SH, Silverman ME. Clinical course and long-term prognosis of spontaneous coronary artery dissection. Am J Cardiol 1989; 64:471–474.

144. Bac DJ, Lotgering FK, Verkaaik APK, et al. Spontaneous coronary artery dissection during pregnancy and post partum. Eur Heart J 1995; 16:136–138.

145. Antoniucci D, Diligenti M. Spontaneous dissection of three major coronary arteries. Eur Heart J 1990; 11:1130–1134.

146. Eltchaninoff H, Cribier A, Letac B. Multiple spontaneous coronary artery dissection in young women. Lancet 1995; 346:310–311.

147. Bybee KA, Kara T, Prasad A, et al. Transient left ventricular apical ballooning: a syndrome that mimics ST-segment elevation myocardial infarction. Ann Intern Med 2004; 141:858–865.

148. Sharkey SW, Lesser JR, Zenovich AG, et al. Acute and reversible cardiomyopathy provoked by stress in women from the United States. Circulation 2005; 111:472–479.

149. Wittstein IS, Thiemann DR, Lima JA, et al. Neurohumoral features of myocardial stunning due to sudden emotional stress. N Engl J Med 2005; 352:539–548.

150. Parodi G, Del Pace S, Carrabba N, et al. Incidence, clinical findings and outcome of women with left ventricular apical ballooning syndrome. Am J Cardiol 2007; 99:182–185.

151. Parodi G, Del Pace S, Salvadori C, et al. for the Tuscany Registry of Tako-Tsubo Cardiomyopathy Investigators. Left ventricular apical ballooning syndrome as a novel cause of acute mitral regurgitation. J Am Coll Cardiol 2007; 50:647–649.

152. Woodfield SL, Lundergan CF, Reiner JS, et al. Angiographic findings and outcome in diabetic patients treated with thrombolytic therapy for acute myocardial infarction: the GUSTO-I experience. J Am Coll Cardiol 1996; 28:1661–1669.

153. The Fibrinolytic Therapy Trialists' (FTT) Collaborative Group.Indications for fibrinolytic therapy in suspected acute myocardial infarction: collaborative overview of early mortality and major morbidity results from all randomised trials of more than 1,000 patients Lancet 1994; 343:311–322.

154. Peterson ED, Shaw LJ, Califf RM, et al. Risk stratification after acute myocardial infarction. Ann Intern Med 1997; 126:561–582.

155. Ryan TJ, Anteman EM, Brooks NH, et al. American College of Cardiology/American Heart Association guidelines for the management of patients with acute myocardial infarction. Executive summary and recommendations. A report of the American College of Cardiology/American Heart Association Task Force on practice guidelines. Circulation 1999; 100:1016–1030.

156. Hasdai D, Granger CB, Srivatsa SS, et al. Diabetes mellitus and outcome after primary coronary angioplasty for acute myocardial infarction: lessons from the GUSTO-IIb angioplasty substudy. J Am Coll Cardiol 2000; 35:1502–1512.

157. Brener SJ, Ellis SG, Sapp SK, et al. Predictors of death and reinfarction at 30 days after primary angioplasty: the GUSTO IIb and RAPPORT trials. Am Heart J 2000; 139:476–481.

158. Mattos LA, Grines CL, de Sousa JE, et al. One-year follow-up after primary coronary intervention for acute myocardial

infarction in diabetic patients. A substudy of the STENT-PAMI trial. Arq Bras Cardiol 2001; 77:556–561.

159. Antoniucci D, Valenti R, Migliorini A, et al. Impact of insulin-requiring diabetes mellitus on effectiveness of reperfusion and outcome of patients undergoing primary percutaneous coronary intervention for acute myocardial infarction. Am J Cardiol 2004; 93:1170–1172.

160. Schroeder R, Wegscheider K, Schroeder K, et al. Extent of early ST segment elevation resolution: a strong predictor of outcome in patients with acute myocardial infarction and a sensitive measure to compare thrombolytic regimens. J Am Coll Cardiol 1995; 26:1657–1664.

161. Van't Hof AW, Liem A, de Boer M-J, et al. Clinical value of 12-lead electrocardiogram after successful reperfusion for acute myocardial infarction. Lancet 1997; 350:615–619.

162. Santoro GM, Valenti R, Buonamici P, et al. Relation between ST-segment changes and myocardial perfusion evaluated by myocardial contrast echocardiography in patients with acute myocardial infarction treated with direct angioplasty. Am J Cardiol 1998; 82:932–937.

163. Nahser PJ, Brown RA, Oskarsson H, et al. Maximal coronary flow reserve and metabolic coronary vasodilation in patients with diabetes mellitus. Circulation 1995; 91:635–640.

164. Abaci A, Oguzhan A, Kahranan, et al. Effect of diabetes mellitus on formation of coronary collateral vessels Circulation 1999; 99:2239–2242.

165. Prasad A, Stone GW, Stuckey TD, et al. Impact of diabetes mellitus on myocardial perfusion after primary angioplasty in patients with acute myocardial infarction. J Am Coll Cardiol 2005; 45:508–514.

166. Marso SP, Miller T, Rutherford BD, et al. Comparison of myocardial reperfusion in patients undergoing percutaneous coronary intervention in ST-segment elevation acute myocardial infarction with versus without diabetes mellitus (from the EMERALD Trial). Am J Cardiol 2007; 100:206–210.

167. Carrabba N, Valenti R, Parodi G, et al. Left ventricular remodeling and heart failure in diabetic patients treated with primary angioplasty for acute myocardial infarction. Circulation 2004; 110:1974–1979.

168. Antoniucci D, Valenti R, Migliorini A, et al. Abciximab therapy improves survival in patients with acute myocardial infarction complicated by early cardiogenic shock undergoing coronary artery stent implantation. Am J Cardiol 2002; 90:353–357.

169. Neumann F-J, Kastrati A, Schmitt C, et al. Effect of glycoprotein IIb/IIIa receptor blockade with abciximab on clinical and angiographic restenosis rate after the placement of coronary stents following acute myocardial infarction. J Am Coll Cardiol 2000; 35:915–921.

170. Montalescot G, Barragan P, Wittenberg O, et al. Platelet glycoprotein IIb/IIIa inhibition with coronary stenting for acute myocardial infarction. N Engl J Med 2001; 344:1895–1903.

171. Antoniucci D, Rodriguez A, Hempel A, et al. A randomized trial comparing primary infarct artery stenting with or without abciximab in acute myocardial infarction. J Am Coll Cardiol 2003; 42:1879–1885.

172. Marso SP, Lincoff AM, Ellis SG, et al. Optimizing the percutaneous interventional outcomes for patients with diabetes mellitus: results of the EPISTENT (Evaluation of Platelet IIb/IIIa Inhibitor for Stenting) trial diabetic substudy. Circulation 1999; 100:2477–2484.

173. Aronson D, Bloomgarden Z, Rayfield EJ. Potential mechanisms promoting restenosis in diabetic patients. J Am Coll Cardiol 1996; 27:528–535.

174. Killip T. Cardiogenic shock complicating myocardial infarction. J Am Coll Cardiol 1989; 14:47–48.

175. Goldberg RJ, Gore JM, Alpert JS, et al. Cardiogenic shock after acute myocardial infarction: incidence and mortality from a community-wide perspective, 1975 to 1988. N Engl J Med 1991; 325:1117–1122.

176. Califf RM, Bengston JR. Cardiogenic shock. N Engl J Med 1994; 330:1724–1730.

177. Goldberg RJ, Samad NA, Yarzebski J, et al. Temporal trends in cardiogenic shock complicating acute myocardial infarction. N Engl J Med 1999; 340:1162–1168.

178. Fox KAA, Steg PG, Eagle KA, et al. Declines in rates of death and heart failure in acute coronary syndromes, 1999–2006. JAMA 2007; 297:1892–1900.

179. Lee L, Bates ER, Pitt B, et al. Percutaneous transluminal coronary angioplasty improves survival in acute myocardial infarction complicated by cardiogenic shock. Circulation 1988; 78:1345–1351.

180. Bengston JR, Kaplan AJ, Pieper KS, et al. Prognosis in cardiogenic shock after acute myocardial infarction in the interventional era. J Am Coll Cardiol 1992; 20:1482–1489.

181. O'Keefe JHJ, Rutherford BD, Mc Conahay DR, et al. Early and late results of coronary angioplasty without antecedent thrombolytic therapy for acute myocardial infarction. Am J Cardiol 1989; 64:1221–1230.

182. Hibbard MD, Holmes DR Jr., Bailey KR, et al. Percutaneous transluminal coronary angioplasty in patients with cardiogenic shock. J Am Coll Cardiol 1992; 19:639–646.

183. Moosvi AR, Khaja F, Villanueva L, et al. Early revascularization improves survival in cardiogenic shock complicating acute myocardial infarction. J Am Coll Cardiol 1992; 19:907–914.

184. Holmes DR, Bates ER, Kleiman NS, et al. Contemporary reperfusion therapy for cardiogenic shock: the Gusto-I trial experience. J Am Coll Cardiol 1995; 26:668–674.

185. Eltchaninoff H, Simpfendorfer C, Franco I, et al. Early and 1-year survival rates in acute myocardial infarction complicated by cardiogenic shock: a retrospective study comparing coronary angioplasty with medical treatment. Am Heart J 1995; 130:459–464.

186. Barron H, Every NR, Parsons LS, et al. The use of intra-aortic balloon counterpulsation in patients with cardiogenic shock complicating acute myocardial infarction: Data from the National Registry of Myocardial Infarction 2. Am Heart J 2001; 141:933–939.

187. Ohman EM, Califf RM, George BS, et al. The use of intraaortic balloon pumping as an adjunct to reperfusion therapy in acute myocardial infarction. Am Heart J 1991; 121:895–901.

188. Ohman EM, George BS, White CJ, et al. Use of aortic counterpulsation to improve sustained coronary patency during acute myocardial infarction. Circulation 1994; 90:792–799.

189. Ishihara M, Sato H, Tateishi H, et al. Intraaortic balloon pumping as adjunctive therapy to rescue coronary angioplasty after failed thrombolysis in anterior wall acute myocardial infarction. Am J Cardiol 1995; 76:73–75.

190. Waksman R, Weiss AT, Gotsman Ms, et al. Intra-aortic balloon counterpulsation improves survival in cardiogenic shock complicating acute myocardial infarction Eur Heart J 1993; 14:71–74.

191. Urban P, Stauffer JC, Bleed D, et al. A randomized evaluation of early revascularization to treat shock complicating acute myocardial infarction. Eur Heart J 1999; 20:1030–1038.

192. Berger PB, Holmes DR, Stebbins AL, et al. Impact of an aggressive invasive catheterization and revascularization strategy on mortality in patients with cardiogenic shock in the GUSTO-I trial. Circulation 1997; 96:122–127.

193. Zeymer U, Vogt A, Zahn R, et al. Predictors of in-hospital mortality in 1333 patients with acute myocardial infarction complicated by cardiogenic shock treated with primary percutaneous intervention (PCI). Eur Heart J 2004; 25:322–328.

194. Berger PB, Ellis SG, Holmes DR Jr., et al. Relationship between delay in performing direct coronary angioplasty and early clinical outcome in patients with acute myocardial infarction Circulation 1999; 100:14–20.

195. Brodie BR, Hansen C, Stuckey TD, et al. Door to balloon time with primary percutaneous coronary intervention for acute myocardial infarction impacts late cardiac mortality in high risk patients presenting early after the onset of symptoms. J Am Coll Cardiol 2006; 47:289–295.

196. Webb JG, Carere RG, Hilton JD, et al. Usefulness of coronary stenting for cardiogenic shock. Am J Cardiol 1997; 79:81–84.

197. Klein LW, Snow RE, Krone RJ, et al. Mortality after emergent percutaneous coronary intervention in cardiogenic shock secondary to acute myocardial infarction and usefulness of a mortality prediction model. Am J Cardiol 2005; 96:35–45.

198. Suguta M, Hoshizaki H, Naito S, et al. Right ventricular infarction with cardiogenic shock treated with percutaneous cardiopulmonary support: a case report. Jpn Circ J 1999; 63:813–815.

199. Bowers TR, O'Neill WW, Grines CL, et al. Effect of reperfusion on biventricular function and survival after right ventricular infarction. N Engl J Med 1998; 338:933–940.

200. Brodie BR, Stuckey TD, Hansen C, et al. Comparison of late survival in patients with cardiogenic shock due to right ventricular infarction versus left ventricular pump failure following primary percutaneous coronary intervention for ST-elevation acute myocardial infarction. Am J Cardiol 2007; 99:431–435.

201. Chauhan A, Zubaid M, Ricci DR, et al. Left main intervention revisited: early and late outcome of PTCA and stenting. Cathet Cardiovasc Diagn 1997; 41:21–29.

202. Quigley RL, Milano CA, Smith LR, et al. Prognosis and management of anterolateral myocardial infarction in patients with left main disease and cardiogenic shock. The left main shock syndrome. Circulation 1993; 88:1165–1170.

203. Marso SP, Steg G, Plokker T, et al. Catheter-based reperfusion of unprotected left main stenosis during an acute myocardial infarction (the ULTIMA experience). Am J Cardiol 1999; 83:1513–1517.

204. Neri R, Migliorini A, Moschi G, et al. Percutaneous reperfusion of left main coronary disease complicated by acute myocardial infarction. Catheter Cardiovasc Interv 2002; 56:31–34.

205. Holmes DR, Berger PB, Hochman JS, et al. Cardiogenic shock in patients with acute ischemic syndromes with and without ST-segment elevation. Circulation 1999; 100:2067–2073.

Section 2
The Technical Perspective

3

Techniques

ANGELA MIGLIORINI AND RENATO VALENTI

Division of Cardiology, Careggi Hospital, Florence, Italy

INTRODUCTION

From a technical point of view, the most relevant characteristic of percutaneous coronary interventions (PCIs) for acute myocardial infarction (AMI) is the need for a quick reestablishment of a normal epicardial flow in a setting where a thrombotic component of the target lesion is nearly invariably present and is frequently the dominant component of the target lesion.

The swiftness of the procedure is a relevant component of its quality and is dependent on the logistic model used for the primary PCI program, the skill of the operator, and the right selection of techniques and materials to carry out the right interventional strategy.

ENTRY SITE

The selection of the entry site in a patient with AMI should be based on the ease and quickness in the introduction of a shaft, placement of the guide catheter, and making one or more exchanges of the guide catheter if needed. The most used approach, the femoral approach, has several advantages over the radial and the brachial approaches. The most important advantage is that the femoral approach allows the routine use of large guide catheters, with the potential for the employment of all types of techniques and devices. In patients without significant aortoiliac disease,

the placement of the guide catheter is easy and quick, while for patients with significant aortoiliac disease, the potential problems related to iliac stenosis or tortuosity may be promptly solved with the use of hydrophilic wires and long shafts. On the contrary, for the same type of problems encountered with the radial or brachial approach, the technical solution may not be easy and the placement of a long shaft more problematic and harmful. These advantages of the femoral approach over the alternative approaches are more evident in the elderly population, where vessel tortuosity and peripheral vessel disease are frequent. The femoral approach allows a more easy and prompt placement of ventricular pacing if needed. The need for two arterial accesses, one for the PCI procedure and the other for intra-aortic balloon counterpulsation, makes the femoral approach as the preferred approach for operator convenience.

The radial approach has the major advantage over the femoral approach of decreased risk of bleeding and vascular complications, while in emergency PCI for AMI its potential for immediate deambulation cannot be considered a significant advantage as in elective procedures. The radial approach may be considered in stable patients, with a good radial pulse allowing the easy placement of at least a 7F shaft. A small randomized trial based on a sample of 114 patients with AMI compared the radial approach with the femoral approach (1). Exclusion criteria included cardiogenic shock, a history of coronary surgery, atrioventricular block, and a negative Allen test. Cross-over to femoral approach was more frequent and fluoroscopy time longer in patients randomized to radial approach, while in-hospital stay was similar in the two groups. As expected, patients randomized to the radial approach had a lower incidence of peripheral arterial complications compared with patients randomized to the femoral approach.

The provisional use of the radial or brachial approaches after failure of the femoral approach attempts deserves some comments. If aortoiliac disease or tortuosity prevents a successful femoral approach, it is likely that the radial or brachial approaches will not be easy. A small amplitude of the radial pulse may suggest the need for the use of a 6F shaft, with subsequent limitations in the use of large devices (atherectomy or thrombectomy devices) or in the treatment of bifurcation lesions. The direct surgical cut down of the brachial artery after surgical isolation should be considered after the failure of radial and femoral approaches. The percutaneous brachial technique carries the potential for major compressive ischemic or neurological complications due to bleeding.

GUIDE CATHETERS

The selection of the guide catheter in the setting of AMI is based on the same criteria used for elective PCI. Large catheters (7F or 8F) should be preferred since they provide a more stable position and backup compared with 6F or 5F catheters. Moreover, in patients with complex coronary anatomy, or unknown anatomy of the totally occluded target vessel, large guide catheters allow the use of all types of devices and are more convenient for the treatment of bifurcation or trifurcation lesions. In the Florence experience, most cases could be successfully and quickly approached with the use of Voda curve guide catheter for the left coronary system and Judkins right curve for the right coronary artery.

The Voda curve catheter has the advantage of superior backup compared with the Judkins left curve (DVD: Case 1). In patients with a normal ascending aorta and origin of the left main, the first option Voda curve is 3.0 for left anterior descending artery and 3.0 or 3.5 for circumflex artery; a longer Voda curve for circumflex artery allows a more direct alignment of the guide catheter, with the vessel favoring the pushability of the coronary devices. For the treatment of middle or distal left main occlusion, a Voda 3.0 or 3.5 is considered the first option curve, while for very proximal left main disease or true left main ostial lesion, the first choice should be the multipurpose curve or alternatively the Amplatz left curve. These types of curves allow the placement of the distal tip of the catheter near to the left main ostium,

avoiding the uncontrolled intubation of left main with the risk of subsequent left main dissection (DVD: Case 4). The Voda and Amplatz left curves are the first-option guide catheter curves if the right radial or brachial approaches are used. As in non-AMI procedures, the left coronary system disease in large ascending aorta can be approached with longer Voda, Amplatz, or Judkins catheter curves or other types of catheters (such as the El-Gamal B type, multipurpose catheters, and others).

Most right coronary arteries can be easily engaged using the Judkins right curve. This type of curve also allows an easy deep catheter intubation if needed. For the "shepherd's crook" takeoff, effective alternatives to the Judkins curve are the "hockey stick" curve, the Amplatz left 1-2 curve, or the multipurpose curve. In patients with a large aorta, or with a right coronary arising from the upper or posterior region of the right coronary sinus, the more effective guide catheter curves are the Amplatz right or left curves or the hockey stick curve.

The anomalous origin of the circumflex artery from the right coronary sinus, or the first segment of the right coronary artery, can be easily approached using the Amplatz right curve or the multipurpose curve guide catheters.

The anomalous origin of the right coronary artery from the left coronary sinus can be approached with a short left coronary catheter (Judkins or Amplatz type) or the multipurpose catheter.

The anomalous origin of the left main from the right coronary sinus can be approached with the multipurpose or the Amplatz curve catheters.

CORONARY WIRES AND ANGIOPLASTY BALLOONS

The use of these devices in the setting of AMI does not deserve specific comments. An intermediate type coronary wire is effective in most cases in crossing "softly" the target lesion and in providing sufficient support to coronary stenting.

TECHNIQUES FOR THE ASSESSMENT OF THE ANATOMY OF A TARGET VESSEL PERSISTENTLY OCCLUDED AFTER CROSSING OF THE WIRE

In a substantial minority of patients, the crossing of the coronary wire is not followed by the reestablishment of infarct artery flow. A persistent TIMI grade 0 to 1 flow after the crossing of the wire prevents the angiographic definition of the anatomy of the vessel and of the characteristics of the target lesion. In these cases, an ultra-selective dye injection beyond the occlusion may be extremely useful for the judgment on the right placement of the wire, the need for a second wire if a major branch is involved in the target lesion, the thrombotic burden, the length of the lesion, and other significant lesions within the infarct artery (DVD: Case 14).

The more convenient approach to this problem is the use of a dual lumen catheter such as the Multifunctional Probing (Boston Scientific, Maple Grove, Minnesota, U.S.) or the Twin-Pass catheter (Vascular Solutions, Minneapolis, Minnesota, U.S.). One lumen is used for the transport of the catheter beyond the occlusion with the monorail system, while the second lumen can be used for dye injection. The multiple functions that the device may discharge include ultraselective administration of drugs, exchange of the coronary wire, and support for the placement of a second wire into a branch with an unfavorable takeoff.

An alternative device is an over-the-wire balloon catheter. However, its use has several disadvantages, such as the need for removal of the coronary wire for dye injection and the fact that it is ultimately a more time-consuming procedure.

An alternative technique to the ultraselective dye injection is the reestablishment of flow avoiding embolization. This goal may be achieved with a thrombectomy device, since in most cases thrombus is a large component of the occlusion in AMI. Other techniques with the potential for major embolization, such as repeat crossings of a deflated angioplasty balloon through the occlusion or angioplasty using undersized balloons, should be avoided.

THROMBECTOMY

Occlusive thrombosis triggered by a disrupted or eroded atherosclerotic plaque is the anatomic substrate of most AMI. Because of this substrate, macro- and microembolization during PCI in AMI is frequent (2) and may result in obstruction of the microvessel network and decreased efficacy of reperfusion and myocardial salvage (DVD: Case 27). Despite the risk of embolization during conventional PCI for AMI being very high, the use of thrombectomy or atherectomy devices has been limited for a long time because of the potential of old devices, such as directional coronary atherectomy device or transluminal extraction atherectomy, for paradoxical increase in the risk of embolization. The high profile of these devices, as well as their poor flexibility and trackability, resulted in very traumatic approach to the target lesion with the dislodgment of thrombus and atheromatous debris in the peripheral coronary network. Recent advancements in the conception and design of these types of devices have dramatically decreased the risk of embolization; these devices should be used in the majority of patients with AMI.

Many types of thrombectomy devices are currently available, from low technology catheters based on manual thrombus aspiration to high technology devices using mechanical energy or other energies such as laser and ultrasounds to disrupt the thrombotic material.

The rheolytic thrombectomy (RT) system (AngioJet, Possis Medical Inc., Minneapolis, Minnesota, U.S.) consists of a dual lumen catheter, with an external pump providing pressurized saline solution via the effluent lumen to the catheter tip. Multiple saline jets from the distal part of the catheter travel backward at 390 mph and create a localized negative pressure zone that draws thrombus where the jets fragment it and propel the small particles to the evacuation lumen of the catheter. The first 5F generation catheter for coronary use (LF 140) was associated with a substantial device failure rate because of the uncrossability of the lesion by the large and poor trackable catheter, embolization, and vessel perforation. In a post hoc analysis in a series of 70 patients with AMI enrolled in the VEGAS 1 and 2 trials, the device failure rate was 22% (3). The second-generation AngioJet catheter for coronary use (XMI) and the more recent third-generation catheter (Spiroflex) that are available either as over-the-wire system or rapid exchange are 4F in size and have an improved design of the profile and of the opening of the jets, allowing easy and nontraumatic navigation through the coronary vessels and more thrombectomy power.

The appropriate technique for an effective and safe thrombectomy is the single-pass anterograde technique (4). A single pass of the RT catheter is sufficient to remove a fresh large thrombus in most patients (DVD: Cases 4, 5, 10, 12, 13, 31, 34, 39, 41, 43, and 45). The RT catheter should be activated at least 1 cm proximal to the thrombus to create a suction vortex prior to advancing the device. Thrombectomy is initiated by advancing the RT catheter slowly (1–3 mm/sec) to and through the thrombosed segment. Typically, the RT catheter can cross the lesion without difficulty, and it should be advanced as far as possible according to lesion location and the length of the vessel distal to the occlusion. Thrombectomy is restarted at the end of the proximal-to-distal pass, with a distal-to-proximal pullback at the same velocity. After the first proximal-to-distal pass, the device is retrieved into the guide catheter. An angiographic check is performed to assess restoration of flow. In the majority of cases, a TIMI grade 3 flow is restored without any evidence of residual thrombus, and treatment with the RT catheter should be stopped at this point. In the event of persistent occlusive thrombosis, a second pass with the RT catheter should be performed (DVD: Cases 9, 16, 17, 20, 21, 25, 32, 38, 44, and 46). Such persistence of thrombus is generally due to old, partially organized thrombus in an aneurysmatic vessel. In this situation, a second pass with the RT catheter may be only partially effective, and the placement of a noncovered or covered stent should be considered to decrease the risk of distal embolization.

In some cases, treatment with the RT catheter may result in the persistence of TIMI flow grade 0 or 1. In such cases, "no-reflow" may be due to occlusive epicardial spasm or exceptionally to microvessel spasm. Intracoronary administration of vasodilatory agents (e.g., nitrate-nitroglycerin or isosorbide dinitrate or nipride- and/or verapamil, or diltiazem or adenosine) may resolve the spasm in a few seconds. If spasm is apparent after the first pass with the RT catheter, subsequent passes should not be made until the spasm is resolved, and only if there is evidence of residual thrombus. If no-reflow persists, it is mandatory to understand the underlying cause before any other attempt with RT catheter, or a balloon catheter, or adjunctive pharmacological therapy is administered. An effective diagnostic approach is an ultraselective injection of contrast medium beyond the occlusion, using a dual lumen catheter. This method will allow assessment of the wire position within the lumen and the diagnosis of persistent microvessel spasm, or persistent massive thrombosis, or an incorrect position of the wire (dissection or perforation). In cases of no-reflow distal to the occlusion, repeat administration of intracoronary vasodilatory drugs should be performed. This precautionary policy may avoid not only severe bradycardia during RT procedure but also other major complications such as extensive dissection, coronary perforation, and cardiac tamponade.

A distal-to-proximal pullback pass is used by some operators, but the retrograde technique should not be performed as the initial thrombectomy run, as the relatively high profile of the RT catheter may produce embolism while crossing the lesion without tip activation, and no-reflow due to distal embolization not only may decrease the effectiveness of reperfusion but also may increase the risk of reflex bradycardia.

If bradycardia occurs during the RT procedure, it is sufficient to stop the activation of the device in most cases: supraventricular or spontaneous ventricular escape beats, or favored by cough or atropine, break off the bradycardia. Thus, in some cases the single-pass procedure may be done with multiple device activation for very short periods.

The efficacy of RT in decrease procedural embolization and subsequent clinical adverse events was already demonstrated by the Vein Graft AngioJet Study (VeGAS 2) trial that enrolled patients with a very high risk of embolization, such as patients with diseased venous grafts or native vessels with angiographic evidence of large thrombus (5). Patients with AMI were excluded. The study, based on a sample of 352 patients, compared RT with intravessel infusion of urokinase and showed a more than 50% reduction in one-month major adverse events in patients randomized to thrombectomy (16% and 33%, respectively, $p < 0.001$).

The Florence-AngioJet randomized trial is a mechanistic small study based on a sample of 100 patients with a first AMI, and the end points of the study were early ST-segment resolution, the corrected TIMI frame count, and the infarct size as assessed by Tc-99m sestamibi scintigraphy at one month (6). Thus, the three end points explored the effectiveness of myocardial reperfusion by three different ways (electrocardiography, angiography, and scintigraphy). All end points were reached. Patients randomized to thrombectomy before direct stenting at a higher incidence of early ST-segment elevation resolution (90% vs. 72%, $p = 0.022$), lower corrected TIMI frame counts (18.2 ± 7.7 vs. 22.5 ± 11.0, $p = 0.032$), and smaller infarcts (13.0% ± 11.6% vs. 21.2% ± 18.0%, $p = 0.010$) compared with patients randomized to direct stenting alone. By multivariate analysis, the only variables related to the early ST-segment resolution were randomization to thrombectomy (OR 3.56, 95% CI 1.11–11.42, $p = 0.032$) and diabetes mellitus (OR 0.24, 95% CI 0.07–0.86, $p = 0.029$). At one month, no patient died or had reinfarction, and the six-month clinical outcome was similar in the two arms: the mortality rate was 2% in both groups and no reinfarctions occurred.

The study tried to avoid the confounding effects of some procedural variables that may affect the efficacy of reperfusion, such as predilation or postdilation after stenting, different types of stents, use or nonuse of IIb/IIIa inhibitors. Direct stenting was attempted in all patients and was successfully performed in 84% of them, while in 16 patients predilation was performed after direct stenting attempt failure. After stenting no patient needed further balloon dilation, and only two types of bare tubular stents were used (one with a closed cell design and the other one with an open cell design; the latter was used in target lesions involving a major branch). Nearly all patients received the same antithrombotic treatment (all but two patients had abciximab treatment), while the crossover to thrombectomy occurred in only four patients of the direct stenting alone arm. The AngioJet device crossed directly the target lesion in nearly all cases, and only two patients needed a predilation with a small balloon before thrombectomy. Early ST-segment resolution and infarct size were assessed in predefined narrow temporal windows (30 minutes from the end of the procedure for ST-segment resolution and 1 month for scintigraphy). The study was powered to detect a difference in early ST-segment resolution, and no differences in clinical outcome could be revealed because of the small number of patients and the criteria used for the enrollment (patients with a history of previous myocardial infarction were excluded). As expected, no impact on mortality could be revealed by this study that enrolled only first AMI patients. However, this was not an empirical trial, but the goal of the study was the demonstration of an improved reperfusion as assessed by surrogate end points.

The AIMI (AngioJet Rheolytic Thrombectomy in Patients Undergoing Primary Angioplasty for Acute Myocardial Infarction) trial is a multicenter randomized trial that compared RT before stenting of the infarct artery with stenting alone and is based on a sample of 480 patients (7). The primary end point of the study was infarct size as assessed by sestamibi scintigraphy at 14 to 28 days after the procedure. The secondary end points were angiographic (TIMI flow grade, TIMI myocardial perfusion grade, corrected TIMI frame count), electrocardiographic ($>70\%$ ST-segment elevation resolution at 90–180 minutes after the procedure), and clinical (the composite of death, myocardial infarction, target vessel revascularization, and stroke at 30 days). The study showed larger infarcts in the thrombectomy arm compared with the control arm ($12.5\% \pm 12.13\%$ and $9.8\% \pm 10.92\%$, respectively, $p = 0.03$), and more importantly, an unexpected higher mortality in the thrombectomy arm at one (4.6% vs. 0.8%, $p = 0.02$) and six months (6.7% vs. 1.7%, $p = 0.01$). Final TIMI grade 3 flow was revealed more frequently in the control arm compared with the thrombectomy arm (97% and 91.8%, respectively, $p < 0.02$). No differences between arms were revealed in the incidence of other angiographic or electrocardiographic markers of reperfusion.

Several concerns in study design and RT technique may explain the negative and harmful results of the study. The enrollment criteria did not include angiographically visible thrombus, and moderate to large thrombus (grade 3 and 4 according to TIMI thrombus score) was present in an unrealistic minority of patients at baseline angiography (21.3% in the thrombectomy arm and 19.6% in the control arm). This figure suggests a selection bias against the enrollment of patients with a large amount of thrombus and who could derive strong benefit from thrombectomy before coronary stenting. Unfortunately, the authors did not provide a screen fail registry, but other characteristics of the study patient cohort strengthen this suspect. More than one-third of patients (35%) already had an open infarct artery at baseline angiography, and more importantly, the infarct size was very small in both arms, with similar normal left ventricular ejection fraction at the time of scintigraphic assessment ($51.3\% \pm 11.53\%$ in the thrombectomy arm and $52.3\% \pm 10.89\%$ in the control arm). Another concern of the study design is the exclusion from enrollment of patients with severe left ventricular dysfunction and cardiogenic shock. The exclusion of these high-risk patients is not easily explained, considering that just in this type of patients a no-reflow due to PCI embolization may be immediately fatal. The nonuniformity of treatment may have introduced confounding effects favoring the control arm. Eight percent of patients randomized to thrombectomy did not have the treatment, procedural variables that may have a significant impact on the risk of no-reflow, such as predilation, or postdilation,

or stent type, were left at discretion of the operator, as well as the thrombectomy technique, with a distal-to-proximal approach used in 48% of cases. The thrombectomy retrograde technique should be considered as inappropriate since with this technique the thrombectomy catheter is activated only after the positioning of the device across the occlusion favoring embolization before thrombectomy.

The ev3 X-SIZER (EndiCor Medical Inc., San Clemente, California, U.S.) thrombectomy device provides direct mechanical thrombus ablation using a distal helical cutter and vacuum-assisted debris removal. The device is available in 1.5-, 2.0-, and 2.3-mm cutter sizes and is compatible with 7F to 9F guide catheters according to the cutter diameter. The device may work mostly within the same radius of the catheter, and efficacy in thrombectomy is dependent on the mismatch between the diameter of the vessel and the size of the device. This limitation is more evident in large or aneurysmatic vessels. The first reported randomized clinical experience with this device in the setting of acute coronary syndromes was based on a cohort of 66 patients (8). Patients randomized to X-SIZER catheter had a better corrected TIMI frame count and ST-segment elevation resolution compared with patients randomized to placebo, and multivariate analysis showed randomization to X-SIZER thrombectomy as the single independent predictor of ST-segment elevation resolution (OR 4.35, $p < 0.04$), and a TIMI grade 3 flow after thrombectomy was achieved in 83% of patients. Another randomized study based on 92 patients with ST-segment elevation AMI has shown better ST-segment elevation resolution and blush grade than in patients randomized to X-SIZER thrombectomy before infarct artery stenting (9). Complete ($>70\%$) ST-segment resolution rate was 58.7% in patients randomized to thrombectomy and 32.6% in those randomized to placebo ($p = 0.001$), while a blush grade 3 was achieved in 71.7% and 36.9% of patients, respectively ($p = 0.006$). A subsequent study, the X-Amine trial, provided similar results (10).

Few data exist about the efficacy and safety of energies alternative to the direct mechanical energy for thrombectomy.

The excimer laser provides ultraviolet emission, resulting in thrombus removal by vaporization and in ablation of the underlying atherosclerotic plaque. The coronary catheter diameters range from 0.9 to 2.0 mm (Vitesse, Spectranetics, Orlando, Florida, U.S.) and may emit concentrically or eccentrically. In a series of 100 patients with acute coronary syndromes (out of these, 49 patients had ST-segment elevation AMI), the laser energy thrombectomy was associated with a 75% reduction of thrombus burden (11). The catheters are not very trackable, and the ablation is poor in large vessels. In a registry based on 56 patients with AMI and evidence of large thrombus (TIMI thrombus grade 5), the procedural success rate was only 86%, with an increase of TIMI flow from 0 to 2.7 ± 0.5

($p < 0.001$) (12). The technique was complicated by embolization in 4% of the cases, no-reflow in 2%, coronary perforation in 0.6%, and major coronary dissection in 4%.

The rationale for the use of an ultrasound catheter for the treatment of thrombus is that ultrasound energy produces a cavitation effect resulting in a vortex that pulls thrombus toward the catheter tip where it is lysed or liquefied to a subcapillary size. Low-frequency ultrasound thrombolysis effectiveness was assessed in a small prospective registry study, including 15 patients with anterior AMI using the Acolysis system (Angiosonics Inc., Morris Ville, North Carolina, U.S.) that fits into a 10F guide catheter (13). In this feasibility study, there were no mechanical complications related to the traumatic, large, and stiff device. However, one patient did not have Acolysis because of diffuse left anterior descending artery disease, and another needed repeat target vessel revascularization because of target vessel reocclusion. The trial was subsequently extended to 126 patients with acute coronary syndrome (out of these, 3 patients had AMI) (14). A TIMI grade 2 or 3 flow was reestablished in 89% of these cases. However, macroembolization was revealed in five patients. The second-generation Acolysis catheter has a lower profile and is compatible with a 7F guide catheter. This device was tested in a randomized study in 181 patients with diseased saphenous grafts (15). Despite the lower profile, the ease of venous graft anatomy, and the use of extra-support wire, the catheter could not reach the target lesion in 14 of 92 patients randomized to ultrasound thrombolysis (device failure rate 15%). In the Acolysis group, the incidence of Q-wave or non-Q-wave myocardial infarction as a consequence of embolization was higher compared to that in the non-Acolysis group (25% vs. 10%), and the primary end point rates (successful procedure without complications) were 53.8% and 73.1% ($p = 0.014$), respectively. Because of these negative and harmful preliminary results, the trial was stopped prematurely.

The majority of the concluded studies on thrombectomy in patients with AMI used simple aspiration catheters (16–21) (DVD: Cases 3 and 11). The manual aspiration catheters used in these study include the Diver CE (Invatec, Brescia, Italy), RESCUE (Boston Scientific, Maple Growe, Minnesota, U.S.), Pronto (Vascular Solutions, Minneapolis, Minnesota, U.S.), and Export (Medtronic, AVE, Santa Rosa, California, U.S.). A major advantage of manual aspiration catheters is that they are easy to use. Two major limitations of these devices are the unpredictability of the completeness of thrombus removal due to the eccentricity of the distal aspiration lumen or the collapse of the vessel produced by the negative pression without simultaneous turbulent flow and the high profile of the catheters that may promote embolization when the occlusion is crossed. All randomized studies used

surrogate end points as the primary end points, and all but one study were positive.

Kaltoft et al. randomized 215 patients to thrombectomy using the RESCUE catheter or control (20). The primary end point of the study was myocardial salvage measured by paired sestamibi scintigraphies before PCI and at 30 days. In the thrombectomy arm, final infarct size was larger compared to that in the control arm (median 15% and 8%, respectively, $p = 0.004$), while there were no differences in myocardial salvage (median 13% and 18%, respectively, $p = 0.12$). These negative results can be explained with the intrinsic limitations of this high-profile catheter (4.5F) that resulted in the need for predilation using 2.0 to 2.5 mm balloons in a substantial minority of patients and in the high incidence (11%) of device failure due to inability to reach the lesion despite predilation. Furthermore, 36 patients (24 in the thrombectomy arm and 12 in the control arm, $p = 0.004$) did not have an early sestamibi scan because of poor clinical condition.

Another study that deserves a specific comment is the Thrombus Aspiration during Percutaneous Coronary Intervention in Acute Myocardial Infarction Study (TAPAS) (21). This study randomized 1071 patients with AMI to thrombus aspiration using the Export catheter or control. The primary end point of the study was myocardial blush, while secondary end points were TIMI grade flow, ST-segment elevation resolution, persistence of ST-segment deviation, target vessel revascularization, myocardial infarction, death, and composite of clinical adverse events at 30 days. The study was positive for all surrogate end points. An ineffective reperfusion as expressed by a myocardial blush grade 0 to 1 was more frequent in the control arm compared with the thrombus aspiration arm (26.3% and 17.1%, respectively; HR 0.65, 95% CI 0.51–0.83, $p < 0.001$). Patients randomized to thrombus aspiration had more frequently complete (>70%) ST-segment resolution (56.6% vs. 44.2%, HR 1.28, 95% CI 1.13–1.45, $p < 0.001$). At 30 days, there was a strong trend of decreased mortality in the thrombus aspiration arm (2.1% vs. 4.0%, $p = 0.07$). The survival curve continued to diverge after one month, and at one year the mortality rate was nearly 8% in the control arm and 4% in the thrombus aspiration arm ($p = 0.04$) (22). Several strengths of this study should be highlighted. First, patients were randomized before angiography, and the study addressed the issue of routine thrombectomy without any bias after coronary angiography, and angiographic evidence of thrombus was revealed in less than half of patients. Second, a key secondary end point, complete early ST-segment elevation resolution, which is a strong marker of the effectiveness of reperfusion, was defined within an early and narrow temporal window after PCI (30–60 minutes, median time of assessment 44 minutes), and the figure of a better ST-segment resolution in the thrombus aspiration together with the higher blush grade link these surrogates with the clinical outcome. Third, the procedures are of high quality and uniformity, which is suggested by the short time from admission to PCI (<30 minutes), the short fluoroscopic time (median 7 minutes), the use of abciximab in most patients (>90%), the low incidence of major bleeding despite the routine use of heparin plus abciximab (<4%), and the high success rate of the device (90%) despite the high profile of the Export catheter (6F).

A meta-analysis of concluded randomized studies using thrombectomy devices shows a positive impact of thrombectomy on surrogate end points (23). However, the negative and harmful results of the AIMI trial (7) and the study by Kaltoft et al. (20) prevented the broad application of thrombectomy before infarct artery stenting, while only one study, the TAPAS trial, showed a significant positive clinical impact of thrombectomy (21,22).

Keeping in mind the limitations and strengths of concluded studies, it can hardly be denied that the removal of atherothrombotic material before infarct artery stenting is a rational approach when considering the pathological vascular substrate of AMI, and the potential benefits of thrombectomy include decreased embolization and microvessel disruption and a more precise angiographic assessment of the characteristics of the culprit lesion that will be treated with a stent with appropriate length and technique. It should be remembered that thrombectomy devices may be associated with increased risk of embolization because of their high profile and the use of an appropriate technique is of crucial importance. Other two critical points that should be considered in the analysis of most concluded randomized studies are related to the confounding effect of many variables related to the clinical outcome other than the PCI-related embolization and limitations of surrogate end points. These concepts may help to explain the conflicting or negative results of studies on thrombectomy before infarct artery stenting and the relative value of evidence-based medicine-generated data.

Again, an early or major clinical benefit from thrombectomy can be expected only in patients with angiographic evidence of thrombus, patients at very high risk of no-reflow, and patients with baseline left ventricular dysfunction with the potential for fatal acute ventricular failure subsequent to a no-reflow. All these studies used surrogate end points and were underpowered to show a possible link between an improved myocardial perfusion and salvage with an improved survival. Thus, all concluded randomized studies cannot provide an evidence-based support to the routine use of thrombectomy in AMI. An empirical trial should include thousands of patients to be sufficiently powered and should have design characteristics that avoid the confounding effects of clinical, angiographic, and procedural variables such as a previous myocardial infarction, the presence or absence of thrombus, the use of the same stenting technique for all patients, and a thrombectomy device with predictable efficacy and safety in thrombus removal. Moreover, the need for a long follow-up can be anticipated, since if thrombectomy is clinically effective, the improvement in survival should be linked to the prevention or reduction of the process of left ventricular remodeling and subsequent congestive heart failure. Meanwhile, it seems reasonable to perform thrombectomy before infarct artery stenting in all patients with visible thrombus and to recommend thrombectomy in patients with thrombus and large area at risk or a preexisting severe left ventricular dysfunction (4).

EMBOLI PROTECTION DEVICES

There is a plethora of this type of devices that are available for coronary use or are under development. The following description will be limited to the prototype devices and based on personal experience with these devices.

There are two types of antiembolic systems: the nonocclusive system based on filters that trap embolic debris and the occlusive systems based on the occlusion of the vessel distally to the target lesion and subsequent retrieval of the embolic debris after the procedure by aspiration catheters. Both systems have the potential major disadvantage that the emboli protection may be complete only if the device can be placed beyond the occlusion in a segment without major branches. Otherwise, debris from the target lesion may embolize into the branches. On the other hand, a very proximal location of the device in tortuous vessels may provide poor support for a successful stenting procedure.

The prototype of the filter devices is the Angioguard XP filter wire (Cordis, Johnson & Johnson, Miami Lakes, Florida, U.S.). The device consists of a guidewire with an integrated filter at the distal end. The available basket sizes range from 4 to 8 mm, and the device should oversize the vessel diameter by 0.5 to 1.0 mm in order to provide a right apposition to the vessel wall of the filter in the open position. Otherwise, a poor circumferential wall apposition between the struts of the basket allows embolization. The basket travels in a closed position into a delivery sheath and is deployed after crossing the target lesion. After the interventional procedure, another shaft allows the retrieval of the device by collapsing and capturing the basket. The device is compatible with 8F guide catheters and is very easy to use. Potential disadvantages are embolization during wiring or during collapse of a basket full of embolic debris that may extrude from the device (DVD: Case 42).

The Microvena TRAP (Microvena, Metamorphic Surgical Devices, Pittsburgh, Pennsylvania, U.S.) filter has a more sophisticated system of capture and collapse of the nitinol basket filter, which is based on the use of a second proximal nitinol basket that allows the capture of the filter in the open position, minimizing the risk of embolization in this phase. The major limitation of this device is its very high profile and the need for a 9F guide catheter.

The Filter Wire device (Boston Scientific, Santa Clara, California, U.S.) consists of a basket delivered with a peel-away delivery sheath and is very simple to use. The profile of the device is 3.9F, and the nitinol loop of the basket adjusts for 3.5 to 5.5 mm vessels. Two major problems frequently encountered with this device are the need for predilation to cross the target lesion due to the high profile of the device and the bad apposition of the loop of the basket in bent vessels, such as coronary arteries. The design of the device was enhanced with a suspension arm of the basket that conforms filter to vessel curvature. A recently concluded trial, the DEDICATION study (the Drug Elution and Distal Protection in ST-Elevation Myocardial Infarction), enrolled 626 patients to filter antiembolic protection [2 devices were used, the Filter Wire in most of the patients and the Spyder-X (eV3, Minneapolis, Minnesota, U.S.) in a small number of patients] (24). The study showed a high percentage of device placement failure despite predilation with 1.5- to 2.0-mm balloon angioplasty and no significant effect on the efficacy of reperfusion as assessed by ST-segment elevation resolution (ST resolution $\geq 70\%$ at 90-minute rate was 76% in the protection group and 72% in the control group, $p = 0.29$).

The GuardWire (Medtronic, AVE, Santa Rosa, California, U.S.) is the prototype of the occlusive protection systems. The system consists of a 0.014-in balloon wire, a microseal adapter for inflation and deflation of the balloon, and a 5F aspiration catheter (Export catheter). The balloon wire has a very low profile (2.1F), allowing a good trackability and a relatively low risk of embolization during wiring the target lesion. The efficacy of this device in protection from embolization was shown in patients with diseased saphenous vein grafts. In the SAFER trial, 801 patients with diseased saphenous vein grafts underwent percutaneous intervention with or without the protection of the GuardWire system in a randomized fashion (25). The device's success rate was 90.1%, and patients randomized to GuardWire had a significant reduction in the rate of adverse events related to embolization compared with the control group (9.6% vs. 16.5%, $p = 0.004$).

The major advantages of this system are the good support of the wire, no limit to the amount of retrieved material, and the low profile as compared with the available filter devices. The correct use of the device in coronary vessels is not too easy and simple as it is in venous grafts or carotid vessels. The right placement of the tip of the GuardWire and the right occlusive balloon diameter are relatively simple in an already open infarct artery. In persisting occluded vessels after crossing of the GuardWire, repeat passages of a low-profile balloon

angioplasty or direct aspiration with the Export catheter may restore the flow at the price of high risk of significant embolization (DVD: Cases 17, 33, and 38). An ultra-selective dye injection beyond the occlusion using the Multifunctional Probing, the profile of which is lower than that of the Export catheter, may minimize the risk of embolization. Oversizing the diameter of the balloon is advisable, since after stenting and restoring of a good flow, the originally selected balloon diameter may be no more occlusive, frustrating the entire protection procedure. However, excessive balloon oversizing may result in vessel trauma and disruption of the intimal tear. The high support of the GuardWire may produce pseudonarrowing of a tortuous infarct artery, preventing any aspiration and retrieval by the Export catheter. The aspiration by the Export catheter of blood and debris may be difficult or impossible. In this case, a large debris may have obstructed the lumen of the catheter. The catheter should be retrieved immediately under negative pressure and the debris may be easily removed, pushing it out of the catheter with a forced saline injection. An excessive negative pressure on the Export catheter may result in the collapse of the vessel and prevention of aspiration. The GuardWire should be handled very carefully, avoiding any damage of the wire by an excessively tight torquer or any kinking that may prevent the inflation of the balloon, or, much worse, its deflation.

The Enhanced Myocardial Efficacy and Recovery by Aspiration of Liberated Debris (EMERALD) trial assessed the efficacy of this device in patients with ST-segment elevation AMI (26). The study is based on a cohort of 501 patients who were randomized to GuardWire PCI or conventional PCI. Exclusion criteria were multivessel intervention, unprotected left main disease, and coronary artery surgery required within 30 days. The primary end points of the study were ST-segment elevation resolution and infarct size as assessed by SPECT Tc-99m sestamibi. Secondary end points included angiographic assessment of reperfusion, major cardiac and cerebral adverse events, including death, myocardial infarction, target vessel revascularization, and stroke at one and six months, and major adverse cardiac events (MACE) related to left ventricular dysfunction (death, new onset of sustained hypotension, new onset of severe heart failure, and hospital readmission for left ventricular dysfunction) at one and six months. Despite the retrieval of visible debris in the majority of cases assigned to antiembolic protection (73%), no end point of the study was reached. Complete ST-segment elevation resolution (63.3% and 61.9%, $p = 0.78$) as well as the infarct size (median 12% vs. 9.5%, $p = 0.15$) and the composite of major adverse events at six months (10% vs. 11%, $p = 0.66$) were similar in both groups. Besides the intrinsic limitation of distal occlusive antiembolic devices, the negative results of the trial may be explained at least in part by the fact that 21% of patients assigned to anti-embolic device did not receive the protection because the placement of the device was impossible (5%) or needed predilation or aspiration (15%). The study design included the visualization of the infarct artery distally to the culprit lesion as a prerequisite to the GuardWire placement. Thus, patients with persistent occluded infarct artery after wiring, an angiographic characteristic that generally suggests a large occlusive thrombus, were predilated to restore a flow, and these maneuvers may obviously promote embolization.

An innovative concept for protection from embolization during intervention is based on the proximal occlusion of the vessel. These systems have the potential for a complete protection of the vessel and the branches before any intervention device crosses the target lesion. The stagnating blood distally to the proximally occluded device or the reversal of flow if there is an effective collateral flow from arteries other than the infarct artery could prevent any embolization to the distal bed, while the catheter can allow the retrieval of atherothrombotic debris after the stenting procedure. Moreover, the large lumen of the occlusive catheter provides an excellent visualization of the target vessel. The revascularization procedure is performed through the large lumen of the occlusive catheter that can easily accommodate the coronary wire and most of the currently available delivery stent system. The only available proximal occlusive device is the Proxis system (Velocimed, Minneapolis, Minnesota, U.S.) (DVD: Cases 2 and 15). The feasibility and safety of the Proxis system in native coronary vessels were assessed in two registry studies and a noninferiority randomized trial in venous graft disease that compared the proximal occlusive system with a distal protection device (27–29). The first registry included only 40 selected patients and showed that occlusion is effective and that debris may be captured through the occlusive catheter (27). The second registry included 172 patients with AMI: in this cohort of patients, the Proxis-supported PCI was associated with complete ST-segment elevation resolution (>70% at 1 hour) in 72% of patients, an incidence of one-year death of 2.3%, and MACE of 10.5% (28). The Proxis system was compared in noninferiority trials with a distal protection device (29). The study showed similar efficacy and safety of the occlusive system compared to the distal protection system.

The placement of the device is easy if the target lesion is located in venous grafts or in the right coronary artery; its simple anatomy allows a quick and nontraumatic access. But the placement of the device is difficult or its use is contraindicated in the left coronary system, with unfavorable take off of the left anterior descending artery or circumflex artery, if the culprit lesion is too proximal to the left main trunk. Moreover, the aspiration is effective when following the occlusion there is a positive pressure sustained by a collateral flow; otherwise, the negative pressure applied to the occlusive catheter may be non-effective for aspiration. In this case a small infusion catheter may be used to augment the reflow toward the occlusive catheter (the infusion catheter is included in the system kit), or alternatively, aspiration and balloon deflation may be started simultaneously.

STENTS

The Historical Perspective

A major pitfall of balloon coronary angioplasty in the setting of AMI was the high incidence of early and late restenosis or reocclusion of the infarct artery (30–35). Early infarct artery reocclusion occurred in 10% to 15% of patients treated successfully by coronary angioplasty, while late target vessel failure rate requiring repeat intervention in the first six months remained disappointingly high. In the PAMI-2 (Primary Angioplasty in Myocardial Infarction 2) trial, the risk of early restenosis or reocclusion of the infarct artery was 8% in low-risk patients and 20.2% in high-risk patients (33). In the PAMI-2 patient cohort, the angiographic predictors of early target vessel failure were a nonoptimal angiographic result of the procedure, defined as a residual stenosis >30% or residual dissection after coronary angioplasty.

The mechanism of early restenosis or reocclusion of the infarct artery is occlusive thrombosis, which is favored by an abnormal flow because of a disrupted atherosclerotic plaque associated with a postangioplasty vessel elastic recoil or, more frequently, vessel dissection.

Despite the high incidence of early infarct artery restenosis and reocclusion, for a long time coronary stenting in the setting of AMI was considered an absolute contraindication, since the thrombotic milieu of an ulcerated coronary plaque complicated by thrombotic occlusion in conjunction with the low-pressure implantation technique and the aggressive anticoagulation regimens were associated with a prohibitive risk of stent thrombosis and bleeding complications. The diffusion of adequate pressure stent implantation technique associated with the efficacy of dual antiplatelet regimens and the omission of aggressive anticoagulation treatment dramatically reduced stent thrombosis and bleeding complications in patients with stable or unstable angina.

The first case of stent implantation in the setting of cardiogenic shock complicating AMI was published in 1991. Cannon et al. described a patient who had bailout stenting for cardiogenic shock complicating acute occlusion of the right coronary artery (36). A balloon-expandable coil stent was implanted for marked vessel recoil after coronary angioplasty, followed by prolonged intracoronary infusion of urokinase for 18 hours. Clinical and angiographic follow-up at six months showed satisfactory results, without any evidence of stent thrombosis or restenosis. In 1996, four small observational studies, including a minority of patients with cardiogenic shock, showed that in the setting of AMI provisional coronary stenting is feasible, the acute angiographic result optimizes, and clinical outcomes improve (37–40). In 1998, the Florence investigators showed in a series of 66 patients with cardiogenic shock complicating AMI that a strategy of provisional coronary stenting resulted in a procedural success rate of 94% and that this high success rate was associated with an overall mortality rate of 29% (41). In this series of patients, 47% of the patients had infarct artery stenting for a poor or suboptimal angiographic result after balloon angioplasty. Patients with a stented infarct artery had a better event-free survival rate compared to those who underwent angioplasty alone (70% vs. 40%, $p = 0.026$).

The postulated mechanisms of the benefit of stent in AMI are the achievement of an initial optimal angiographic result and the correction of any residual dissection by stenting to decrease the incidence of recurrent ischemia as well as the clinical events related to recurrent ischemia, such as fatal and nonfatal reinfarction and angina. It is important to point out that most patients with recurrent ischemia due to target vessel failure experience only angina or nonfatal reinfarction, while death as a consequence of recurrent ischemia accounts for only a minority of deaths (10% in the PAMI-2 trial cohort) (33), since the large majority of deaths after successful coronary angioplasty are due to refractory cardiogenic shock despite a patent infarct artery. The CADILLAC (Controlled Abciximab and Device Investigation to Lower Late Angioplasty Complications) trial investigators have shown that patients with early recurrent ischemia due to thrombosis had a mortality rate similar to that of patients without early thrombosis (1-year mortality, 5% and 4.2%, respectively, $p = 0.81$), while, as expected, patients with early thrombosis had a greater incidence of reinfarction (32% vs. 2.1%, $p < 0.0001$) and target vessel revascularization (92% vs. 12.6%, $p < 0.0001$) (42). As a consequence, the expected benefit of stent in terms of reduction of mortality is limited only to patients with a large area at risk or severe left ventricular dysfunction. In these patients, reocclusion of the infarct artery may result in fatal reinfarction. For patients "not at high risk," the benefit of stent may result only in a significant reduction of the incidence of nonfatal reinfarction and mainly of repeat target vessel revascularization. Obviously, target vessel revascularization is a "soft" end point compared to death. Nevertheless, this soft end point has very important economic and clinical implications when considering the adjunctive costs of a repeat revascularization procedure that include in most cases bailout stenting, longer hospital stay, and quality of life of the patients. Seven concluded randomized trials compared primary coronary stenting with conventional angioplasty alone or conventional angioplasty and provisional stenting in AMI (43–49). All studies showed a benefit of primary stenting in terms of decreased incidence of early and late repeat target vessel revascularization, while, as expected, no benefit of stenting in terms of decreased mortality could be demonstrated.

At first sight, the results of these trials seem very similar. However, several major differences in study designs should be emphasized to put these results into proper perspective. Moreover, a critical appraisal of the studies helps to explain the true potential benefit of routine infarct artery stenting and why the definition of this benefit required so many studies.

The GRAMI (Gianturco-Roubin in Acute Myocardial Infarction) trial was based on a sample of 104 patients with AMI randomized to angioplasty or stenting within 24 hours of symptom onset (43). The primary end point (in-hospital death, reinfarction, target vessel revascularization, and stroke) rate was 3.8% in the stent arm and 19.2% in the angioplasty arm ($p = 0.03$). The late event-free survival rate was 83% in the stent arm and 65% in the angioplasty arm. The benefit of elective stenting of the infarct artery could be demonstrated despite the inclusion of high-risk patients, or previously fibrinolytic-treated patients, and the high incidence of crossover to stent of patients randomized to angioplasty alone (25% of patients randomized to angioplasty had coronary stenting).

The Zwolle trial, based on a sample of 227 patients, enrolled exclusively low-risk patients in whom the infarct artery was considered ideal for stenting (44) Patients with cardiogenic shock as well as those with left main disease, bifurcation lesions, diffuse disease of the infarct artery, tortuous target vessels, no flow after angioplasty, and angiographic evidence of large thrombotic burden were excluded. Early target vessel failure occurred in five patients of the angioplasty group and one patient of the stent group. The six-month event-free survival was better in the stent group compared with the angioplasty group (95% vs. 80%, respectively, $p = 0.001$), and randomization to angioplasty was independently related to the risk of major adverse events (RR 3.2, 95% CI 1.2–8.5). The generalization of the trial results of all patients with AMI is problematic, considering that the inclusion criteria of the trial design prevented at least half of patients deemed suitable for coronary angioplasty from being randomized. The higher in-hospital mortality of non-randomized patients compared with that of randomized patients (7% vs. 2%) suggests that the study population was biased.

The FRESCO (Florence Randomized Elective Stenting in Acute Coronary Occlusion) trial was based on a sample of 150 patients (45). The study design has several unique features. Firstly, the study compares optimal coronary angioplasty with primary infarct artery stenting and takes for granted the benefit of provisional stenting for a nonoptimal angiographic result after coronary angioplasty. This design characteristic prevented the crossover to stenting of patients randomized to angioplasty and rendered the intention-to-treat analysis similar to the treatment analysis. Secondly, patients at high risk were included, resulting in a sample of patients representative of the real world of AMI. Finally, the primary end point of the study was consistent with the rationale for stenting, which is the prevention of recurrent ischemia resulting in death, reinfarction, or repeat revascularization procedure due to restenosis or reocclusion of the infarct artery within six months of the procedure. The primary end point rate was 9% in the stent arm and 28% in the angioplasty arm ($p = 0.003$). The benefit of stenting was evident both in the early phase (1-month recurrent ischemia rate was 3% in the stent arm and 15% in the angioplasty arm) and the late phase (from 1 month to 6 months, the recurrent ischemia rate was 7% in the stent arm and 16% in the angioplasty arm). Consistent with the results of the study, patients who could not be randomized because of a nonoptimal angiographic result after conventional angioplasty and treated by provisional or bailout stenting had six-month target vessel failure rate similar to that of patients randomized to primary stenting (12%).

The PASTA (Primary Angioplasty versus Stent Implantation in Acute Myocardial Infarction) trial is based on a sample of 136 patients with AMI (46). This trial also included high-risk patients and confirmed the benefit of stenting. The primary end point (composite of death, reinfarction, and target vessel revascularization) rate at 12 months was 21% in the stent arm and 46% in the angioplasty arm ($p < 0.0001$). The six-month angiographic restenosis rate was 17% in the stent arm and 37.5% in the angioplasty arm ($p = 0.02$).

The Stent-PAMI trial is based on a sample of 900 patients with AMI and compared primary stenting with angioplasty alone or angioplasty plus provisional stenting (47). The primary end point of the study was the composite of death, reinfarction, target vessel revascularization, and stroke at six months from the procedure. The primary end point rate was lower in the stent group compared with the angioplasty group (12.6% vs. 17.0%, $p < 0.01$). This difference was driven by a decreased incidence of the six-month target vessel failure (7.7% vs. 17.0%, $p < 0.001$). The six-month mortality rate was slightly higher in the stent arm compared with the angioplasty arm (4.2% vs. 2.7%,), while a postprocedure TIMI grade 3 flow was reached more frequently in the angioplasty arm (92.7% vs. 89.4%). At one year, the survival rate was 94.6% in the stent arm and 97% in the angioplasty arm ($p = 0.054$). Despite the fact that this

difference was not significant, the PAMI investigators considered the trend toward an increased mortality as a "disturbing" result and concluded that another trial had to be conducted to confirm stenting as the routine treatment for patients with AMI undergoing primary percutaneous intervention. Some major limitations of this study should be highlighted. The study design prevented the enrollment of nearly 40% of eligible patients with AMI. Patients with cardiogenic shock were excluded from randomization as well as those with high-risk coronary anatomy (left main disease, ostial lesion of left anterior descending artery, or circumflex artery, target vessel tortuosity, calcification, and side branch involved in the culprit lesion). Moreover, the crossover to stent of patients randomized to conventional angioplasty (15%) might have reduced the benefit of primary stenting, as showed by the lower-than-expected in-hospital recurrent ischemia rate in the angioplasty arm (4%), similar to that of the stent arm (2.9%, $p = 0.30$). The selection of the patients for enrollment may also explain the lack of benefit of stenting in women, as revealed by this study.

The STENTIM-2 (STENTing in Acute Myocardial Infarction) trial is based on a sample of 211 patients with AMI (48). Differently from previous trials that used clinical end points, the primary end point of this study was six-month angiographic restenosis. The restenosis rate was significantly lower in patients randomized to stenting compared with patients randomized to angioplasty (25.3% vs. 39.6%, $p = 0.04$). No differences could be revealed between stenting and angioplasty in clinical outcome, including the need for a repeat procedure (5.0% vs. 5.4%). However, the very high incidence of crossover to stent of patients randomized to angioplasty (36.4%) rendered the analysis based on intention to treat unacceptable.

The CADILLAC trial compared coronary angioplasty with stenting, with and without abciximab (49). This study was designed by the same investigators as that of the Stent-PAMI trial. Patients ($n = 2082$) were randomly assigned in a balanced fashion to one of the four interventional strategies of reperfusion: angioplasty, angioplasty plus abciximab, stenting, and stenting plus abciximab. The primary end point (composite of death, myocardial infarction, target vessel revascularization, and stroke at six months) rates were 20.0% in the angioplasty alone arm, 16.5% in the angioplasty plus abciximab arm, 11.5% in the stenting alone arm, and 10.2% in the stenting plus abciximab arm. The multivariate analysis showed stenting to be inversely related to the risk of the primary end point (OR 0.54, 95% CI 0.42–0.68, $p < 0.001$). The results of the study definitely showed the benefit of stenting compared with that of angioplasty alone, without any adjunctive benefit of abciximab. The benefit was driven by the decrease in the need for target vessel revascularization, while the disturbing trend toward increased mortality, as revealed in the Stent-PAMI trial, was not confirmed. Moreover, the analysis of predefined subgroups revealed that the benefit was similar in men and women. The exclusion of patients with cardiogenic shock or high-risk anatomy resulted in the exclusion from randomization of more than 20% of patients, while the crossover to stent of patients randomized to angioplasty was 16%.

Furthermore, in all but 1 study, 46 patients were randomized before coronary angioplasty. This study design feature resulted in a comparison of planned stenting with optimal as well as nonoptimal conventional angioplasty and also in the crossover to stenting of a substantial percentage of patients randomized to angioplasty.

The Current Perspective

Before the conclusion of the CADILLAC trial routine, infarct artery stenting was already considered as a mainstay therapy for patients undergoing primary PCI. In 2001, the guidelines of ACC/AHA highlighted the positive results of the concluded trials (50), and a recent meta-analysis of randomized trials comparing stent with balloon angioplasty confirmed that the benefit of infarct artery stenting is limited to the need for target vessel revascularization (51).

Currently, the studies focus on the use of drug-eluting stents (DESs) for AMI because of the conflicting results of randomized trials and large registries comparing DESs with bare-metal stents.

The TYPHOON (Trial to Assess the Use of the Cypher Stent in Acute Myocardial Infarction Treated with Balloon Angioplasty) trial included 742 patients and compared the sirolimus-eluting stent (Cypher, Cordis, Johnson & Johnson, Miami Lake, Florida, U.S.) with any commercially available uncoated stent (52). The primary end point of the study was one-year target vessel failure defined as target vessel–related death, myocardial infarction, and target vessel revascularization. The primary end point rate was 7.3% in the DES arm and 14.3% in the uncoated stent arm ($p = 0.004$). The difference between groups was driven by target vessel revascularization, since there were no differences in death (2.3% and 2.2%, respectively) or reinfarction (1.1% and 1.4%, respectively). The thrombosis rates were nearly identical in the two groups (3.4% in the DES arm and 3.6% in the bare-metal stent arm). A major concern of this study is the very low-risk population enrolled in the trial confirmed by the very low mortality rate at one year, and this characteristic is explained by the criteria used for exclusion from randomization (left ventricular dysfunction, previous myocardial infarction, and complex coronary anatomy). A second concern is that the investigators were unblinded to treatment, and it cannot be excluded as a bias favoring

DES patients for target vessel revascularization that drove the differences between groups.

The PAclitaxel-eluting stent in myocardial infarction with ST-Segment elevatION (PASSION) trial randomly assigned 619 patients to paclitaxel-eluting stent (TAXUS Express 2, Boston Scientific, Boston, Massachusetts, U.S.) or to an uncoated stent (Express or Liberté, Boston Scientific, Boston, Massachusetts, U.S.) (53). The primary end point was the composite of cardiac death, recurrent myocardial infarction, and ischemia-driven revascularization of the target lesion. The study showed only a trend favoring DES for the composite of major adverse events at one year (8.8% vs. 12.8%, HR 0.63, 95% CI 0.37–1.07, $p = 0.09$). No difference between groups was revealed in the incidence of stent thrombosis (1% in both arms). The risk profile of this population is higher than that in the population enrolled in the TYPHOON trial. However, also in this study, patients with cardiogenic shock or who had undergone intubation or ventilation were excluded from randomization.

A study with a more complex design is the Single High Dose Bolus Tirofiban and Sirolimus Eluting Stent vs. Abciximab and Bare Metal Stent in Myocardial Infarction (STRATEGY) that compared a strategy of an expensive stent (Cypher, Cordis, Johnson & Johnson, Miami Lake, Florida, U.S.) plus a cheap glycoprotein IIb/IIIa inhibitor with the strategy of an expensive antithrombotic drug (abciximab) plus a bare-metal stent in 175 patients with AMI (54). The primary end point of the study was a composite of clinical and angiographic components: death, myocardial infarction, stroke, or binary restenosis at eight months. The primary end point rate was 19% in the sirolimus-eluting stent plus tirofiban group and 50% in the abciximab plus bare-metal stent group ($p < 0.001$). There were no differences in mortality or reinfarction rates between the groups, while target vessel revascularization rate was 20% in the bare-metal stent group and 7% in the sirolimus-eluting stent group ($p = 0.01$). A major concern of this study is the very high incidence of target vessel revascularization in the bare-metal stent arm (20%), while the incidence of target vessel revascularization in the DES arm was similar to that reported by previous primary PCI trials using bare-metal stents [the target vessel revascularization rate was 9% in the CADILLAC trial (49), 8% in the Stent-PAMI trial (47), and 6% in the EMERALD trial (26)], and this finding suggests a possible bias favoring DES owing to the fact that operators were unblinded to treatment. In the MULTISTRATEGY (MULTIcentre evaluation of Single high-dose bolus TiRofibAn and sirolimus eluting STEnt versus abciximab and bare metal stent in acute mYocardial infarction) trial, the same study design but with different end points was applied to a larger patient sample size (745 patients) (55). The use of sirolimus-eluting stent was associated with a decrease in adverse events mainly driven by a decrease in target vessel revascularization: 3.2% in the DES arm and 10.2% in the bare-metal stent arm. At first sight the results of the STRATEGY trial were confirmed by the MULTI-STRATEGY trial. However, it should be highlighted that in the latter the incidence of target vessel revascularization in both arms was halved compared with that of the former trial.

The MISSION! trial is a single-blind randomized study that compared sirolimus-eluting stents with bare-metal stents in 310 patients with AMI (56). The study design included nine-month angiographic and IVUS follow-up, and the primary end point was late luminal loss. The one-year clinical outcome favored DES with an event-free survival rate of 86% in patients randomized to sirolimus-eluting stent and 73.6% in patients randomized to bare-metal stent ($p = 0.01$), and this difference was driven by target vessel revascularization, since the rates of death, myocardial infarction, and stent thrombosis were similar in the two groups. As expected, late luminal loss was lower in the sirolimus-eluting stent group compared with the uncoated stent group (0.12 ± 0.43 mm vs. 0.68 ± 0.57 mm, $p < 0.001$). Late stent malapposition, as assessed by nine-month IVUS, was revealed in 37.5% of patients randomized to sirolimus-eluting stent and in 12.5% of patients randomized to bare-metal stent ($p < 0.001$). Acquired late stent malapposition was found in 25% of the sirolimus-eluting stent patients and could be explained by the positive remodeling of the vessel (57). Despite the proven benefit in decreasing target vessel revascularization rate at 12-month follow-up, the very high incidence of positive remodeling and subsequent stent malapposition raise concern about the long-term safety of sirolimus-eluting stent in AMI patients.

Two other small trials comparing sirolimus-eluting stent with bare-metal stents showed results favorable to DES. Diaz de la Llera et al. in a study of 120 patients showed a trend toward a decrease in the composite of death, myocardial infarction, and target vessel revascularization in the DES arm compared with that in the uncoated stent arm (6.7% and 11%, respectively, $p = 0.402$) (58). Menichelli et al. in a trial including 320 patients showed a significant decrease in target vessel revascularization and in the composite of MACE in patients receiving sirolimus-eluting stents compared with patients receiving uncoated stents (59).

The DEDICATION trial randomized 626 patients to distal filter protection or standard PCI and after the first randomization to bare-metal stents or DESs (in these trials, 3 types of DESs were used: sirolimus-eluting, paclitaxel-eluting, and zotarolimus-eluting stents) (24). In the mixed DES group, the incidence of major adverse events at eight months was lower compared to that in bare-metal stent group (8.9% and 14.4%, $p < 0.05$), and the difference was driven by the decrease in target lesion

revascularization in the DES arm (5.1% and 13.1%, respectively, $p < 0.001$), while there was a trend toward a higher cardiac mortality in the DES group (4.2% and 1.6%, respectively, $p = 0.09$) (data presented by Kelbaek H at the TCT 2007, Washington DC, October 2008).

All randomized trials comparing DES with uncoated stent did not raise safety concerns, specifically stent thrombosis. Stent thrombosis rate in these studies ranged from 0 of the STRATEGY trial (54) to 3.4% of the TYPHOON trial (53).

However, the evidence provided by concluded randomized trials in terms of either efficacy or safety cannot be considered as strong, considering the small sample size of the studies, the short follow-up, and more importantly, the low-risk profile of the enrolled populations. Thus, it is not surprising that registry studies have not provided results consistent with those of randomized trials, and many of these studies raised very important safety concerns.

The three-year clinical efficacy of sirolimus-eluting stents and paclitaxel-eluting stents versus bare-metal stents in AMI was assessed in the RESEARCH and T-SEARCH (Rapamycin-Eluting Stent Evaluated at Rotterdam Cardiology Hospital, RESEARCH, and Taxus-Stent Evaluated at Rotterdam Cardiology Hospital, T-SEARCH) registries (60). The two registries include 505 patients (183 bare-metal stent, 186 sirolus-eluting stent, and 136 paclitaxel-eluting stent). At three years, the mortality rates were similar in the three groups, as well as the cumulative incidence of death, myocardial infarction, and target vessel revascularization (25.5% in the bare-metal stent group, 17.9% in the sirolimus-eluting stent group, and 20.6% in the paclitaxel-eluting stent group). Definite stent thrombosis was more frequent in the two DES groups compared with the bare-metal stent group (sirolimus group 2.7%, paclitaxel group 2.9%, bare-metal group 1.6%).

The PREMIER (Prospective Registry Evaluating Myocardial Infarction: Events and Recovery) registry is a prospective multicenter U.S. registry enrolling patients with AMI (61). The study analyzed the compliance to dual antiplatelet treatment and its impact on outcome in 500 patients who received DES for AMI. A substantial minority of patients, 13.6%, discontinued the dual antiplatelet treatment within 30 days. At one-year follow-up, the mortality rate was 7.5% in patients who discontinued the dual antiplatelet treatment and 0.7% who continued dual antiplatelet treatment ($p < 0.0001$).

The GRACE (Global Registry of Acute Coronary Events) investigators compared the mortality rates of patients receiving DESs and uncoated stents for AMI: in a series of 2298 patients (569 treated with DESs and 1729 treated with uncoated stents), the mortality rate at six months to two years was 8.6% in the DES group and 1.6% in the uncoated stent group (HR 6.69, $p = 0.002$) (data presented at the 2007 ESC session).

Conversely, no significant difference in 90-day mortality was revealed in the APEX-AMI trial cohort, including 5124 patients (2221 treated with DESs and 2909 treated with uncoated stents): mortality rate 3.0% in DES-treated patients and 4.6% in uncoated stent patients, with an adjusted OR of 0.69 favoring DES (95% CI 0.48–1.09, $p = 0.062$) (Patel R at 2007 ESC session).

Hannan et al. revealed a decreased mortality in patients with AMI receiving DESs (1154 patients) compared with those receiving uncoated stents (772 patients): adjusted mortality rates 5.0% and 8.6%, respectively, $p = 0.007$ (62). However, patients receiving DESs had a different risk profile compared with patients receiving bare-metal stents, and it is uncertain that the statistical methods will provide a true adjustment for differences in patient baseline characteristics, considering also that this study was not a matched case control analysis.

Sianos et al. assessed the incidence and predictors of DES thrombosis in a series of 812 patients (63). The two-year mortality rate was 10.4%, myocardial infarction rate 5.9%, and target vessel revascularization rate 6.7%. DES thrombosis rate was 1.1% at 30 days, increased to 3.2% at two years, and continued to increase beyond two years. A baseline large thrombotic burden was a strong independent predictor both of death (HR 1.76, 95% CI 1.08–2.87, $p = 0.023$) and of stent thrombosis (HR 8.73, 95% CI 3.39–22.47, $p < 0.001$).

This study shows that in a real-world AMI population the problem of stent thrombosis is not negligible, considering the rigid criteria used in this study for the definition of stent thrombosis that included angiographic evidence of occlusive thrombosis and concomitant ischemic event. Thus, all cases of probable or possible stent thrombosis according to the Academic Research Consortium definition (64) were excluded, resulting in an underestimation of the true incidence of stent thrombosis.

In the ASAN registry that included 1911 patients with stable angina, unstable angina, and AMI treated with DES and followed up for two years, the incidence of definite or probable stent thrombosis was 0.8%. In this registry, AMI was a strong predictor of stent thrombosis: HR 12.24, 95% CI 1.67–88.71, $p = 0.014$ (65).

Similarly, the RECLOSE (Responsiveness to CLOpidogrel and Stent-Related Events) trial confirmed a very high incidence of definite or probable DES thrombosis in patients with AMI at six months (4.6%), and AMI was a strong predictor of thrombosis (HR 2.41, 95% CI 1.04–5.63, $p = 0.041$) (66).

A large multicenter registry from Spain, the ESTROFA registry (Estudio ESpañol sobre TROmbosis de stents Farmacoactivos), which included 23,199 patients treated with DESs, of whom 2652 were ST-elevation AMI patients, showed at three years an incidence of definite stent thrombosis of 4.2% in AMI patients (67). AMI was a

strong independent predictor of both subacute (HR 6.9, 95% CI 4–12, $p < 0.0001$) and late (HR 5.2, 95% CI 5.5–7.6, $p < 0.0001$) stent thrombosis.

The conflicting results of randomized trials and registries make impossible a definite recommendation about the use of DES as alternative to bare-metal stents in AMI. It should be remembered that the only potential benefit of DES in AMI is the reduction in the incidence of late restenosis and that it is a consequence of late repeat target vessel revascularization, which is in most cases an elective procedure, while several concerns should be considered, such as the potential for an increased risk of stent thrombosis and subsequent clinical events including death. Despite the lack of robust data, it is very likely that the risk is increased in patients with AMI, considering that AMI is a setting that limits the physician's ability to ascertain the patient's compliance to long-term dual antiplatelet treatment as showed by the results of the PREMIER registry (61), with an increased risk of early as well as late stent malapposition (57).

It seems reasonable to use DES only in very selected cases that include patients with anticipated compliance to long-term dual antiplatelet treatment, a complex coronary anatomy associated with a large area at risk and high risk of restenosis, typically patients with distal left main disease, or last patent vessel. The DES procedure should be supported by the use of thrombectomy and/or antiembolic devices and IVUS in order to decrease the risk of embolization and no-reflow and allow a correct assessment of stent size and apposition.

Direct IRA Stenting Without Predilation

In the Stent-PAMI trial, infarct artery stenting was associated with a trend toward a lower incidence of TIMI grade 3 flow at the end of the procedure and an increased mortality compared with that in angioplasty alone (47). On the other hand, an acute reduction of a normal angiographic flow after balloon angioplasty may be observed after stent deployment and expansion, suggesting that the negative effect on distal flow may be the consequence of increased atherosclerotic and thrombotic material embolization in the microvasculature (DVD: Cases 30 and 47). The rate of arterial embolization in the microvasculature after PCIs is unexpectedly high (2). In patients with angina, the rate of arterial embolization complicated by myocardial infarction induced by stenting using a conventional technique appears to be greater than the one occurring with balloon angioplasty. It is likely that the pathological substrate of AMI, including in many cases an already disrupted atherosclerotic plaque with superimposed thrombosis, may potentiate the bulk atherosclerotic-platelet embolization promoted by catheter-based reperfusion therapy. Direct stenting without predilation could be expected to reduce embolization of plaque constituents and the deterioration of flow, thereby increasing perfusion and myocardial salvage in patients with AMI. It has been hypothesized that with the conventional stenting technique, the single or multiple high-pressure balloon inflations after stent deployment, associated with a bulky effect of the expanding stent, may promote the embolization of atherosclerotic debris and thrombotic material extruded through the struts during initial stent expansion. Moreover, in animal models it has been shown that stent deployment and expansion with a single-balloon inflation is associated with less vessel wall injury (68), and as a consequence, one may infer, less disruption to distal microvessel network produced by the embolic material. Potential disadvantages of the direct stenting technique are embolization promoted during target lesion crossing attempt, stent loss, and incomplete stent expansion in a "hard" calcified lesion. Enhanced stent design with increased trackability as well as enhanced crimping techniques and the very low risk of an undilatable lesion in the setting of AMI make many patients eligible for direct infarct artery stenting.

A randomized study based on 206 patients with AMI comparing direct stenting with conventional stenting confirmed a better reperfusion after direct stenting with decreased incidence of the no-reflow phenomenon and macroembolization, and a higher rate of early ST-segment resolution, that is a marker of effectiveness of reperfusion (69). Direct stenting was associated with a better clinical outcome, but the improvement in outcome did not reach significance because of the small sample of the studied population.

In a cohort of 423 consecutive patients with AMI who underwent infarct artery stenting, conventional stenting, and direct stenting techniques were compared (70). At baseline, patients who underwent direct stenting had a better risk profile than those with conventional stenting. The incidence of angiographic no-reflow was 12% in the conventional stenting group and 5% in the direct stenting group ($p = 0.040$). The one-month mortality rate was 8% in the conventional stenting group and 1% in the direct stenting group ($p = 0.008$). The mortality rate was 11% in patients with no-reflow after stenting and 5.6% in patients with a normal flow. Multivariate analysis showed that age, preprocedural patent infarct artery, and lesion length were related to the risk of no-reflow. In the subset of patients with a more favorable anatomy (target lesion length $\leq$ 15 mm), the variables independently related to the risk of no-reflow were age, direct stenting, and final balloon inflation pressure. The absence of correlation between direct stenting and no-reflow may be explained by the predominant impact of plaque burden and extensive atherosclerotic disease on no-reflow. In fact, when the multivariate

logistic regression analysis was performed in the subset of patients with a target lesion length $\leq$ 15 mm, the variables independently related to no-reflow were age, direct stenting, and final balloon inflation pressure. According to the results of previous studies (71–75), no-reflow had a negative prognostic significance, being associated with a twofold increased one-month mortality compared with patients with a TIMI grade 3 immediately after the revascularization procedure. In this study, patients who were not considered eligible for direct stenting had more adverse baseline clinical and angiographic characteristics and the potential for a higher mortality rate compared with patients who underwent direct stenting. This selection bias should be taken into account to assess the potential advantages of direct stenting correctly. The unfavorable anatomic characteristics for direct stenting, such as diffuse disease or multiple focal lesions within the infarct artery and heavy calcification, may explain the higher incidence of the no-reflow phenomenon in patients deemed nonsuitable for direct stenting, since the diffusion of atherosclerotic disease is a risk factor for embolization in the microvasculature (76,77).

Despite the lack of robust data from randomized controlled trials, direct stenting is performed frequently in current clinical practice. The MULTISTRATEGY (55) trial that compared an everolimus-eluting stent with any uncoated stent encouraged the direct stenting technique whenever possible, even though the incidence of direct stenting was not reported. Again, in the Rotterdam registry, direct infarct artery stenting was performed in 55.8% of cases (63).

There is no doubt that the increased invasiveness of the conventional stenting technique, with repeat balloon dilations, with respect to vessel wall injury may also be considered a dominant risk factor for embolization. Paradoxically, the advantage of the direct stenting technique in the reduction of embolization could be superior in those anatomical settings currently considered unfavorable, such as long lesions, bifurcation lesions, or multiple lesions within the infarct artery. However, in these complex anatomical settings, the percutaneous coronary approach should consider primarily technical aspects (thrombus removal, antiembolic protection devices, good lesion preparation before stenting) other than direct infarct artery stenting.

Type of Stent and Early Target Vessel Failure

The occurrence of target vessel failure after stenting was dramatically reduced but not abolished, despite the fact that most studies excluded patients with diffuse disease, multiple focal lesions, and massive thrombosis.

The early recurrent ischemia rate was 3% in the FRESCO trial (45), 2.9% in the Stent-PAMI trial (47), and 5% in the STENTIM-2 trial (48). Definite subacute stent thrombosis was revealed in 3% of patients enrolled in the FRESCO trial (45), 0.9% in Stent-PAMI trial (47), and 1% in the Zwolle trial (44).

Most stents used in these pioneering randomized trials are no more available. These trials used coil stents or first-generation tubular stents that had a lower performance compared with second-generation tubular stents, which provide more flexibility, more uniform stent expansion with the putative potential for less intimal injury, more uniform vessel wall coverage, and less recoil.

In the CADILLAC trial, a second-generation (corrugated ring) tubular stent was used (49). The subacute stent thrombosis rate was 1.3% in the stent alone arm and 0% in the stent plus abciximab arm ($p = 0.01$), suggesting a strong protective effect of abciximab also in a low-risk population.

In the ACE (Abciximab and Carbostent Evaluation) trial, a randomized study comparing stenting alone with stenting plus abciximab, a carbon-coated stent (Carbostent Sorin, Saluggia, Italy) was used (78). Overall, the stent thrombosis rate was 2.7%. In this study, a potent protective effect of abciximab against stent thrombosis was revealed: the stent thrombosis rate was 0.5% in patients randomized to stent plus abciximab and 5% in patients randomized to stent alone ($p = 0.010$). All patients with stent thrombosis had one or more of the following unfavorable clinical and procedural characteristics: multiple stents, diabetes, cardiogenic shock, crossover to bailout abciximab, and final inflation pressure > 18 atmospheres. Thus, in patients with diabetes or cardiogenic shock or complex anatomy and procedural characteristics, the risk of stent thrombosis is not negligible, despite the high thromboresistance of the carbon-coating stent.

In concluded randomized trials comparing bare-metal stent with balloon angioplasty, the reported six-month restenosis rate is quite variable, ranging from 17% (40) to 31% (43–49,79). It is likely that this variability is more related to the patient and lesion characteristics than to the type of stent used.

Concluded randomized trials comparing DESs with bare-metal stents have shown a decrease in the incidences of angiographic restenosis and late target vessel revascularization in patients treated with DES and no increase in early stent thrombosis (52–59). However, as highlighted previously, this expected positive effect of DES should be considered cautiously, considering the impossibility to generalize the results obtained in selected low-risk population to all patients with AMI.

Technical Issues

In lesions with angiographic evidence of large thrombotic burden, thrombectomy using one of the available devices should be considered as the more appropriate approach before angioplasty or stenting. Thrombectomy may reestablish a grade TIMI 3 flow in most cases, allowing a more exact definition of the length of the lesion and a correct direct placement of the stent.

The stent size should match the vessel diameter proximally to the occlusion, since in most cases the post occlusion vessel diameter may underestimate the actual vessel size because of low pressure or spasm. An undersized stent is associated with a high incidence of thrombosis and restenosis because of incomplete stent apposition and disturbed flow. The MISSION! investigators have shown that early stent malapposition is frequent with either bare-metal stents or DESs (56).

For occlusion involving a major branch, it is mandatory to obtain a correct definition of the geometry of the disrupted atherosclerotic plaque before stenting (DVD: Cases 14 and 43). The occlusion may be a true bifurcation lesion, or the branch may be involved only by the thrombotic component of the plaque. In the first case, as in patients with angina, the more effective approach includes the placement of two wires, angioplasty of both vessel, elective stenting of the main vessel, and provisional stenting of the branch. In the second case, the more effective strategy includes thrombectomy of the main vessel, followed by thrombectomy of the branch, if necessary, and stenting of the main vessel. Also, in DES era, bifurcation stenting is contraindicated for a pseudobifurcation lesion, for the high risk of macro- and microembolization, thrombosis, and restenosis. For a branch not too large, the goal is the reestablishment of a good flow whatever the residual stenosis, since a late positive remodeling is relatively frequent, while the risk of in-stent restenosis is high. A specific comment deserves the treatment for distal left main occlusion. In this setting, the percutaneous technical approach requires a very short time to reperfusion and a high probability of an optimal acute angiographic result. Thrombectomy should be considered as mandatory to decrease the risk of an immediately fatal no-reflow. The restoration of a normal flow after thrombectomy allows a correct definition of the anatomy of the lesion and adoption of the more appropriate technique, from the fast and relatively simple kiss stent technique to the more complex techniques requiring two or more stents.

For occlusion involving the ostium, or the very proximal portion, of the left anterior descending artery or circumflex artery, the most relevant technical problem is the prevention of retrograde shift of atherothrombotic material after angioplasty or stenting of the target vessel (DVD: Cases 4, 12, 13, and 43). The risk of retrograde plaque shift is very high in patients with AMI, and this fact may be explained by the characteristics of the occlusive plaque, which in most cases is a low-density large-volume mass with the potential for high strain under low stress. Thrombectomy is the best primary mechanical approach in case of the thrombotic component of the plaque being prominent. If the residual stenosis after thrombectomy is severe, suggesting a prominent atherosclerotic component of the occlusion, the risk of plaque shift and also the possibility of a distal left main equivalent procedure is high. In all cases, the placement of a protection wire into the nontarget vessel is indicated and should be considered mandatory when the characteristics of takeoff of the nontarget vessel suggest a potential difficult engagement of the vessel by a coronary wire.

Similar to the treatment of diffuse lesions in patients with angina, for diffuse lesions in AMI, the spot stenting technique should be considered as the more effective approach with conventional stents, while total lesion coverage should be considered if DESs are used.

In all cases, very high balloon inflation pressures should be avoided, since the high mechanical trauma may promote embolization, deterioration of flow, and exuberant hyperplastic response and restenosis.

OTHER TECHNIQUES

Hyperoxemic Reperfusion

Hyperoxemic reperfusion using hyperoxygenated blood has shown to have a protective effect against ischemic and reperfusion myocardial injury in the canine model (80). A device currently under investigation (TherOx Inc., Irvine, California, U.S.) in humans may soprasature the blood at high pressure using aqueous oxygen. A nonrandomized feasibility study based on 29 patients with AMI has shown the high feasibility of a 90-minute hyperoxemic reperfusion after stenting of the infarct vessel (81). The AMIHOT trial is a randomized study based on a sample of 269 patients with anterior or large inferior AMI that compared hyperoxemic reperfusion with normoxemic blood autoperfusion (82).

The primary end points were final infarct size at 14 days as assessed by sestamibi scintigraphy, ST-segment elevation resolution at three hours, and the echographic Δ regional wall motion score index at three months. No end point was reached. Hyperoxemic reperfusion did not improve ST-segment elevation resolution, or decrease infarct size, or improve regional wall motion. In a post-hoc analysis, the subset of patients with anterior AMI and reperfused < six hours reached the three end points. After the conclusion of the study, the AMIHOT investigators implemented the study results with a further sample of patients with anterior AMI < six hours. Because of the limitations of a post-hoc analysis, the definition of the primary end point that included three coprimary surrogate end points, and the statistical assumption for pooling the data of the first study with the second one, there is not sufficient evidence to consider hyperoxemic reperfusion as an effective reperfusion technique.

REFERENCES

1. Brasselet C, Tassan S, Nazeyrollas P, et al. Randomised comparison of femoral versus radial approach for percutaneous coronary intervention using abciximab in acute myocardial infarction: results of the FARMI trial. Heart 2007; 93:1556–1561.
2. Topol EJ, Yadav JS. Recognition of the importance of embolization in atherosclerotic vascular disease. Circulation 2000; 101:570–580.
3. Rinfret S, Katsiyiammis PT, Ho KK, et al. Effectiveness of rheolytic coronary thrombectomy with the AngioJet catheter. Am J Cardiol 2002; 90:470–476.
4. Antoniucci D, Valenti R, Migliorini A. Thrombectomy during PCI for acute myocardial infarction: are the randomized controlled trial data relevant to the patients who really need this technique? Catheter Cardiovasc Interv 2008; 71:863–869.
5. Kuntz RE, Baim DS, Cohen DJ, et al. A trial comparing rheolytic thrombectomy with intracoronary urokinase for coronary and vein graft thrombus (the Vein Graft Angiojet Study [VeGAS 2]). Am J Cardiol 2002; 89:326–330.
6. Antoniucci D, Valenti R, Migliorini A, et al. Comparison of rheolytic thrombectomy before direct infarct artery stenting versus direct stenting alone in patients undergoing percutaneous coronary intervention for acute myocardial infarction. Am J Cardiol 2004; 93:1033–1035.
7. Ali A, Cox D, Dib N, et al. Rheolytic thrombectomy with percutaneous coronary intervention for infarct size reduction in acute myocardial infarction: 30-day results from a multicenter randomized study. J Am Coll Cardiol 2006; 48:244–252.
8. Beran G, Lang I, Schreifer W, et al. Intracoronary thrombectomy with the X-Sizer catheter system improves epicardial flow and accelerates ST-segment resolution in patients with acute coronary syndromes. Circulation 2002; 105:2355–2360.
9. Napodano M, Pasquetto G, Saccà S, et al Intracoronary thrombectomy improves myocardial reperfusion in patients undergoing direct angioplasty for acute myocardial infarction. J Am Coll Cardiol 2003; 42:1395–1402.
10. Lefèvre T, Garcia E, Reimers B, et al. X-sizer for thrombectomy in acute myocardial infarction improves ST-segment resolution: results of the X-sizer in AMI for negligible embolization and optimal ST resolution (X AMINE ST) trial. J Am Coll Cardiol 2005; 46:246–252.
11. Topaz O, Minisi AJ, Bernardo N, et al. Comparison of effectiveness of excimer laser angioplasty in patients with acute coronary syndromes in those with versus without normal left ventricular function. Am J Cardiol 2003; 91:797–802.
12. Dahn JB, Ebersole D, Das T, et al. Prevention of distal embolization and no-reflow in patients with acute myocardial infarction and total occlusion in the infarct related artery. A subgroup analysis of the cohort of acute

revascularization in myocardial infarction with excimer laser—CARMEL multicenter study. Catheter Cardiovasc Interv 2005; 64:67–74.

13. Rosenchlin U, Roth A, Rassin T, et al. Analysis of coronary ultrasound thrombolysis end point in acute myocardial infarction ACUTE trial. Results of the feasibility phase. Circulation 1997; 95:1411–1416.

14. Halkin A, Rosenchein V. Catheter-delivered ultrasound therapy for native coronary arterial thrombosis and occluded saphenous vein grafts. Echocardiography 2001; 18:225–231.

15. Singh M, Rouseschen U, Kalon KL, et al. Treatment of saphenous vein bypass grafts with ultrasound thrombolysis. A randomized study (ATLAS). Circulation 2003; 107: 2331–2336.

16. Dudek D, Mielecki W, Legutko J, et al. Percutaneous thrombectomy with the RESCUE system in acute myocardial infarction. Kardiol Pol 2004; 61:523–533.

17. Burzotta F, Trani C, Romagnoli E, et al. Manual thrombus-aspiration improves myocardial reperfusion: the randomized evaluation of the effect of mechanical reduction of distal embolization by thrombus-aspiration in primary and rescue angioplasty (REMEDIA) trial. J Am Coll Cardiol 2005; 46:371–376.

18. Silva-Orrego P, Colombo P, Bigi R, et al. Thrombus aspiration before primary angioplasty improves myocardial reperfusion in acute myocardial infarction: the DEAR-MI (Dethrombosis to Enhance Acute Reperfusion in Myocardial Infarction) study. J Am Coll Cardiol 2006; 48:1552–1559.

19. De Luca L, Sardella G, Davidson CJ, et al. Impact of intracoronary aspiration thrombectomy during primary angioplasty on left ventricular remodelling in patients with anterior ST elevation myocardial infarction. Heart 2006; 92:951–957.

20. Kaltoft A, Bøttcher M, Nielsen SS, et al. Routine thrombectomy in percutaneous coronary intervention for acute ST-segment-elevation myocardial infarction: a randomized, controlled trial. Circulation 2006; 114: 40–47.

21. Svilaas T, Vlaar PJ, van der Horst IC, et al. Thrombus aspiration during primary percutaneous intervention. N Engl J Med 2008; 358:557–567.

22. Vlaar PJ, Svilaas T, van der Horst IC, et al. Cardiac death and reinfarction after 1 year in the Thrombus Aspiration during Percutaneous coronary intervention in Acute myocardial infarction Study (TAPAS): a 1-year follow-up study. Lancet 2008; 371:1915–1920.

23. De Luca G, Suryapranata H, Stone GW, et al. Adjunctive mechanical devices to prevent distal embolization in patients undergoing mechanical revascularization for acute myocardial infarction: a meta-analysis of randomized trials. Am Heart J 2007; 153:343–353.

24. Kelbaek H, Terkelsen CJ, Helquist S, et al. Randomized comparison of distal protection versus conventional treatment in primary percutaneous coronary intervention. The Drug Elution and DIstal protection in ST-elevation myoCArdial infarcTION trial. J Am Coll Cardiol 2008; 51:899–905.

25. Baim D, Wahr D, George B, et al. Randomized trial of distal embolic protection device during percutaneous intervention of saphenous vein aortocoronary bypass grafts. Circulation 2002; 105:1285–1290.

26. Stone GW, Webb J, Cox DA, et al. Distal microcirculatory protection during percutaneous coronary intervention in acute ST-segment elevation myocardial infarction. JAMA 2005; 293:1063–1072.

27. Sievert H, Wahr DW, Schuler G, et al. Effectiveness and safety of the Proxis system in demonstrating retrograde coronary blood flow during proximal occlusion and in capturing embolic material. Am J Cardiol 2004; 94:1134–1139.

28. Kock KT, Haek JD, van der Schaaf RJ, et al. Proximal embolic protection with aspiration in percutaneous coronary intervention using the Proxis device. Rev Cardiovasc Med 2007; 8:160–166.

29. Mauri L, Cox D, Hermiller J, et al. The PROXIMAL trial: proximal protection during saphenous vein graft intervention using the Proxis embolic system. J Am Coll Cardiol 2007; 50:1442–1449.

30. O'Neill WW, Brodie BR, Ivanhoe R, et al. Primary coronary angioplasty for acute myocardial infarction (the Primary Angioplasty Registry). Am J Cardiol 1994; 73:627–634.

31. Brodie BR, Grines CL, Ivanhoe R, et al. Six-month clinical and angiographic follow-up after direct angioplasty for acute myocardial infarction: final results from the Primary Angioplasty Registry. Circulation 1994; 25:156–162.

32. Nakagawa Y, Iwosaky Y, Kimura T, et al. Serial angiographic follow-up after successful direct angioplasty for acute myocardial infarction. Am J Cardiol 1996; 78:980–984.

33. Stone GW, Marsalese D, Brodie BR, et al. A prospective, randomized evaluation of prophylactic intraaortic balloon counterpulsation in high risk patients with acute myocardial infarction treated with primary angioplasty. Second Primary Angioplasty in Myocardial Infarction (PAMI II) Trial Investigators. J Am Coll Cardiol 1997; 29:1459–1467.

34. Brener SJ, Barr LA, Burchenal J, et al. Randomized, placebo-controlled trial of platelet glycoprotein IIb/IIIa blockade with primary angioplasty for acute myocardial infarction: Reopro and Primary PTCA Organization and Randomized trial (RAPPORT) Investigators. Circulation 1998; 98:734–741.

35. The RESTORE Investigators. Effect of platelet glycoprotein IIB/IIIa blockade with tirofiban and adverse cardiac events in patients with unstable angina or myocardial infarction undergoing coronary angioplasty. Circulation 1997; 96:1445–1453.

36. Cannon AD, Roubin GS, Macander PJ, et al. Intracoronary stenting as an adjunct to angioplasty in acute myocardial infarction. J Invasive Cardiol 1991; 3:255–258.

37. Garcia-Cantu E, Spaulding C, Corcos T, et al. Stent implantation in acute myocardial infarction. Am J Cardiol 1996; 77:451–454.

38. Rodriguez AE, Fernandez M, Santaera O, et al. Coronary stenting in patients undergoing percutaneous coronary angioplasty during acute myocardial infarction. Am J Cardiol 1996; 77:685–689.

39. Antoniucci D, Valenti R, Buonamici P, et al. Direct angioplasty and stenting of the infarct-related artery in acute myocardial infarction. Am J Cardiol 1996; 78:568–571.

40. Saito S, Hosokawa G, Kunikane K, et al. Primary stent implantation without coumadin in acute myocardial infarction. J Am Coll Cardiol 1996; 28:74–81.

41. Antoniucci D, Valenti R, Santoro GM, et al. Systematic direct angioplasty and stent-supported angioplasty therapy for cardiogenic shock complicating acute myocardial infarction: in-hospital and long-term survival. J Am Coll Cardiol 1998; 31:294–300.

42. Dangas G, Aymong ED, Mehran R, et al. Predictors and outcomes of early thrombosis following balloon angioplasty versus primary stenting in acute myocardial infarction and usefulness of abciximab (the CADILLAC trial). Am J Cardiol 2004; 94:983–988.

43. Rodriguez A, Bernardi V, Fernandez M, et al. In-hospital and late results of coronary stents versus conventional balloon angioplasty in acute myocardial infarction (GRAMI trial). Am J Cardiol 1998; 81:1286–1291.

44. Suryapranata H, van't Hof AWJ, Hoorntje JCA, de Boer MJ, Zijlstra F. Randomized comparison of coronary stenting with balloon angioplasty in selected patients with acute myocardial infarction. Circulation 1998; 97:2502–2505.

45. Antoniucci D, Santoro GM, Bolognese L, et al. A clinical trial comparing primary stenting of the infarct-related artery with optimal primary angioplasty for acute myocardial infarction. J Am Coll Cardiol 1998; 31:1234–1239.

46. Saito S, Hosokawa G, Tanaka S, et al. Primary stent implantation is superior to balloon angioplasty in acute myocardial infarction: final results of the Primary Angioplasty versus Stent Implantation in Acute Myocardial Infarction (PASTA) trial. Catheter Cardiovasc Interv 1999; 48:262–268.

47. Grines CL, Cox DA, Stone GW, et al. Coronary angioplasty with or without stent implantation for acute myocardial infarction. N Engl J Med 1999; 341:1949–1956.

48. Maillard L, Hamon M, Khalife K, et al. A comparison of systematic stenting with conventional balloon angioplasty during primary percutaneous transluminal coronary angioplasty for acute myocardial infarction. J Am Coll Cardiol 2000; 35:1729–1736.

49. Stone GW, Grines CL, Cox DA, et al. Comparison of angioplasty with stenting, with or without abciximab, in acute myocardial infarction. N Engl J Med 2002; 346:957–966.

50. ACC/AHA guidelines for percutaneous coronary intervention (revision of the 1993 PTCA guidelines) Executive summary. J Am Coll Cardiol 2001; 37:2215–2238.

51. De Luca G, Suryapranata H, Stone GW, et al. Coronary stenting versus balloon angioplasty for acute myocardial infarction: a meta-regression analysis of randomized trials. Int J Cardiol 2008; 126:37–42.

52. Spaulding C, Henry P, Teiger E, et al. Sirolimus-eluting stent versus uncoated stents in acute myocardial infarction. N Engl J Med 2006; 355:1093–1104.

53. Laarman GJ, Suttorp MJ, Dirksen MT, et al. Paclitaxel-eluting versus uncoated stents in primary percutaneous intervention. N Engl J Med 2006; 355:1105–1113.

54. Valgimigli M, Percoco G, Malagutti P, et al. Tirofiban and sirolimus-eluting stent vs abciximab and bare metal stent for acute myocardial infarction. JAMA 2005; 293:2109–2117.

55. Valgimigli M, Campo G, Percoco G, et al. Comparison of angioplasty with tirofiban or abciximab and with implantation of sirolimus-eluting stent or uncoated stetnts for acute myocardial infarction: the MULTISTRATEGY randomized trial. JAMA 2008; 299:1788–1799.

56. van der Hoeven BL, Liem SS, Jukema JW, et al. Sirolimus-eluting stents versus bare metal stents in patients with ST-segment elevation myocardial infarction: 9-month angiographic and intravascular ultrasound results and 12-month clinical outcome results from the MISSION! Intervention Study. J Am Coll Cardiol 2008 51:618–626.

57. van der Hoeven BL, Liem SS, Dijkstra J, et al. Stent malapposition after sirolimus-eluting stent and bare-metal stent implantation in patients with ST-segment elevation myocardial infarction. J Am Coll Cardiol Intv 2008; 1: 192–201.

58. Diaz de la Lera LS, Ballesteros S, Nevado J, et al. Sirolimus-eluting stents compared with standard stents in the treatment of patients with primary angioplasty. Am Heart J 2007; 154:164.e1–164.e6.

59. Menichelli M, Parma A, Pucci E, et al. Randomized trial of sirolimus-eluting stent versus bare-metal stent in acute myocardial infarction (SESAMI). J Am Coll Cardiol 2007; 49:1924–1930.

60. Daemen J, Tanimoto S, Garcìa-Garcìa HM, et al. Comparison of the three-year clinical outcome of sirolimus- and paclitaxel-eluting stents versus bare metal stents in patients with ST-segment elevation myocardial infarction (from the RESEARCH and T-SEARCH Registries). Am J Cardiol 2007; 99:1027–1032.

61. Spertus JA, Kettelkamp R, Vance c, et al. Prevalence, predictors, and outcome of premature discontinuation of thienopiridine therapy after drug-elutng stent placement: results from the PREMIER Registry. Circulation 2006; 133:2803–2809.

62. Hannan EL, Racz M, Walford G, et al. Drug-eluting versus bare-metal stents in the treatment of patients with ST-segment elevation myocardial infarction. J Am Coll Cardiol Intv 2008; 1:129–135.

63. Sianos G, Papaflakis MI, Daemen J, at al. Angiographic stent thrombosis after routine use of drug-eluting stents in ST-segment elevation myocardial infarction. The importance of thrombus burden. J Am Coll Cardiol 2007; 50: 573–583.

64. Mauri L, Hsieh W, Massaro JM, et al. Stent thrombosis in randomized clinical trials of drug-eluting stents. N Engl J Med 2007; 356:1020–1029.

65. Park DW, Park SW, Park KH, et al. Frequency and risk factors for stent thrombosis after drug-eluting stent implantation during long-term follow-up. Am J Cardiol 2006; 98:352–356.

66. Buonamici P, Marcucci R, Migliorini A, et al. Impact of platelet reactivity after clopidogrel administration on drug-eluting stent thrombosis. J Am Coll Cardiol 2007; 49: 2312–2317.

67. de la Torre-Hernandez JM, Alfonso F, Hernandez F, et al. Drug-eluting stent thrombosis. Results from the multicenter Spanish registry ESTROFA (Estudio ESpañol sobre TROmbosis de stents Farmacoactivos). J Am Coll Cardiol 2008; 51:986–990.

68. Rogers C, Parikh S, Seifert P, et al. Remnant endothelium after stenting enhances vascular repair. Circulation 1996; 94:2909–2914.

69. Loubeyre C, Morice MC, Lefevre T, et al. A randomized comparison of direct stenting with conventional stent implantation in selected patients with acute myocardial infarction. J Am Coll Cardiol 2002; 39: 15–21.

70. Antoniucci D, Valenti R, Migliorini A, et al. Direct infarct artery stenting without predilation and no-reflow in patients with acute myocardial infarction. Am Heart J 2001; 142:684–690.

71. The GUSTO Angiographic Investigators. The effects of tissue plasminogen activator, streptokinase, or both on coronary-artery patency, ventricular function, and survival after acute myocardial infarction. N Engl J Med 1993; 329:1615–1622.

72. Feld H, Lichstein E, Schachter J, et al. Early and late angiographic findings of the no-reflow phenomenon following direct angioplasty as primary treatment for acute myocardial infarction. Am Heart J 1992; 123:782–784.

73. Piana NR, Paik GY, Moscucci M, et al. Incidence and treatment of no-reflow phenomenon after percutaneous coronary intervention. Circulation 1994; 89:2514–2518.

74. Abbo KM, Dooris M, Glazier S, et al. Features and outcome of no-reflow after percutaneous coronary intervention. Am J Cardiol 1995; 75:778–782.

75. Laster SB, O'Keefe JH, Gibbons RJ. Incidence and importance of thrombolysis in myocardial infarction grade 3 flow after primary percutaneous transluminal coronary angioplasty for acute myocardial infarction. Am J Cardiol 1996; 78:623–626.

76. Abdelmeguid AE, Topol EJ, Whitlow PL, et al. Significance of mild transient release of creatine kinase-MB fraction after percutaneous coronary interventions. Circulation 1996; 94:1528–1536.

77. Califf RM, Abdelmeguid AE, Kuntz R, et al. Myonecrosis after revascularization procedures. J Am Coll Cardiol 1998; 31:241–251.

78. Antoniucci D, Rodriguez A, Hempel A, et al. A randomized trial comparing infarct artery stenting with or without abciximab in acute myocardial infarction. J Am Coll Cardiol 2003; 42:1879–1885.

79. Neumann F-J, Kastrati A, Schmitt C, et al. Effect of glycoprotein IIb/IIIa receptor blockade with abciximab on clinical and angiographic restenosis rate after the placement of coronary stents following acute myocardial infarction. J Am Coll Cardiol 2000; 35:915–921.

80. Spears JR, Wang B, Wu X, et al. Aqueous oxygen: a highly O2-supersaturated infusate for regional correction of hypotermia and production production of hyperoxemia. Circulation 1997; 96:4385–4391.

81. Dixon SR, Bartorelli AL, Marcovitz PA, et al. Initial experience with hyperoxemic reperfusion after primary angioplasty for acute myocardial infarction. J Am Coll Cardiol 2002; 39:387–392.

82. O'Neill WW, Martin JL, Dixon S, et al. Acute myocardial infarction with hyperoxemic therapy (AMIHOT). A prospective randomized trial of intracoronary hyperoxemic reperfusion after percutaneous coronary intervention. J Am Coll Cardiol 2007; 50: 397–405.

4

Platelet Glycoprotein IIb-IIIa Inhibitors

RENATO VALENTI, GUIDO PARODI, AND ANGELA MIGLIORINI

Division of Cardiology, Careggi Hospital, Florence, Italy

ABCIXIMAB

Observational outcome studies (1–5) have invariably shown that abciximab, the prototypic GP IIb/IIIa inhibitor, as adjunctive therapy to infarct artery stenting provides a significant decrease in the incidence of major cardiac adverse events that is not attributable exclusively to the reduction of ischemic events related to target vessel failure. On the contrary, concluded randomized trials comparing stenting alone with stenting plus abciximab have produced conflicting results (6–10), and the largest study, the CADILLAC (Controlled Abciximab and Device Investigation to Lower Late Angioplasty Complications) trial, apparently did not show any benefit of abciximab as adjunctive treatment to infarct artery stenting.

The effect of abciximab on the clinical events related to the failure of the target vessel could clearly be demonstrated in the RAPPORT (ReoPro and Primary PTCA Organization and Randomized Trial) trial that compared coronary angioplasty alone and coronary angioplasty plus abciximab in 483 patients with acute myocardial infarction (AMI) (11). Similar to the results of the first largest trials on the basis of thousands of patients undergoing elective or high-risk percutaneous coronary intervention (PCI) (12,13), the RAPPORT trial showed a better early outcome of patients randomized to abciximab, with a >70% relative reduction in the composite of death, myocardial infarction, and target vessel revascularization (TVR) at one month

$(2.8\%$ vs. $10.6\%, p < 0.006)$, and this benefit was driven by the reduction of ischemic events related to target vessel failure. The benefit was no more evident at six months, with similar event-free survival curves of the two groups $(28.1\%$ vs. $28.2\%)$. When nonurgent target vessel revascularizations were excluded, the incidence of the composite of death, myocardial infarction, and urgent TVR rate at six months was 17.8% in the placebo group and 11.6% in the abciximab group $(p = 0.05)$. However, it is important to highlight that in this trial, the use of stents was strongly discouraged, and only 70 patients had unplanned coronary stenting. This characteristic of the study design resulted in the easy demonstration of a reduction of ischemic events in abciximab-treated patients due to the very high incidence of early target vessel failure after balloon angioplasty, and at the same time, in the impossibility to identify potential mechanisms of benefit other than the protection from ischemic events related to target vessel failure.

Only a minority of deaths after successful PCI for AMI is due to target vessel failure, and the relationship between death and target vessel failure may emerge only in patients with large area at risk, or severe ventricular dysfunction, or cardiogenic shock, thus, just in high-risk patients who were not fully represented or excluded from enrollment. The spread of the stenting as a routine therapy for AMI, and the subsequent dramatic reduction of ischemic events related to early target vessel failure, apparently decreased the protection by abciximab from target vessel failure, allowing the emergence of the other potential benefits of abciximab beyond the patency of the target vessel. Similar to other effective therapies, whose benefit parallels the risk of the patient, the potential benefits of abciximab on the effectiveness of PCI may be revealed more easily only in high-risk AMI patients, since it may be difficult or even impossible to show the benefit of a strong treatment such as abciximab in low-risk patients. This is a crucial issue for a correct interpretation of the results of concluded trials, and the assessment of the efficacy of abciximab in patients undergoing routine infarct artery stent implantation for AMI.

In the ISAR (Intracoronary Stenting and Antithrombotic Regimen)-2 trial, 200 patients with AMI were randomized to infarct artery stenting alone, and 201 to stenting plus abciximab (6). At one month, the incidence of the composite of death, nonfatal reinfarction, and TVR was lower in the abciximab group as compared to the stent-alone group (5.0% and 10.5%, respectively, $p = 0.038$). However, at one month, there were no differences between the two groups in the incidence of the individual components of the composite clinical end point, including mortality (2.0% in the abciximab group, and 4.5% in the stent-alone group, $p = 0.16$). Despite a relative reduction in mortality in >50%, this difference was not significant due to the small sample population. However, mortality was not the prespecified primary end point of the study, and sample size was defined according to the hypothesis on the basis of a decrease in late loss in abciximab-treated patients at six months. The one-month clinical benefit was not maintained at the six-month follow-up, and this figure may be explained by the high incidence of late TVR in both groups. TVR was the largely dominant component of the composite end point and overcame the other two hard end points, mortality and nonfatal reinfarction, preventing a significant difference in the outcome between groups.

In the ADMIRAL (Abciximab before Direct Angioplasty and Stenting in Myocardial Infarction Regarding Acute and Long-term Follow-up) trial, 149 patients with AMI were randomized to abciximab plus infarct artery stenting, and 151 to stenting alone (8). The one-month mortality rate was 3.4% in the abciximab group and 6.6% in the stent-alone group. Again, despite a relative reduction in mortality of nearly 50%, this difference did not reach significance ($p = 0.19$), and this was due to the small patient cohort. It is important to highlight that the population enrolled in this study had a more "realistic" risk profile as compared to those of previous randomized trials of primary coronary angioplasty in AMI. In fact, in the ADMIRAL trial the mortality rate was significantly higher as compared to those in previous studies. Nevertheless, nearly 90% of patients were in Killip class 1 on enrollment, the majority of them had non-anterior myocardial infarction, and the study design excluded patients with cardiogenic shock on admission. The trial design is

very complex and deserves specific comments to put the results of the study into a proper perspective. Patients were randomized early after presentation and before coronary angiography, and 76 patients were administered abciximab or placebo before their arrival at the catheterization laboratory. After coronary angiography, PCI was performed in 137 patients of the abciximab group, and in 143 patients of the placebo group. Overall, infarct artery stenting was accomplished in 258 of the 300 enrolled patients. Thus, 14% of patients included in the analysis did not receive stent or PCI. The primary end point of the study was the composite of death, reinfarction, or urgent TVR at 30 days. Urgent TVR was defined as repeat PCI performed within 24 hours after a new ischemic episode. The difference in the primary end point rate (6.0% abciximab group, and 14.6% placebo group, $p = 0.01$) was driven by the difference in the incidence of urgent target revascularization (1.3% abciximab group, and 6.6% in the placebo group, $p = 0.01$). The differences in the other two components of the end point, death and reinfarction, both favored abciximab but did not reach significance. Different from the ISAR-2 trial, the exclusion of late nonurgent TVR in the end point allowed the benefit of abciximab treatment maintained at the six-month follow-up: the primary end point rate resulted halved in the abciximab group as compared to the placebo group (7.4% vs. 15.9%, respectively, $p = 0.02$) with a relative risk value of 0.46 (95% CI 0.22–0.93, $p = 0.02$). A major benefit of abciximab treatment could also be demonstrated in the small subset of diabetic patients ($n = 57$): the six-month mortality was 0 in abciximab treated patients and 16.7% in placebo patients ($p = 0.02$), and the primary end point rates were 20.7% and 50.0%, respectively ($p = 0.02$). However, these differences were no more significant at multivariate analysis because of the small number of patients. Again, the small number of women enrolled in the study ($n = 55$) prevented the demonstration of abciximab benefit in this subset of patients. The benefit was superior in those patients who received early abciximab administration (RR = 0.12, 95% CI 0.01–0.98, $p < 0.05$) as compared to patients randomized in the coronary care unit or the catheterization laboratory. The ADMIRAL investigators explain this relation with a higher incidence of a preprocedural TIMI grade 3 flow in patients randomized to abciximab (16.8% vs. 5.4%, $p = 0.01$), suggesting an effect of abciximab on the early reopening of the target vessel. Caution is required in the interpretation of the trial results when considering some characteristics of the enrolled population, and the procedural results. The mean age of patients is less than expected in a "real world" population (59.6 years and 62.1 years in the abciximab group and the placebo group, respectively), as well as the incidence of women, while the incidence of patients with a history of previous coronary intervention is more than expected (28.1% in the abciximab group, and 23.3% in the placebo group). Again, the incidence of repeat TVR within one month of the index procedure in the placebo group (11.3%) may be considered unexpectedly high.

The largest randomized trial comparing primary coronary angioplasty and primary coronary stenting with and without abciximab administration is the CADILLAC trial (9). This trial included 2082 patients who were randomized to four arms: conventional angioplasty and provisional stenting with and without adjunct abciximab treatment, and primary infarct artery stenting with and without adjunct abciximab treatment. The primary end point of the study was the six-month composite incidence of death, reinfarction, disabling stroke, and ischemic TVR. The comparison between the two groups of stent alone (516 patients) and stent plus abciximab (529 patients) did not show any clinical benefit of abciximab in patients undergoing routine infarct artery stent implantation. The incidence of the primary end point was 10.2% in the abciximab-treated patients, and 11.5% in the stent-alone group, and no differences were revealed for each individual component of the composite end point. The main criticism raised from the results of this trial is the low risk of the enrolled population. The six-month mortality rate was very low for all four arms (4.5% in the angioplasty-alone arm, 2.5% in the angioplasty plus abciximab arm, 3.0% in the stent-alone arm, and 4.2% in the stent plus abciximab arm), as was the median age of the four groups (59, 60, 60, and 59 years, respectively). Furthermore, patients with cardiogenic shock were excluded, and the baseline left ventricular function of the enrolled patients was nearly normal (median value >56% in all groups). Finally, only in a minority of patients the left anterior descending artery was the infarct vessel (38.7%). All these figures make the enrolled population poorly representative of the real world of AMI. In fact, 599 patients with AMI eligible for the study were excluded from enrollment (22% of all eligible patients), and had a worse baseline risk profile as compared to enrolled patients, and most patients ($n = 565$) had high-risk coronary anatomy.

However, also in this low-risk population the protective effect of abciximab against early ischemic events was evident. The early thrombosis rate was decreased in both arms of patients randomized to abciximab: 0.8% vs. 1.9% ($p = 0.05$) in the two balloon angioplasty arms, and 0 vs. 1.3% ($p = 0.01$) in the two stent arms. Patients who experienced early thrombosis had similar mortality at one year to the one of patients without early thrombosis (5% and 4.2%, respectively, $p = 0.81$). This finding is expected since with a baseline left ventricular ejection fraction >56%, the possibility of death due to recurrence of ischemia is remote unless a free wall rupture occurs.

However, patients with early thrombosis had a very high incidence of reinfarction (32%) and of urgent TVR (92%). Obviously, due to the low incidence of early thrombotic events, the initial efficacy of abciximab is offset by the much more frequent late TVR events (14).

The ACE (Abciximab and Carbostent Evaluation) trial assigned 400 patients with ST-segment elevation AMI to undergo infarct artery stenting alone or stenting plus abciximab (10). The primary end point of this study was a composite of death, reinfarction, TVR and stroke at one month. Key secondary end points of the study were effectiveness of reperfusion as assessed by early ST-segment resolution, infarct size as assessed by one-month Tc-99m sestamibi scintigraphy, and six-month clinical outcome. The incidence of the primary end point was lower in the abciximab group as compared to the stent-alone group (4.5% and 10.5%, respectively, $p = 0.023$), and randomization to abciximab was independently related to the risk of the primary end point (OR 0.41, 95% CI 0.17–0.97, $p = 0.041$). Early ST-segment resolution was more frequent in the abciximab group (85% vs. 68%, $p < 0.001$). Infarct size, as assessed by one-month Tc-9m sestamibi scintigraphy, revealed smaller infarcts in the abciximab group. At six months, the cumulative difference in mortality between groups increased, with a 44% reduction in mortality in the abciximab group (4.5% in the abciximab group vs. 8.0% in the stent-alone group, $p = 0.148$). At one-year follow-up, the difference in survival rates increased and became significant: $95 \pm 2\%$ in the abciximab arm and $88 \pm 2\%$ in the control arm ($p = 0.017$) (15). The incidence of the composite of six-month death and reinfarction was lower in the abciximab group as compared to stent-alone group (5.5% and 13.5%, respectively; $p = 0.006$). Six-month repeat TVR and restenosis rates were similar in the two groups.

In this study, more than one-third of patients were aged >70, 66% were at "not-low-risk" according to the TIMI criteria, the more frequent location of the AMI was anterior, diffuse disease or multiple lesions within the infarct artery resulted in multiple stent implantation in 25% of patients, patients with cardiogenic shock on admission were included, as well as patients with coronary anatomy at high risk. Moreover, the overall compliance with the protocol was excellent: coronary stenting was attempted in all patients, and in nearly all cases stenting was successful using a last generation passive coating stent, while the incidence of the crossover to bailout abciximab in patients randomized to stenting alone was very low (11%). The study design resulted in the enrollment of a population whose characteristics are consistent with those of large survey studies on AMI (16,17). Thus, the study sample can be considered representative of the entire population of patients with ST-segment elevation AMI.

The mechanistic secondary end points related to the effectiveness of reperfusion and myocardial salvage (ST-segment elevation resolution and infarct size) suggest a benefit of abciximab beyond the effects on the epicardial vessel, and are consistent with the results of a mechanistic randomized trial from the Munich group based on a sample of 200 patients treated by stenting and randomized to abciximab or placebo (7).

This study showed that abciximab may prevent or reduce microvascular damage after reperfusion and improve coronary flow, coronary reserve, and left ventricular function after reperfusion, assessed by intracoronary Doppler measurements and left ventricular angiography. These effects may be related to the prevention or reduction of platelet microvascular plugging by inhibition of glycoprotein IIb-IIIa receptors, as well as neutrophil activation by inhibition of $\alpha M\beta 2$ receptors and $B\beta 3$ receptors that are present on granulocytes and monocytes (18,19). The inhibitory effect of abciximab also includes one of the most important platelet mediators, the CD40 ligand, which is principally expressed in monocytes, macrophages, and endothelial cells and plays a major role in the unleashing of inflammation and production of interleukins and chemochines (20).

Two meta-analyses of randomized trials comparing abciximab with control in patients undergoing primary PCI show a significant reduction in mortality provided by abciximab.

De Luca et al. assessed the effect of abciximab on survival, using data from pharmacological or mechanical reperfusion trials. The comprehensive analysis of PCI trials that includes nearly 4000 patients shows that abciximab randomized patients had a lower 6- to 12-month mortality as compared to control patients (4.4% and 6.2%, respectively, $p = 0.01$) (21).

In a more recent meta-analysis that includes the three European trials (22), Montalescot et al. have found a strong impact of abciximab on long-term survival. This study included 1101 patients and used data on individual patient from each trial, keeping to a minimum any potential effect of reporting bias. The population resulting from the three trials had a high risk profile: 41% of patients had anterior AMI, 30% a history of myocardial infarction, 8.4% cardiogenic shock, and 3.1% a history of coronary artery surgery. The study revealed an absolute 3.6% reduction in mortality and 5.6% in the composite of death and myocardial infarction, a three-year follow-up with a relative risk reduction of 31% in mortality and 37% in the composite of death and myocardial infarction in patients randomized to abciximab. These benefits were more pronounced in the subset of diabetic patients. The absolute increase of 0.6% in major bleeding in patients randomized to abciximab did not offset the strong clinical benefit of the drug at long-term follow-up (22).

EPTIFIBATIDE AND TIROFIBAN

Eptifibatide and tirofiban are specific for the IIb/IIIa receptor, and have no effect on the adhesion of platelet and endothelial cells and of platelets and white cells. Eptifibatide has been shown to be useful in the management of acute coronary syndromes without ST-segment elevation and when combined with tissue plasminogen activator in AMI (23,24).

There are very few data on the utility of eptifibatide as adjunctive treatment to infarct artery stenting for AMI. The emergency room administration of the drug before primary PCI for AMI may facilitate PCI and provide early infarct artery recanalization (25). A small feasibility and efficacy study on the basis of 55 patients with ST-segment elevation AMI treated by infarct artery stenting and double bolus and 24-hour infusion of eptifibatide was stopped prematurely because of an unacceptable subacute stent thrombosis rate (9.1%) (26). It has been speculated that the short glycoprotein IIb/IIIa inhibition provided by the drug could lead to a rebound prothrombotic state favoring stent thrombosis. Despite the lack of data from randomized data, eptifibatide is used as alternative to abciximab in the primary PCI setting, and two large registries have shown that there is no apparent difference in outcome of patients treated with eptifibatide compared with patients treated with abciximab. Additional randomized studies are warranted to confirm these results (27,28).

The RESTORE (Randomized Efficacy Study of Tirofiban for Outcomes and REstenosis) trial was based on a sample of 2212 patients with acute coronary syndromes or AMI (29) The study population included 6% of primary PCI for ST-segment elevation AMI, but no data have been reported with regard to this subset of patients. However, in the overall population, tirofiban treatment was not associated with a significant reduction in the composite of death, myocardial infarction, coronary surgery or repeat PCI, or bailout stenting (10.3% in the tirofiban group and 12.2% in the placebo group; $p = 0.160$). The efficacy of tirofiban administration before primary PCI for AMI was assessed in the TIGER-PA (TIrofiban Given in the Emergency Room before Primary Angioplasty) pilot trial based on a sample of 100 patients who were randomized to early drug administration in the emergency room, or later administration in the catheterization laboratory (30). Early drug administration resulted in improved preprocedural infarct artery TIMI grade 3 flow (32% vs. 10%).

The High dose boluS TiRofibAn and sirolimus eluting STEnt vs. abciximab and bare metal stent in acute mYocardial Infarction (STRATEGY) (31) and the MULTI-STRATEGY (MULTIcentre evaluation of Single high-dose bolus TiRofibAn and sirolimus eluting STEnt vs. abciximab and bare metal stent in acute mYocardial infarction) (32) trials compared in a randomized fashion tirofiban and abciximab in the setting of primary stenting for AMI. The unique features of these two trials are (*i*) the study designs compared a strategy of a sirolimus-eluting stent plus tirofiban with a bare metal stent plus abciximab and (*ii*) tirofiban was administered as a high off-label dose (bolus of 25 µg/kg followed by a 18 to 24-hour infusion at 0.15 µg/kg/min). The sample size of 745 patients of the MULTISTRATEGY trial allowed the comparison between the two drugs. For drug comparison, the hypothesis was the noninferiority of tirofiban as compared to abciximab assuming early ST-segment elevation resolution (>50% at 90 minutes) as surrogate end point of efficacy. The study showed similar early ST-segment resolution rates in the two groups, as well as similar ischemic and hemorrhagic complications.

BIVALIRUDIN

Because of the growing evidence that periprocedural bleeding is a strong predictor of adverse outcome, the reduction of bleeding complications has emerged as a priority in patients undergoing PCI. The study REPLACE (Randomized Evaluation of Pci Linking Angiomax to reduced Clinical Events) 2 and ACUITY (Acute Catheterization and Urgent Intervention Triage strategY) trial have shown that in patients undergoing PCI for stable angina or non-ST-segment-elevation acute coronary syndrome, the direct thrombin inhibitor bivalirudin is associated with similar ischemic event rates as unfractionated heparin plus glycoprotein IIb/IIIa inhibitors while significantly reducing major bleeding (33,34). Whether bivalirudin plus bailout glycoprotein IIb/IIIa inhibitors have comparable safety and efficacy in patients with ST-segment elevation is currently under investigation in the HORIZONS (Harmonizing Outcome with Revascularization and Stents in AMI) trial (35). This prospective randomized trial compares bivalirudin plus bailout glycoprotein IIb/IIIa inhibitors with unfractioned heparin plus routine glycoprotein IIb/IIIa inhibitors (abciximab or eptifibatide as per investigator discretion) in 3602 patients undergoing primary PCI for AMI. A second randomization (stent arm) compares the safety and efficacy of a paclitaxel-eluting stent with the equivalent uncoated stent. The two primary end points of the pharmacological study are major bleeding and net clinical outcome at 30 days. Net clinical outcome is defined by the sum of major bleeding and major adverse clinical events (death from any cause, infarction, ischemic TVR, and stroke), while major adverse clinical event is a secondary end point. Bailout glycoprotein IIb/IIIa inhibitors were recommended in the bivalirudin-alone arm in case of giant thrombus or refractory no-reflow. The adjunctive treatment included preangiography loading of 300 or 600 mg of clopidogrel in all patients. The 30-day results of the pharmacological arm of

the study showed a benefit of the strategy of bivalirudin monotherapy. Two primary end points were reached: the major bleeding rate was 8.3% in the glycoprotein IIb/IIIa inhibitor arm and 4.9% in the bivalirudin arm (*p* <0.0001), and the net clinical outcome rate 12.1% and 9.2%, respectively (*p* = 0.006). The major clinical adverse event rates were similar in the two groups (5.5% and 5.4%), while the cardiac mortality rate was lower in the bivalirudin-alone arm as compared to the glycoprotein IIb/IIIa inhibitor arm: 1.8% and 2.9%, respectively (*p* = 0.035). Ischemic TVR was more frequent in the bivalirudin arm as compared to the glycoprotein IIb/IIIa inhibitor arm (2.6% vs. 1.9%, *p* = 0.18), as well as acute stent thrombosis (1.3% vs. 0.3%, *p* = 0.009). The 30-day survival curve shows an excess of mortality in the bivalirudin arm in the first five days, which was related to the increase in stent thrombosis in this group. Several issues suggest caution in the interpretation of these preliminary results. First, the two primary end points were reached using the major bleeding definition of the ACUITY trial. The differences in major bleeding between the groups are less relevant or absent when using the corresponding TIMI definition of major bleeding (5.0% in the glycoprotein arm and 3.1% in the bivalirudin arm, *p* = 0.003) or the GUSTO definition (0.6% and 0.4%, *p* = 0.65), respectively. Second, the study was underpowered for major adverse ischemic events. Thus, the unexpected finding of a lower 30-day mortality in the bivalirudin arm should be considered critically, while the true clinical impact of bivalirudin-alone treatment will be determined by the planned ongoing long-term follow-up.

THIENOPYRIDINES

The PCI-CURE (PCI-Clopidogrel in Unstable angina to prevent Recurrent Events) trial showed the efficacy in preventing adverse events of dual antiplatelet treatment with aspirin and clopidogrel for patients undergoing PCI (36). Dual antiplatelet treatment is an established therapy also for patients undergoing primary coronary stenting for AMI, and after the PCI-CURE trial, all trials on primary PCI included in their designs dual antiplatelet treatment for at least one month. The CREDO (Clopidogrel for the Reduction of Events During Observation) trial (37) and the CHARISMA (Clopidogrel for High Atherothrombotic Risk, Ischemic Stabilization, Management, and Avoidance) (38) trial have shown that long-term therapy with clopidogrel and aspirin provides clinical benefit in all subsets of patients with atherosclerotic disease. Early discontinuation of clopidogrel is a strong predictor of stent thrombosis and mortality after drug-eluting stent implantation for AMI [Prospective Registry Evaluating Myocardial Infraction: Events and Recovery (PREMIER)] (39).

There is a paucity of data assessing specifically the efficacy of clopidogrel in the setting of primary PCI for AMI.

Lev et al. have shown in a retrospective study including 292 patients that clopidogrel loading before PCI for AMI provides better angiographic and clinical outcomes. TIMI perfusion grade 3 was achieved in 85% of pretreated patients and in 71% of patients who received clopidogrel after PCI (OR 2.2, 95% CI 1.2–3.9, $p = 0.01$), and the incidence of reinfarction at 30-day follow-up was 0 and 3.2%, respectively ($p = 0.04$) (40).

High residual platelet reactivity in vitro after a loading dose of clopidogrel in patients with AMI is highly predictive of adverse events. In a study of 60 patients treated with primary PCI for AMI, the in vitro residual platelet reactivity after clopidogrel was stratified into quartiles according to the percentage reduction of ADP-induced platelet aggregation. The incidence of six-month adverse events was 40% in the first quartile that included one-fourth of patients, 6.7% in the second (1 patient), while no event occurred in the third and the four ($p = 0.007$) (41). Despite the small number of patients, this elegant study highlights the relevance of an appropriate platelet inhibition on clinical outcome, and this fact is still more important in patients receiving drug-eluting stent in the setting of AMI as shown by the RECLOSE (REsponsiveness to CLOpidogrel and Stent-related Events) trial (42) and the ESTROFA (Estudio ESpañol sobre TROmbosis de stents FArmacoactivos) registry (43).

The Bavarian Reperfusion AlternatiVe Evaluation (BRAVE) 3 trial assessed the effect of abciximab after a 600 mg clopidogrel loading pretreatment in 800 patients undergoing primary PCI for AMI (Mehilli J, ACC session, Chicago 2008, oral presentation). The primary end point of the study was final infarct size as assessed by sestamibi scintigraphy at five to seven days, while the secondary end points were death, reinfarction, urgent TVR, stroke, and major and minor bleeding defined according to the TIMI criteria. The final infarct size was not reduced by abciximab (median value 10% and 9%, $p = 0.76$), while there were no differences in 30-day mortality (4.2% in the abciximab arm and 3.3% in the control arm, $p = 0.46$) or major (1.8 in both arms) or minor (3.7 and 1.8, $p = 0.09$) bleedings. The lack of a further benefit of abciximab after 600 mg clopidogrel pretreatment could be explained not only by the high platelet inhibition provided by the high clopidogrel loading but also by the low-risk enrolled population (only 1.4% of patients were in Killip class > 2 on admission). Longer follow-up and further studies are needed to confirm the possibility that high-dose clopidogrel pretreatment alone without adjunct abciximab can be considered as a valid antithrombotic strategy in patients undergoing primary PCI.

Conversely, no doubt exists of the benefit of clopidogrel pretreatment in patients with AMI undergoing PCI after fibrinolytics. The PCI-CLARITY (PCI-CLopidogrel as Adjunctive ReperfusIon TherapY) study that included 1863 patients and used a loading dose of 300 mg of clopidogrel showed an impressive reduction of the incidence of 30-day adverse ischemic events in pretreated patients as compared to control: the incidence of the composite of death, myocardial infarction, stroke was 3.6% in pretreated patients and 6.2% in nonpretreated patients (OR 0.54, 95% CI 0.35–0.85, $p = 0.008$), while pretreated patients did not have excessive bleeding (44).

It is easy to predict a quick shift from clopidogrel to prasugrel therapy in patients with ST-segment elevation AMI when the drug will be available, because of the narrow spectrum of response and the quicker and more pronounced effect of prasugrel on platelets as compared to clopidogrel (45,46).

PREVENTION AND TREATMENT OF BLEEDING

Strong antithrombotic treatments may decrease the risk of recurrent ischemic events in patients with acute coronary syndromes, and as adjunctive therapy to PCI, they have shown a strong clinical benefit. However, a significant decrease in the risk of ischemic complications is invariably associated with an increased risk of bleeding, and there is growing evidence that bleeding in patients with acute coronary syndromes has a strong impact on survival. It is not easy to ascertain the true impact of bleeding on clinical outcome due to the need of large sample of patients to avoid the confounding effect of the worst baseline risk profile of patients who suffer bleeding, the need for an appropriate definition of the severity of bleeding complications, the confounding effect of many variables that are linked to bleeding and that are unexplored in most studies, such as the dose and duration of an antithrombotic treatment, the maintainment of femoral sheath in PCI patients after the procedure, the cut-off of hematological parameters used for blood transfusion, the criteria used for discontinuation of antithrombotic treatment. Again, most deaths are not directly due to a fatal bleeding, and the link between bleeding and mortality is not easily or fully explained in most studies, and the mechanism or mechanisms of death remain largely speculative.

The association between major bleeding and mortality was assessed by Eikelboom et al. in a cohort of 34,146 patients with acute coronary syndromes enrolled in the OASIS (Organization for the Assessment of Strategies for Ischemic Syndromes) registry, in the OASIS-2 trial, and in the CURE trial (47). In this sufficiently powered study, major bleeding occurred in 783 patients (2.3%) and was associated with increased mortality. The 30-day mortality rate was 12.8% in patients who suffered bleeding and 2.5%

in patients without bleeding (HR 5.37, 95% CI 3.97–7.26, p <0.0001). After 30 days, relation between bleeding and mortality was weaker (HR 1.54, 95% CI 1.01–2.36, p = 0.047). The predictors of major bleeding were use of fibrinolitics, glycoprotein IIb/IIIa inhibitors, unfractionated heparin, low-molecular-weight heparin, oral anticoagulant, intra-aortic balloon pump, coronary angiography, and coronary surgery. PCI was not associated with an increased risk of major bleeding. Major bleeding was also associated with an increased risk of ischemic events including death, myocardial infarction, and stroke. The incidence of major ischemic events was 20% in patients with bleeding and 5% in patients without bleeding. This figure suggests that bleeding leading to inappropriate antithrombotic treatment discontinuation may be considered as a major cause of ischemic events.

The discontinuation of antithrombotic treatment as the main link between bleeding and ischemic mortality was clearly shown by the GRACE (Global Registry of Acute Coronary Events) investigators (48). In a registry including 40,087 patients with AMI (53% ST-elevation AMI, 47% non-ST-elevation AMI), the incidence of major bleeding was 2.8%. Patients with major bleeding were older, more severely ill, and more likely to undergo invasive procedures. The in-hospital mortality was 20.9% in patients with major bleeding and 5.6% in patients without major bleeding (p <0.001). After controlling for confounding baseline variables, the risk for increased mortality in patients with major bleeding was lower than the one reported from controlled randomized trials and limited to the in-hospital mortality (HR for in hospital mortality 1.9, 95% CI 1.6–2.2; after hospital discharge HR 0.8, 95% CI 0.6–1).

Among patients who suffered a major bleeding, the in-hospital mortality was considerably higher in those who had antithrombotic treatment discontinued as compared to patients with bleeding and who continued antithrombotic treatment. The mortality rate was 52% in patients who discontinued aspirin and 13% in patients who continued the drug (p <0.001), 58% in patients who discontinued thienopyridine and 13% in patients who continued the drug (p <0.001), and 26% in patients who discontinued heparin and 16% in patients who continued anticoagulant treatment (p = 0.03).

Thus, the findings of the GRACE registry suggest that the association between major bleeding and increased death is lower than reported by controlled randomized trials, limited to the in-hospital stay and no more evident after hospital discharge, and more evident in patients who had discontinuation of at least one antithrombotic drug.

The REPLACE-2 trial compared a strategy of bivalirudin plus provisional IIb/IIIa inhibitors with a strategy of unfractionated heparin plus routine IIb/IIIa inhibitors in 6001 patients undergoing PCI (49). Major bleeding occurred in 195 patients (3.2%) and was more frequent in the heparin plus IIb/IIIa inhibitors. Major bleeding was associated with increased mortality at one month (5.1% vs. 0.2%, p <0.001), and one year (8.7% vs. 1.9%, p <0.001). The hazard risk of death for patients who experienced bleeding was 2.66 (95% CI 1.44–4.92, p = 0.002). Overall, 19 deaths occurred; 10 deaths occurred in 195 patients with major bleeding, and 6 of the 10 deaths were due to a fatal bleeding. This study identified randomization to heparin plus IIb/IIIa inhibitors, provisional use of IIb/IIIa inhibitors in the bivalirudin arm, a time to sheath pull >6 hours, a procedural length >1 hour, and the use of intra-aortic balloon as predictors of major bleeding. Major bleeding definition included a decrease in hemoglobin of at least 3 gr/dL, while TIMI criteria for major bleeding are more stringent (hemoglobin decrease ≥5gr/dL). If TIMI criteria for major bleeding were adopted, there were no more differences in major bleeding between the bivalirudin arm and the heparin plus IIb/IIIa inhibitor arm (0.9% and 0.6%, p = 0.30).

The ACUITY trial is a three-arm study comparing three antithrombotic strategies in patients with acute coronary syndromes: bivalirudin plus provisional IIb/IIIa inhibitors, bivalirudin plus routine IIb/IIIa inhibitors, and heparin plus routine IIb/IIIa inhibitors (34,50). Major bleeding rates were higher in patients randomized to heparin plus II/b/IIIa inhibitors as compared to bivalirudin monotherapy (5.7% vs. 3.0%, p <0.001) and similar to the bivalirudin plus IIb/IIIa inhibitor arm (5.7% vs. 5.3%, p = 0.38). Randomization to heparin plus IIb/IIIa inhibitors was associated with an increased risk of major bleeding, and major bleeding was associated with an increased one-month mortality as compared to patients without major bleeding: 7.3% vs. 1.2%, p <0.0001 (HR 7.55, 95% CI 4.68–12.18, p <0.0001). The incidence of fatal or life-threatening bleeding was very low (<1%), but patients with major bleeding experienced a higher incidence of thrombotic/ischemic events, including death, myocardial infarction, urgent TVR, and stent thrombosis for patients who underwent PCI, confirming that the ultimate cause of death in most patients with major bleeding who die is a thrombotic complication. The latter may be due to platelet activation subsequent to hemorrhage or to blood transfusion, but, it is more likely that discontinuation of antithrombotic treatment plays a major role in the genesis of ischemic complications, as shown by the GRACE investigators (48). The definition of the criteria for major bleeding is not a marginal point. The hypothesis that an antithrombotic treatment that is not noninferior to standard treatment in terms of recurrent ischemic events and that is superior in terms of safety due to a minor incidence of bleeding and subsequent adverse events is not proven. In the ACUITY-PCI (34) a better short-term clinical outcome (the quadruple end point including death, infarction, TVR, and bleeding) provided by bivalirudin monotherapy is not associated with a better one-year survival despite a decrease in major bleeding: one-year mortality rate 3.8 in the bivalirudin-alone arm, 3.9% in the bivalirudin plus IIb/IIIa inhibitor arm, and 3.9% in the heparin plus IIb/IIIa inhibitor arm. On the other hand, it has been demonstrated that the increase in the risk of death parallels the severity of bleeding (47). Thus, the adoption of broad criteria for major bleeding definition may not show any significant impact of an antithrombotic treatment on long-term survival. The HORIZONS trial that compared bivalirudin-alone with heparin plus routine IIb/IIIa inhibitors in ST-elevation AMI reached the primary end points of decreased bleeding and better net clinical outcome at 30 days (35). Whether these results will translate in improvement in survival will be ascertained by the ongoing long-term follow-up. Meanwhile the routine use of IIb/IIIa inhibitors that is supported by a strong evidence of an improved survival (10,21,22) and the use of all measures that may dramatically decrease the entry site complications, including a radial approach in patients with high risk of bleeding and unfavorable femoral-iliac anatomy and the appropriate use of intra-aortic balloon pump and other left ventricle support devices, seems reasonable, while the discontinuation of the antithrombotic treatment should be avoided in all cases but life-threatening bleeding that cannot be corrected quickly by an endoluminal or surgical approach.

EDITOR'S COMMENT

Abciximab plus infarct artery stenting may be considered as the best reperfusion strategy in patients with AMI undergoing primary percutaneous mechanical revascularization. The role of IIb/IIIa inhibitors other than abciximab in the setting of coronary stenting for AMI is less defined. However, a potential benefit of the small molecules only for the events related to the percutaneous procedure and acute target vessel failure can be anticipated, in view of the nearly exclusive effect on platelets of these drugs. The ongoing randomized HORIZONS trial will define if bivalirudin plus provisional glycoprotein IIb/IIIa inhibition may be a more effective pharmacological alternative to the routine use of glycoprotein IIb/IIIa inhibitors. Conversely, periprocedural routine 600 mg loading dose of clopidogrel may be considered as an established effective adjunctive therapy in primary PCI patients.

REFERENCES

1. Giri S, Mitchel JF, Hirst JA, et al. Synergy between intracoronary stenting and abciximab in improving angiographic and clinical outcomes of primary angioplasty in acute myocardial infarction. Am J Cardiol 2000; 86:269–274.

2. Antoniucci D, Valenti R, Migliorini A, et al. Abciximab therapy improves one-month survival in unselected patients with acute myocardial infarction undergoing routine infarct artery stent implantation. Am Heart J 2002; 144:315–322.

3. Beohar N, Davidson CJ, Weigold G, et al. Predictors of long-term outcomes following direct percutaneous coronary intervention for acute myocardial infarction. Am J Cardiol 2001; 88:1103–1107.

4. Chan AW, Chew DP, Bhatt DL, et al. Long-term mortality benefit with the combination of stents and abciximab for cardiogenic shock complicating acute myocardial infarction. Am J Cardiol 2002; 89:132–136.

5. Antoniucci D, Valenti R, Migliorini A, et al. Abciximab therapy improves survival rate in patients with acute myocardial infarction complicated by early cardiogenic shock undergoing routine infarct artery stent implantation. Am J Cardiol 2002; 90:353–357.

6. Neumann F-J, Kastrati A, Schmitt C, et al. Effect of glycoprotein IIb/IIIa receptor blockade with abciximab on clinical and angiographic restenosis rate after the placement of coronary stents following acute myocardial infarction. J Am Coll Cardiol 2000; 35:915–921.

7. Neumann FJ, Blasini R, Schmitt C et al. Effect of glycoprotein IIb/IIIa receptor blockade on recovery of coronary flow and left ventricular function after the placement of coronary-artery stents in acute myocardial infarction. Circulation 1998; 98:2695–2701.

8. Montalescot G, Barragan P, Wittenberg O, et al. Platelet glycoprotein IIb/IIIa inhibition with coronary stenting for acute myocardial infarction. N Engl J Med 2001; 344: 1895–1903.

9. Stone GW, Grines CL, CoxDA, et al. Comparison of angioplasty with stenting, with or without abciximab, in acute myocardial infarction. N Engl J Med 2002; 346:957–966.

10. Antoniucci D, Rodriguez A, Hempel A, et al. A randomized trial comparing primary infarct artery stenting with or without abciximab in acute myocardial infarction. J Am Coll Cardiol 2003; 42:1879–1885.

11. Brener SJ, Barr LA, Burchenal J, et al. Randomized, placebo-controlled trial of platelet glycoprotein IIb/IIIa blockade with primary angioplasty for acute myocardial infarction. ReoPro and Primary PTCA Organization and Randomized trial (RAPPORT) Investigators. Circulation 1998; 98:734–741.

12. EPIC investigators. Use of the monoclonal antibody directed against the platelet glycoprotein IIb/IIIa receptor in high risk coronary angioplasty. N Engl J Med 1994; 330:956–961.

13. EPILOG investigators. Platelet glycoprotein IIb/IIIa receptor blockade and low-dose heparin during percutaneous coronary revascularization. N Engl J Med 1997; 336: 1689–1696.

14. Dangas G, Aymong ED, Mehran R, et al. Predictors and outcomes of early thrombosis following balloon angioplasty versus primary stenting in acute myocardial infarction and usefulness of abciximab (the CADILLAC Trial). Am J Cardiol 2004; 94:983–988.

15. Antoniucci D, Migliorini A, Parodi G, et al. Abciximab-supported infarct artery stent implantation for acute

myocardial infarction and long-term survival. Circulation 2004; 109:1704–1706.

16. Barron HV, Bowlby LJ, Breen T, et al. Use of reperfusion therapy for acute myocardial infarction in the United States: data from the National Registry of Myocardial Infarction 2. Circulation 1998; 97:1150–1156.

17. Oka RK, Fortmann SP, Varady AN. Differences in treatment of acute myocardial infarction by sex, age, and other factors (the Stanford Five-City Project). Am J Cardiol 1996; 78:861–865.

18. Neumann FJ, Zohlnhofer D, Fakhoury L, et al. Effect of glycoprotein IIb/IIIa receptor blockade on platelet-leukocyte interaction and surface expression of the leukocyte integrin Mac-1 in acute myocardial infarction. J Am Coll Cardiol 1999; 34:1420–1426.

19. Reininger AJ, Agneskirchner J, Bode PA, et al. c7E3 Fab inhibits low shear flow modulated platelet adhesion to endothelium and surface-absorbed fibrinogen by blocking platelet GP IIb/IIIa as well as endothelial vitronectin receptor—results from patients with acute myocardial infarction and healthy controls. Thromb Haemost 2000; 83:217–223.

20. André P, Prasad KSS, Denis CV, et al. CD40L ligand stabilizes arterial thrombi by a 3 integrin-dependent mechanism. Nature 2002; 8:247–252.

21. De Luca G, Suryapranata H, Stone GW, et al. Abcximab as adjunctive therapy to reperfusion in acute ST-segment elevation myocardial infarction. A meta-analysis of randomized trials. JAMA 2005; 293:1759–1765.

22. Montalescot G, Antoniucci D, Kastrati A, et al. Abciximab in primary coronary stenting of ST-elevation myocardial infarction: a European meta-analysis on individual patients' data with long-term follow-up. Eur Heart J 2007; 28:443–449.

23. ESPRIT investigators. Novel dosing regimen of eptifibatide in planned coronary stent implantation (ESPRIT): a randomised placebo controlled trial. Lancet 2000; 356:2037–244.

24. O'Shea JC, Hafley GE, Greenberg S, et al. Platelet glycoprotein integrin IIb/IIIa blockade with eptifibatide in coronary stent intervention: the ESPRIT trial-a randomized controlled trial. JAMA 2001; 285:2468–2473.

25. Cultlip DE, Core CJ, Irons D, et al. Emergency room administration of eptifibatide before primary angioplasty for ST elevation acute myocardial infarction and its effect on baseline coronary flow and procedural outcome. Am J Cardiol 2001; 88:62–64.

26. Kaul U, Gupta RK, Haridas KK, et al. Platelet glycoprotein IIb/IIIa inhibition using eptifibatide with primary coronary stenting for acute myocardial infarction: a 30-day follow-up study. Catheter Cardiovasc Interv 2002; 57:497–503.

27. Raveendran G, Ting HH, Best PJ, et al. Eptifibatide vs abciximab as adjunctive therapy during primary percutaneous coronary intervention for acute myocardial infarction. Mayo Clin Proc 2007; 82:196–202.

28. Gurm HS, Smith DE, Collins JS, et al. The relative safety and efficacy of abciximab and eptifibatide in patients undergoing primary percutaneous coronary intervention: insights from a large regional registry of contemporary

percutaneous coronary intervention. J Am Coll Cardiol 2008; 51:529–535.

29. The RESTORE Investigators. Effects of platelet glycoprotein IIB/IIIa blockade with tirofiban and adverse cardiac events in patients with unstable angina or myocardial infarction undergoing coronary angioplasty. Circulation 1997; 96:1445–1453.

30. Lee DP, Herity NA, Hiatt BL, et al. Adjunctive platelet glycoprotein IIb/IIIa receptor inhibition with tirofiban before primary angioplasty improve angiographic outcomes: results of the Tirofiban Given in the Emergency Room before Primary Angioplasty (TIGER-PA) pilot trial. Circulation 2003; 107:1497–1501.

31. Valgimigli M, Percoco G, Malagutti P, et al. Tirofiban and sirolimus-eluting stent vs abciximab and bare metal stent for acute myocardial infarction. JAMA 2005; 293:2109–2117.

32. Valgimigli M, Campo G, Percoco G, et al. Comparison of angioplasty with tirofiban or abciximab and with implantation of sirolimus-eluting stent or uncoated stetnts for acute myocardial infarction: the MULTISTRATEGY randomized trial. JAMA 2008; 299:1788–1799.

33. Lincoff AM, Bittl JA, Harrington RA, et al. Bivalirudin and provisional glycoprotein blockade compared with heparin and planned glycoprotein blockade during percutaneous coronary intervention: REPLACE-2 randomized trial. JAMA 2003; 289:853–863.

34. Stone GW, McLaurin BT, Cox DA, et al. Bivalirudin for patients with acute coronary syndromes. N Engl J Med 2006; 355:2203–2216.

35. Stone GW, Witzenbichler B, Guagliumi G, et al. Bivalirudin during primary PCI in acute myocardial infarction. N Engl J Med 2008; 358:2218–2230.

36. Metha SR, Yusuf S, Peters RJ, et al. Effects of pretreatment with clopidogrel and aspirin followed by long-term therapy in patients undergoing PCI. The PCI-CURE study. Lancet 2001; 358:527–533.

37. Steinhubl SR, Berger PB, Mann JT III, et al. Early and sustained dual oral antiplatelet therapy following percutaneous coronary intervention: a randomized controlled trial. JAMA 2002; 288: 2411–2420.

38. Bhatt DL, Fox KA, Hacke W, et al. Clopidogrel and aspirin versus aspirin alone for the prevention of atherothrombotic events. N Engl J Med 2006; 354:1706–1717.

39. Spertus JA, Kettelkamp R, Vance C, et al. Prevalence, predictors, and outcomes of premature discontinuation of thienopyridine therapy after drug-eluting stent placement: results from the PREMIER registry. Circulation 2006; 113:2803–2809.

40. Lev EI, Kornowski R, Vakmin-Assa H, et al. Effect of clopidogrel pretreatment in patients undergoing primary percutaneous coronary intervention for ST-elevation acute myocardial infarction. Am J Cardiol 2008; 101: 435–439.

41. Matetzky S, Shenkman B, Guetta V, et al. Clopidogrel resistance is associated with increased risk of recurrent antithrombotic events in patients with acute myocardial infarction. Circulation 2004; 109:3171–3175.

42. Buonamici P, Marcucci R, Migliorini A, et al. Impact of platelet reactivity after clopidogrel administration on

drug-eluting stent thrombosis. J Am Coll Cardiol 2007; 49:2312–2317.

43. de la Torre-Hernández JM, Alfonso F, Hernández F, et al. Drug-eluting stent thrombosis: results from the multicenter Spanish registry ESTROFA (Estudio ESpañol sobre TROmbosis de stents FArmacoactivos). J Am Coll Cardiol 2008; 51:986–990.

44. Sabatine MS, Canon CP, Gibson CM, et al. Effect of clopidogrel pretreatment before percutaneous coronary intervention in patients with ST-elevation myocardial infarction treated with fibrinolytics: the PCI-CLARITY study. JAMA 2005; 294:1224–1232.

45. Wiviott SD, Braunwald E, McCabe CH, et al. Prasugrel versus clopidogrel in patients with acute coronary syndromes. N Engl J Med 2007; 357:2001–2015.

46. Wiviott SD, Trenk D, Frelinger AC, et al. Prasugrel compared with high loading- and maintenance-dose clopidogrel in patients with planned percutaneous coronary intervention: the prasugrel in comparison to clopidogrel for inhibition of platelet activation and aggregation-Thrombolyis In Myocardial Infarction 44 trial. Circulation 2007; 116:2923–2932.

47. Eikelboom JW, Mretha SR, Anand SS, et al. Adverse impact of bleeding on prognosis in patients with acute coronary syndromes. Circulation 2006; 114:774–782.

48. Spencer FA, Moscucci M, Granger CB, et al. Does comorbidity account for the excess mortality in patients with major bleeding in acute myocardial infarction? Circulation 2007; 116:2793–2801.

49. Feit F, Voeltz MD, Attubato MJ, et al. Predictors and impact of major hemorrhage on mortality following percutaneous coronary intervention from the REPLACE-2 trial. Am J Cardiol 2007; 100:1364–1369.

50. Stone GW, Ware JH, Bertrand ME, et al. Antithrombotic strategies in patients with acute coronary syndromes undergoing early invasive management. One-year results from the ACUITY trial. JAMA 2007; 298:2497–2506.

5

Mechanical Support

RENATO VALENTI AND GUIDO PARODI

Division of Cardiology, Careggi Hospital, Florence, Italy

INTRA-AORTIC BALLOON PUMPING

Intra-aortic balloon pumping (IABP) supports both ventricles, increasing the diastolic perfusion pressure and decreasing afterload. The latter mechanism may play a pivotal role in patients who have severe multivessel disease, with limited vascular reserve, impaired autoregulation, and consequent pressure-dependent coronary flow in several perfusion territories. These beneficial effects occur without an increase in oxygen demand. On the contrary, the decrease in cardiac workload improves myocardial energy balance up to 15% (1).

IABP is the most widely applied mechanical circulatory support method. It is highly feasible and associated with a low incidence of complications as compared with the other mechanical support devices. The Benchmark Registry was developed to examine IABP indications and outcome of patients with acute myocardial infarction (2). The registry prospectively collected data from 250 centers worldwide and included 5495 patients with acute myocardial infarction. IABP placement was successful in nearly all patients (97.7%). The IABP-related complication rate was 8.1%, and mostly driven by access-site bleeding (4.3%) and limb ischemia (2.3%). The major complication rate was 2.7%, and included severe limb ischemia requiring surgical or endoluminal mechanical treatment, severe bleeding requiring blood transfusion or mechanical intervention, balloon leak, or death directly due to IABP. This complication rate is lower as compared with previous reports (3–6), despite the fact that in the majority of patients (65%) the old large (9.5F) catheters were used. The same investigators, in a post hoc analysis, showed that there was less limb ischemia with the 8F size catheter compared with the 9.5F catheter (7).

In the GUSTO (Global Utilization of Streptokinase and t-PA for Occluded coronary arteries) trial, patients who presented with shock and had early intra-aortic balloon placement showed a trend toward lower one-month and one-year mortality rates, even after the exclusion of patients who had revascularization (8–10). A similar trend was seen in the SHOCK (SHould we emergently revascularize Occluded coronaries in Cardiogenic shocK) trial registry, although it did not persist after adjustment for age and catheterization (11). In a retrospective evaluation of the National Registry of Myocardial Infarction-2, use of IABP in combination with thrombolytic treatment was associated with a marked reduction in the mortality rate; conversely, a benefit was not seen in patients undergoing coronary angioplasty (12).

Similar to the inverse relation between PCI volume and mortality, the National Registry of Myocardial Infarction-2 investigators have shown that high hospital volume IABP is associated with a decreased mortality as compared to low hospital volume IABP. Data collected for 12,730 IABP procedures from 750 hospitals have shown a 30% reduction in mortality in high-volume centers as compared to low-volume centers (crude mortality rates 50.6% and 65.4%, respectively, $p < 0.001$) (13).

Several studies have shown a synergistic interaction between percutaneous mechanical reperfusion and IABP. The synergism may be explained by the improvement in coronary flow subsequent to perfusion pressure augmentation and restoration of flow with mechanical treatment of the target lesion. IABP has been shown to decrease early infarct artery reocclusion after emergency percutaneous coronary intervention for acute myocardial infarction. In a randomized trial including 182 patients with acute myocardial infarction successfully recanalized, patients assigned to prophylactic aortic balloon pumping had a lower incidence of early infarct artery reocclusion (8% vs. 21%, $p < 0.03$) and of major cardiac adverse events (13% vs. 24%, $p < 0.04$) (14). Moreover, the use of IABP in patients with cardiogenic shock complicating acute myocardial infarction may significantly decrease the incidence of major complications during mechanical revascularization in the catheterization laboratory. Brodie et al., in a retrospective analysis of a series of 119 patients with cardiogenic shock, reported a 59% reduction in the incidence of total catheterization laboratory events (ventricular fibrillation and cardiopulmonary arrest) in patients with IABP support before primary coronary angioplasty was performed (15).

OTHER PERCUTANEOUS MECHANICAL CIRCULATORY SUPPORT DEVICES

Clinically, there are very few experiences with mechanical circulatory support devices other than pumping, and it is likely that their use will continue to be limited by the complexity of installation, such as extracorporeal membrane oxygenation (ECMO) devices and relevant procedure-related morbidity. Moreover, to be successful, a program of mechanical support using devices other than IABP requires competent medical and nursing staff in the intensive care unit.

The percutaneous transeptal left ventricular assistance (Tandem Heart pVAD, Cardiac Assist Technologies Inc., Pittsburgh, Pennsylvania, U.S.) is an innovative approach based on the removal of oxygenated blood from left atrium via a 21F transeptal cannula inserted through the femoral vein and returned to the systemic circulation via the femoral artery. A preliminary experience in 18 patients shows that the Tandem Heart may decrease the preload, the workload, and the oxygen demand and increase systemic perfusion (16). A small, randomized study including 33 patients compared the Tandem Heart with IABP and showed that the former achieved significant greater increases in cardiac index and mean arterial pressure and significant decreases in pulmonary wedge pressure (17). Because of the small number of patients, it was not possible to show any difference in clinical outcome. However, patients randomized to Tandem Heart (19 patients) had a high incidence of cardiac tamponade (2 patients), major bleeding (8 patients), and cannulation site infection (3 patients). The Tandem Heart was compared with IABP in a randomized study including 41 patients with AMI complicated by cardiogenic shock (18). The Tandem Heart increased the cardiac power index more than IABP. Unfortunately, the rate of device-related complications was very high: severe bleeding occurred in all but two patients, and severe limb ischemia in one-third of the cases, while the 30-day mortality was similar to the one of the IABP arm.

Finally, it should be highlighted that the longer procedural time needed for the placement of the system may have a detrimental effect in patients with cardiogenic shock complicating acute myocardial infarction.

The Impella Recover LP 2.5 (Abiomed Inc., Danvers, Massachusetts, U.S.) is a novel ventricular unloading assist device. The device is a microaxial rotary blood pump that expels blood from left ventricle into the aorta, and it can be introduced percutaneously through a 12F sheath. It can achieve an output up to 2.5 L/min. Specific relatively frequent complications are related to the dislodgment in aorta rendering the device ineffective, or frequent complex ventricular arrhythmias, or mechanical interference with the movement of the anterior mitral leaflet that may result in a significant obstacle to the emptying of the left atrium. Different from IABP, the device does not need the synchronization with ventricular activity and can be used in patients with aortic regurgitation. It was used with encouraging results in a small series of 19 patients who underwent elective high-risk PCI (19).

The Reitan catheter pump (CardioBridge GmbH, Germany) is another approach based on the removal of blood directly from aorta by a propeller pump, with the advantage of a very easy placement of the catheter, which profile needs a 14F sheath for insertion. The other potential advantages of this system include the creation of a gradient in the aorta with an increased perfusion pressure of the kidneys, the lack of necessity for synchronization to the left ventricular activity, and the lack of complications due to dislodgement of the other devices. The results of a first safety study based on 10 patients showed no complications due to the device, including lack of significant hemolysis (Rothmans MT, data presented at the EuroPCR 2008; Barcelona 2008).

EDITOR'S COMMENT

Several devices have the promise to enhance support in cardiogenic shock complicating AMI. IABP may be considered a mainstay adjunctive therapy for patients with cardiogenic shock undergoing percutaneous coronary intervention.

REFERENCES

1. Bolooki H. Physiology of balloon pumping. In: Bolooki H, ed. Clinical Application of Intraaortic Balloon Pump. Mount Kisko, NY: Futura, 1984:57–126.
2. Stone GW, Ohman EM, Miller MF, et al. Contemporary utilization and outcomes of intra-aortic balloon counterpulsation in acute myocardial infarction. J Am Coll Cardiol 2003; 41:1940–1945.
3. Mahaffey KW, Kruse KR, Ohman EM. Perspectives on the use of intra-aortic balloon counterpulsation in the 1990s. In: Topol EJ, ed. Textbook of Interventional Cardiology, Update Series, Update n.21. Philadelphia, PA: WB Saunders, 1996:303–320.
4. Alderman JD, Gabliani GI, McCabe CH, et al. Incidence and management of limb ischemia with percutaneous wire-guided intra-aortic balloon catheters. J Am Coll Cardiol 1987; 9:524–530.
5. Iverson LI, Herfindahal G, Ecker RR, et al. Vascular complications of intra-aortic balloon counterpulsation. Am J Surg 1987; 154:99–103.
6. Skillman JJ, Ducksoo K, Baim DS. Vascular complications of percutaneous femoral cardiac intervention: incidence and operative repair. Arch Surg 1988; 123:1207–1212.
7. Cohen M, Fergusson JJ, Fredman RJ, et al. Comparison of outcomes after 8 vs. 9.5 French size catheters based on 9332 patients in the prospective Benchmark Registry. Catheter Cardiovasc Interv 2002; 56:200–206.
8. Holmes DR, Bates ER, Kleiman NS, et al. Contemporary reperfusion therapy for cardiogenic shock: the Gusto-I trial experience. J Am Coll Cardiol 1995; 26:668–674.
9. Anderson RD, Ohman EM, Holmes DR, et al. Use of intraaortic balloon counterpulsation in patients presenting with cardiogenic shock: observations from the GUSTO-I trial. J Am Coll Cardiol 1997; 30:708–715.
10. Berger PB, Holmes DR, Stebbins AL, et al. Impact of an aggressive invasive catheterization and revascularization strategy on mortality in patients with cardiogenic shock in the GUSTO-I trial. Circulation 1997; 96:122–127.
11. Hochman JS, Boland J, Sleeper LA, et al. Current spectrum of cardiogenic shock and effect of early revascularization on mortality: results of an international registry. Circulation 1995; 91:873–881.
12. Barron HV, Every NR, Parsons LS, et al. The use of intra-aortic balloon counterpulsation in patients with cardiogenic shock complicating acute myocardial infarction. Am Heart J 2001; 141:933–939.
13. Chen EW, Canto JG, Parsons LS, et al. Relation between hospital intra-aortic balloon counterpulsation volume and mortality in acute myocardial infarction complicated by cardiogenic shock. Circulation 2003; 108:951–957.
14. Ohman EM, George BS, White CJ, et al. Use of aortic counterpulsation to improve sustained coronary patency during acute myocardial infarction. Circulation 1994; 90:792–799.
15. Brodie BR, Stuckey TD, Hansen C, et al. Intra-aortic balloon counterpulsation before primary percutaneous transluminal coronary angioplasty reduces catheterization laboratory events in high-risk patients with acute myocardial infarction. Am J Cardiol 1999; 84:18–23.
16. Thiele H, Lauer B, Hamprecht R, et al. Reversal of cardiogenic shock by percutaneous left atrial-to-femoral arterial bypass assistance. Circulation 2001; 104:2917–2922.
17. Burkhoff D, Cohen H, Brunckhorst C, et al. A randomized multicenter clinical study to evaluate the safety and efficacy of the Tandem Heart percutaneous ventricular assist device versus conventional therapy with intra-aortic balloon pumping for treatment of cardiogenic shock. Am Heart J 2006; 152:469.e1–469.e8.
18. Thiele H, Sick P, Boudriot E, et al. Randomized comparison of intra-aortic balloon support with a percutaneous left ventricle assist device in patients with revascularized acute myocardial infarction complicated by cardiogenic shock. Eur Heart J 2005; 26:1276–1283.
19. Hennriques JPS, Remellink M, Baan J, et al. Safety and feasibility of elective high-risk percutaneous coronary intervention procedures with left ventricular support of the Impella Recover LP 2.5. Am J Cardiol 2006; 97:990–992.

Section 3

The Vessel Perspective

6

Right Coronary Artery (RCA)

RENATO VALENTI AND ANGELA MIGLIORINI
Division of Cardiology, Careggi Hospital, Florence, Italy

CASE 6.1 THE CLASSIC

This case is paradigmatic for the angiographic aspect of the disrupted plaque associated with mild stenosis and superimposed occlusive thrombosis and the simplicity and efficacy of the technical approach.

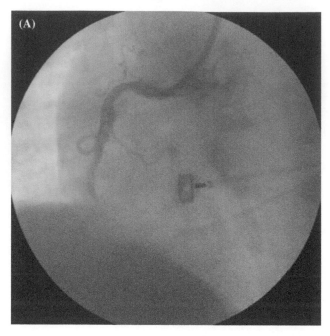

Figure 6.1A Total occlusion of the RCA at the middle segment.

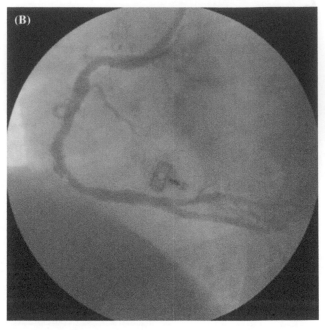

Figure 6.1B After crossing the wire recanalization of the vessel, the angiographic aspect of target lesion is paradigmatic of plaque rupture.

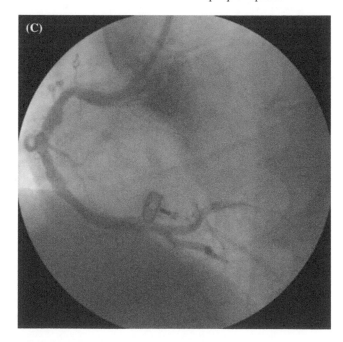

Figure 6.1C After direct stenting no more angiographic evidence of the rupture; the technique is able to correct the rough surface of the target lesion and normalize the shear stress decreasing the risk of recurrent thrombosis.

CASE 6.2 THE ROLLING THROMBUS

One of the complications of a disrupted plaque is migration of the superimposed thrombus distally; the mechanical lysis of the embolus by angioplasty may be considered the more simple and effective approach considering the distal location of the occlusion, and the relatively low risk of no-flow due to microvessel embolization after angioplasty in spontaneous macroembolization of a pure fresh thrombus without atheromatous debris.

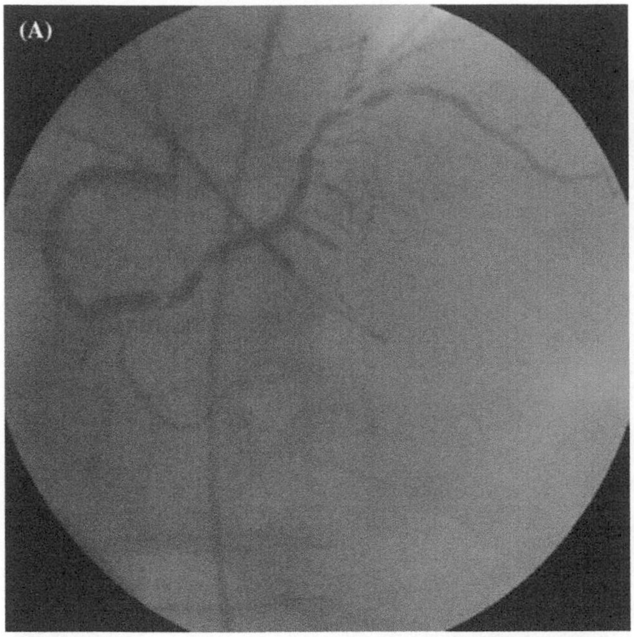

Figure 6.2A Multiple lesions within the RCA; in the third tract there is the evidence of an ulcerated plaque; severe stenoses in the retroventricular branch; occlusion of the mid-portion of posterior descending branch; the location of the occlusion suggests occlusive embolization from the ulcerated plaque in the third tract.

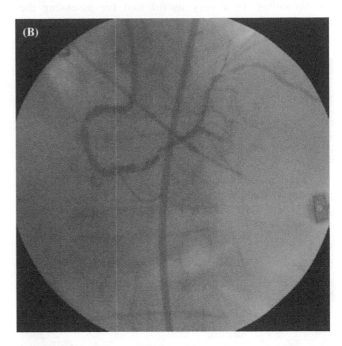

Figure 6.2B After crossing the wire.

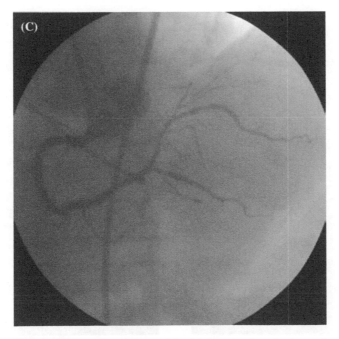

Figure 6.2C After stenting of the third tract and angioplasty of posterior descending and retroventricular branches.

CASE 6.3 THE THROMBUS TRACE

Occlusive thrombosis may occur without angiographic evidence of atherosclerotic plaque (see chap. 1). The staining of dye, due to the sponge-like configuration of the thrombus, is a very useful tool for assessing the dimension of the thrombus and the risk of no-flow after a conventional mechanical approach.

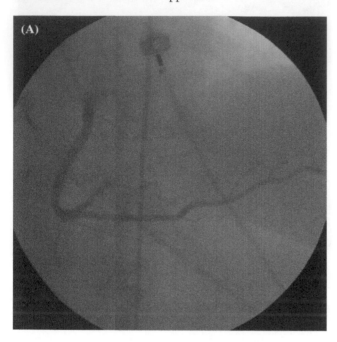

Figure 6.3A Occlusion of distal portion of the RCA.

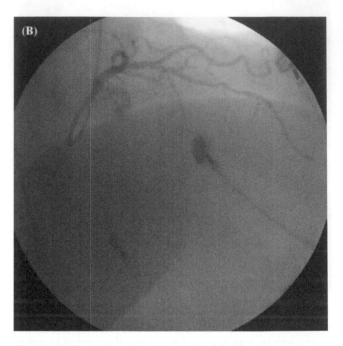

Figure 6.3B Left coronarography; evidence of a large dye staining in the distal portion of the RCA, suggesting the presence of massive thrombosis.

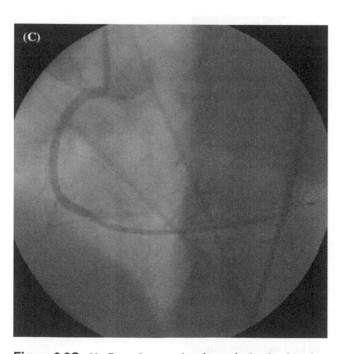

Figure 6.3C No flow after crossing the occlusion by the wire.

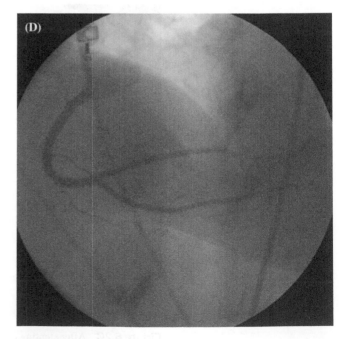

Figure 6.3D After thrombectomy no angiographic evidence of atherosclerotic plaque.

CASE 6.4 ONLY WHERE IT IS NECESSARY

The spot stenting technique should be considered the preferred approach in vessels with diffuse disease.

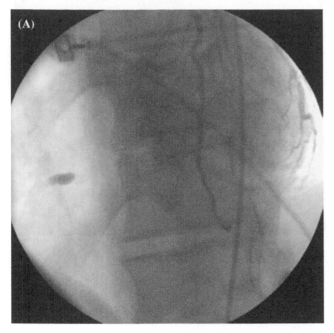

Figure 6.4A Left coronary angiogram; evidence of dye staining in the distal portion of the RCA.

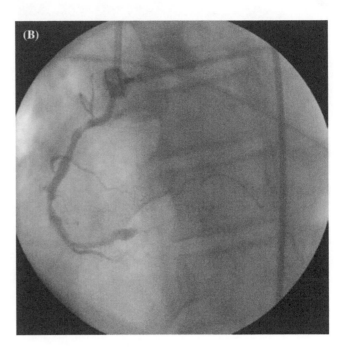

Figure 6.4B No flow after crossing the wire.

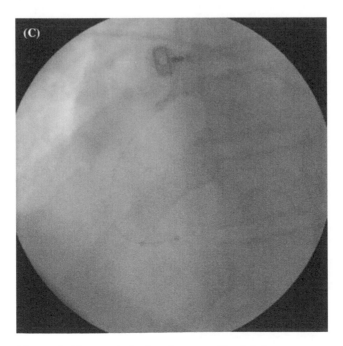

Figure 6.4C Rheolytic thrombectomy (AngioJet).

(*Case 6.4 continued on page 88*)

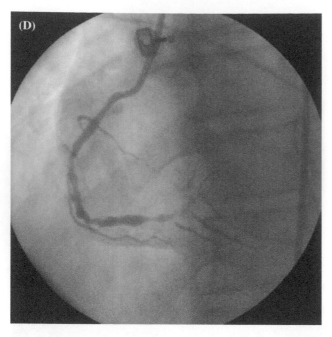

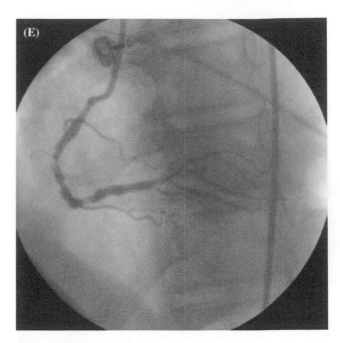

Figure 6.4D After recanalization diffuse disease, and multiple lesions of small branches after the occlusion.

Figure 6.4E After angioplasty and spot stenting.

CASE 6.5 SEEING IS BELIEVING

Macroembolization may be a complication after crossing the wire through the thrombotic occlusion. In this case, the large thrombotic burden and the location of the embolic occlusion suggest a primary thrombectomy approach. The use of a dual lumen catheter allows the ultraselective dye injection beyond the occlusion and the correct diagnosis of macroembolization and the subsequent correct technical approach.

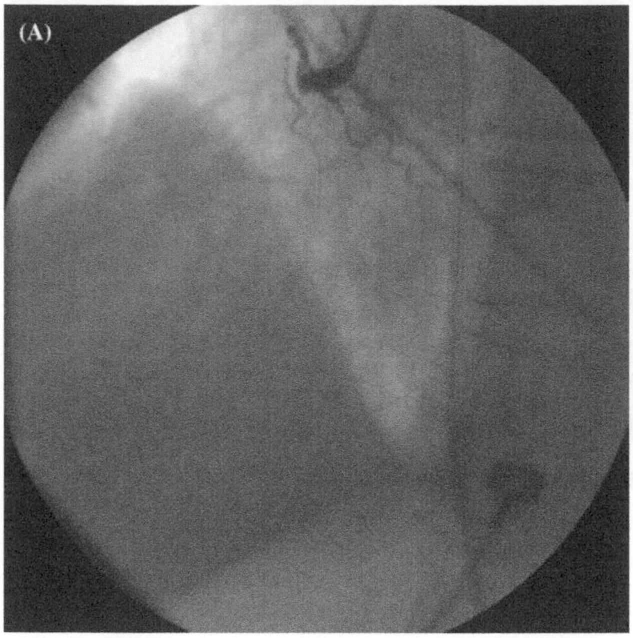

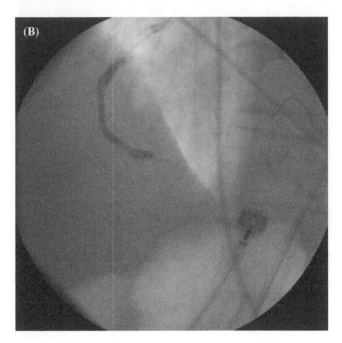

Figure 6.5B No flow after crossing the wire; an ultraselective dye injection, beyond the occlusion, using a dual lumen catheter (Multifunctional Probing) shows a second occlusion at the distal portion of the second tract, suggesting macroembolization from the target lesion.

Figure 6.5A Proximal occlusion of the RCA.

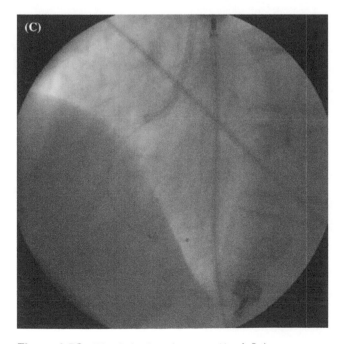

Figure 6.5C Rheolytic thrombectomy (AngioJet).

(*Case 6.5 continued on page 90*)

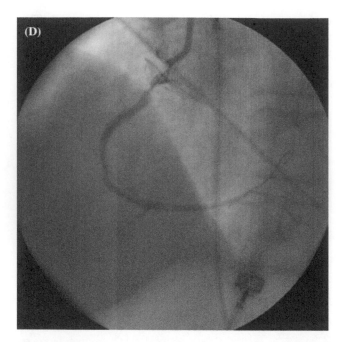

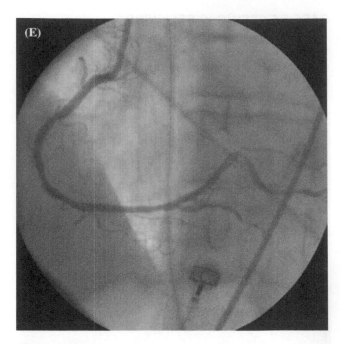

Figure 6.5D Complete recanalization after thrombectomy, without evidence of lesions other than the first tract target lesion determining severe stenosis after the removal of thrombus.

Figure 6.5E Direct stenting of the target lesion.

CASE 6.6 THE FALL INTO THE NET

This impressive example of no-flow after an apparently uncomplicated easy procedure shows the devastating effect of microembolization into the microvessel.

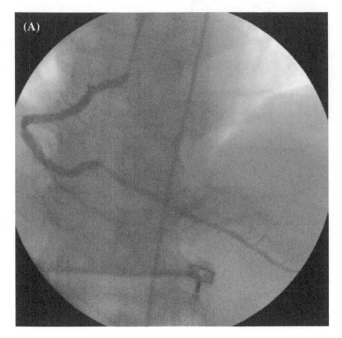

Figure 6.6A Occlusion of the third tract of the RCA.

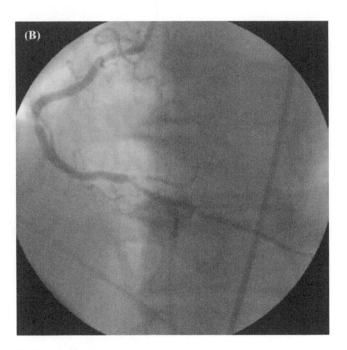

Figure 6.6B No flow after crossing the wire.

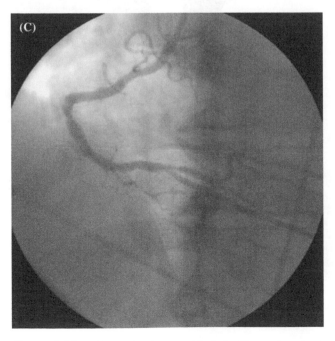

Figure 6.6C After angioplasty, residual significant stenosis at the level of the occlusion.

(*Case 6.6 continued on page 92*)

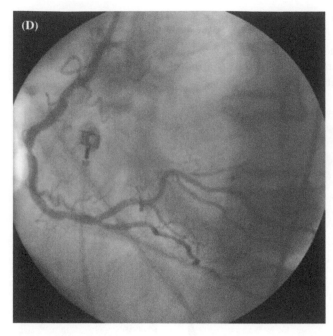

Figure 6.6D Stenting.

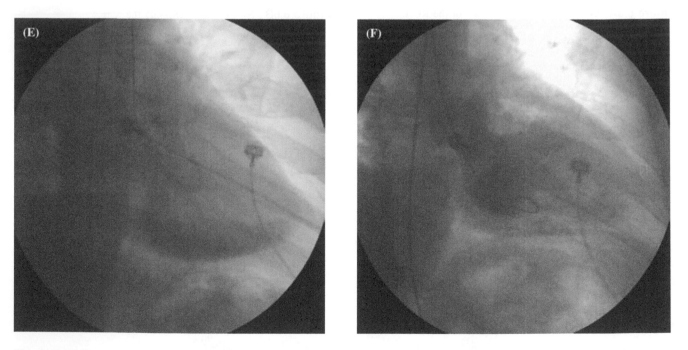

Figure 6.6E,F Staining of contrast dye into the inferoposterior left ventricular wall, persisting minutes after left ventricular emptying.

CASE 6.7 THE CORONARY ACCORDION

The pseudonarrowing phenomenon may have a negative impact on procedural outcome; in this setting, thrombus aspiration may be totally ineffective, while the efficacy of a filter may be superior. The use of a "soft" approach with a soft wire to reduce the pseudonarrowing is not necessarily the best approach considering the potential for a troublesome coronary stenting using a very low support wire in a very tortuous vessel.

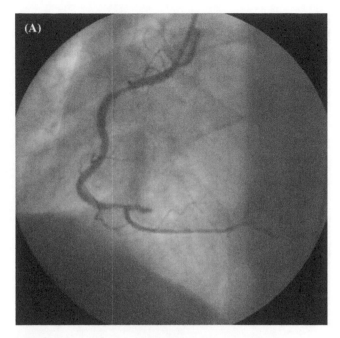

Figure 6.7A Occlusion of the third tract of the RCA.

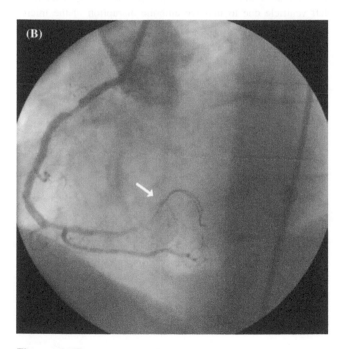

Figure 6.7B Placement of a coronary wire and of an antiembolic occlusive device in the distal portion of the vessel; the arrow indicates the inflated balloon of the antiembolic device (GuardWire); moreover an initial pseudonarrowing is evident in the proximal portion of the RCA due to the tortuosity of the vessel.

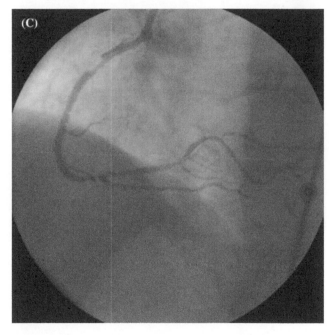

Figure 6.7C After direct stenting at level of the occlusion, the diffuse pseudonarrowing is more evident in all segments of the RCA; the pseudonarrowing prevented aspiration of blood by the export catheter; however, a normal epicardial flow was restored after removal of the antiembolic device.

(*Case 6.7 continued on page 94*)

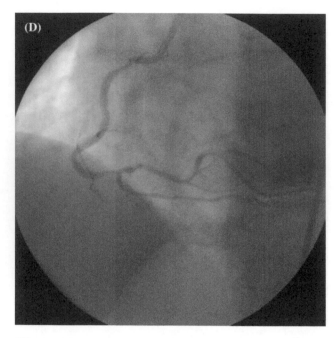

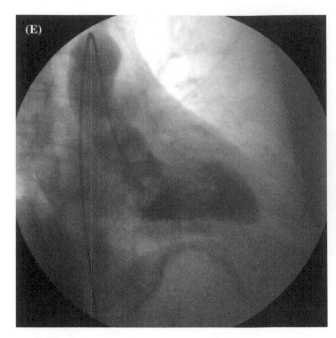

Figure 6.7D Reversal of the pseudonarrowing after removal of the coronary wire.

Figure 6.7E Postprocedure left ventriculography shows intra-myocardial staining of dye in the posteroinferior segments of the left ventricle due to massive embolic disruption of the micro-vessel network.

CASE 6.8 APPEARANCE CAN BE DECEPTIVE

The reference diameter beyond a total occlusion may significantly undersize the physiologic diameter of the vessel because of absence of a significant perfusion pressure. After the reestablishment of a perfusion pressure, the increase in the diameter of the vessel results in a mismatch with the balloon-wire diameter, and the device is no more effective in protection from embolism. To obviate this "operator-dependent device failure," the considered reference diameter should be the one proximal to the occlusion (see case 6.9).

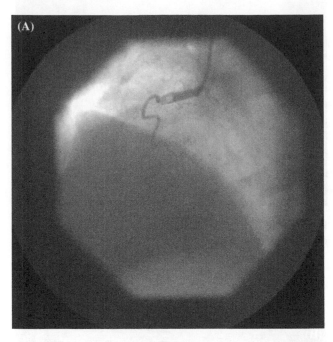

Figure 6.8A Occlusion of the proximal portion of the RCA; evidence of massive thrombosis.

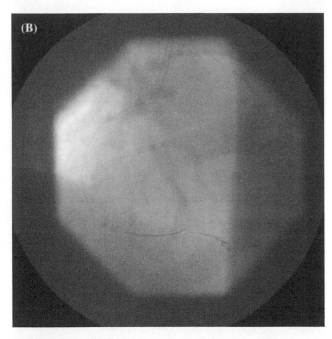

Figure 6.8B Crossing of the wire and placement of an occlusive antiembolic device system (GuardWire).

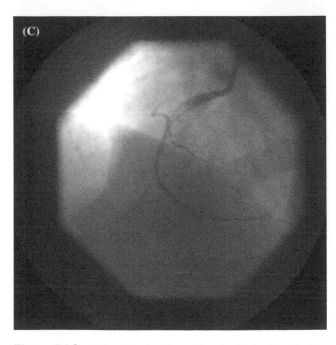

Figure 6.8C A dye injection shows that the device is occlusive.

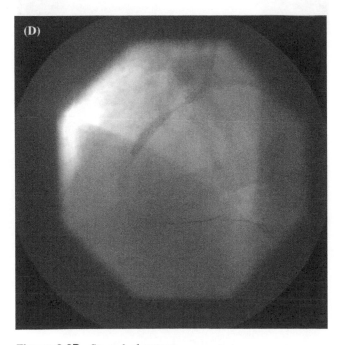

Figure 6.8D Stent deployment.

(*Case 6.8 continued on page 96*)

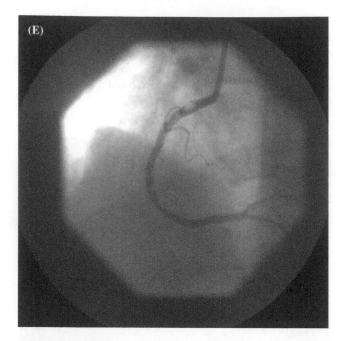

Figure 6.8E Massive thrombosis before the stent, and evidence of distal flow showing that the antiembolic device is no more occlusive.

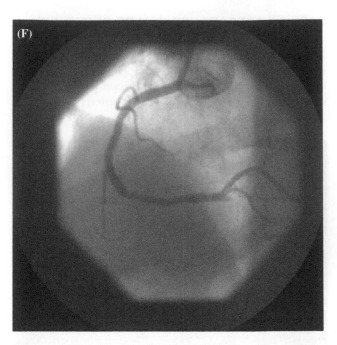

Figure 6.8F Macroembolization occluding the posterior descending branch.

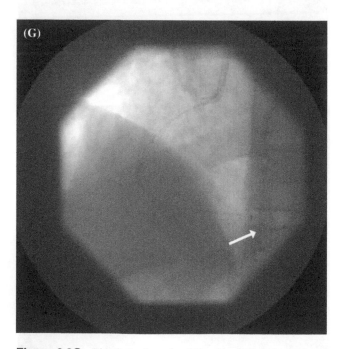

Figure 6.8G Rheolytic thrombectomy (AngioJet) (*arrow*).

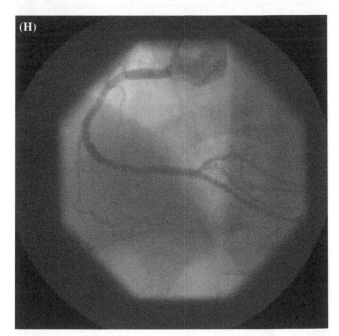

Figure 6.8H No more evidence of thrombus and complete recanalization of the posterior descending branch.

CASE 6.9 GOOD FISHING

A correct use of the occlusive antiembolic protection device may be really effective in preventing embolization.

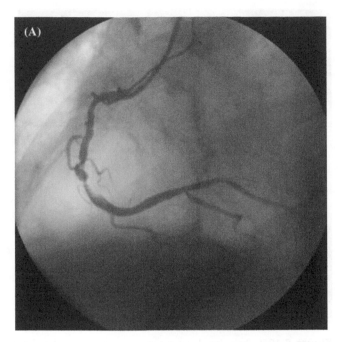

Figure 6.9A Disrupted plaque and superimposed thrombosis at the second tract of the RCA.

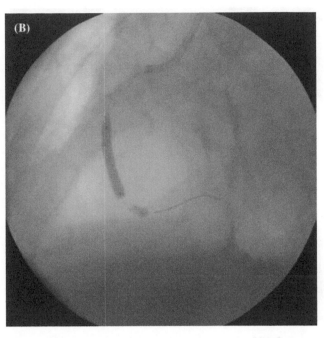

Figure 6.9B Direct stenting after placement of the occlusive protection device (GuardWire).

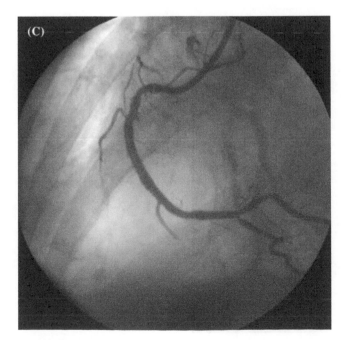

Figure 6.9C After aspiration and the deflation of the balloon of the protection device.

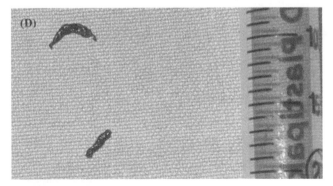

Figure 6.9D Evidence of thrombus and debris after aspiration.

CASE 6.10 THE JAIL

If rheolytic thrombectomy in a large vessel is ineffective in complete thrombus removal, a superior efficacy of the other thrombectomy devices is unlikely. In this case the entrapment of the thrombus by a mesh stent or a covered stent may be the right approach.

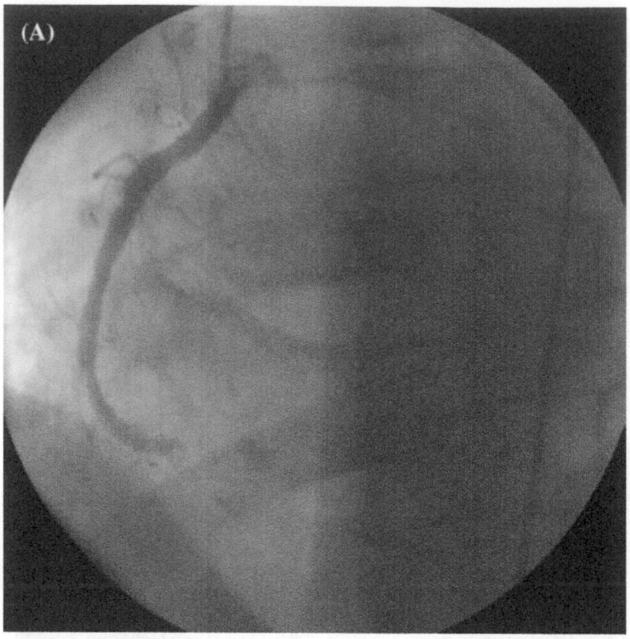

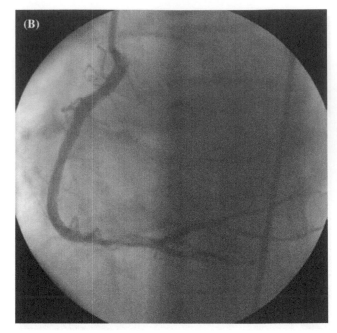

Figure 6.10A Occlusion at the middle tract of the RCA.

Figure 6.10B Massive distal thrombosis after recanalization by the wire.

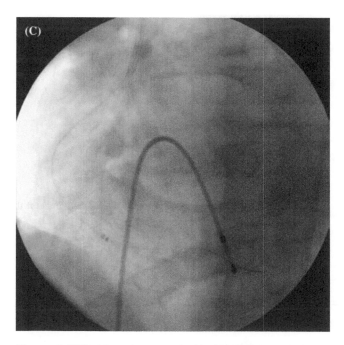

Figure 6.10C Thrombectomy device (AngioJet).

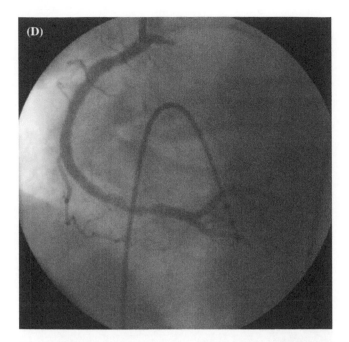

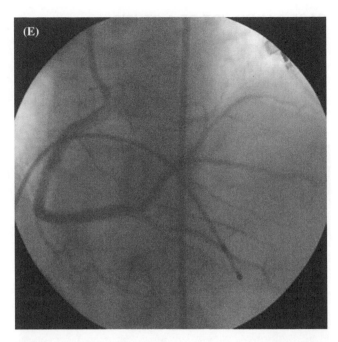

Figure 6.10D Residual massive thrombosis after repeat passage with the thrombectomy device.

Figure 6.10E Autoexpandable mesh stent implantation.

CASE 6.11 DO NOT BE A STUPID

The possibility that the thrombotic burden exceeds widely the length of the target lesion is relatively frequent in the RCA occlusion. The anatomic characteristics of the RCA, a conduit vessel type, and the absence of marginal branches for long tracts may explain the frequent occur-rence of postocclusion massive thrombosis due to staining of blood. In the past balloon angioplasty–alone era, the risk of no-flow and macroembolization in treatment of RCA-acute occlusions with large postocclusion thrombus was very high, and this fact accounted for the fame of the RCA as a "stupid vessel" (see case 6.12).

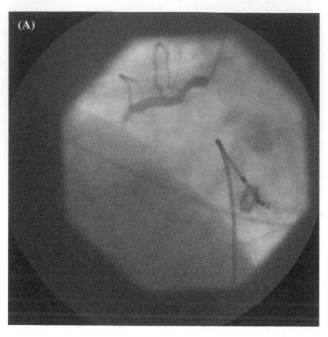

Figure 6.11A Occlusion at the second tract of the RCA.

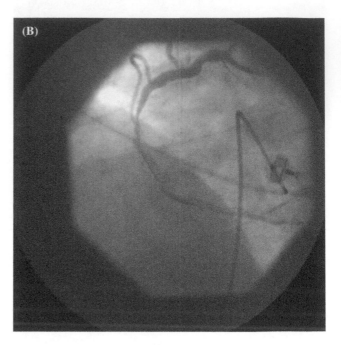

Figure 6.11B After recanalization achieved by crossing the wire, the target lesion is a focal severe stenosis in the second tract of the RCA, but the feature that makes the case challenging is a post-target lesion thrombus extending distally to the third tract of the RCA.

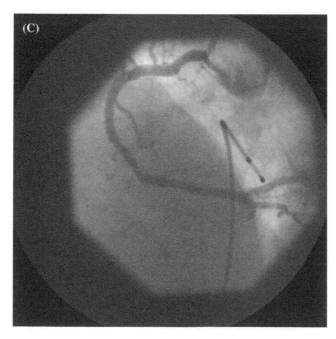

Figure 6.11C After rheolytic thrombectomy (AngioJet) and placement of a short stent at the level of the target lesion.

CASE 6.12 DO NOT BE A STUPID-2

This prethrombectomy old balloon angioplasty clearly illustrates the "stupidity" of the operator in persisting to treat such a case with inadequate technology.

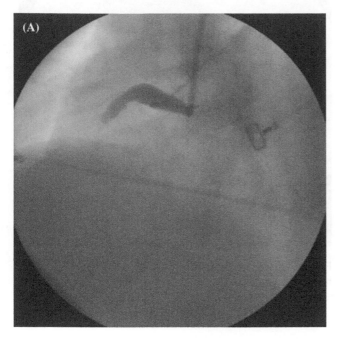

Figure 6.12A Occlusion of the proximal ectatic portion of RCA.

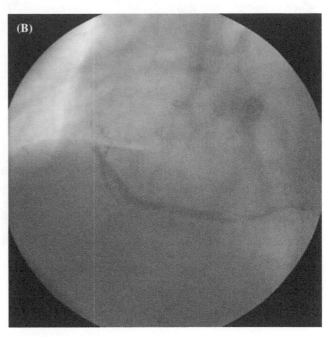

Figure 6.12B After crossing of the wire, the selective injection using a dual lumen catheter (Multifunctional Probing) shows peripheral macroembolization occluding the third tract and major branches of the vessel.

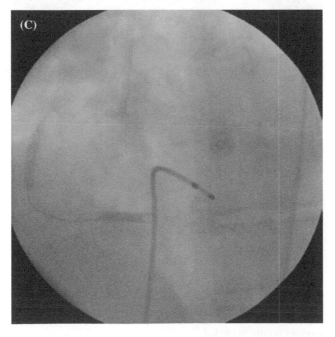

Figure 6.12C Balloon inflation at level of the occlusion.

(Case 6.12 continued on page 102)

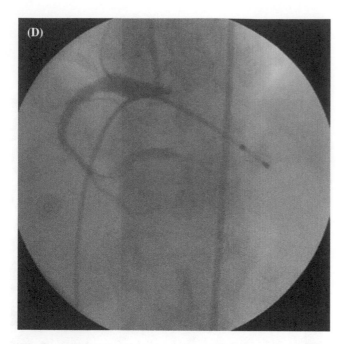

Figure 6.12D No evidence of perfusion of the distal tract of the vessel.

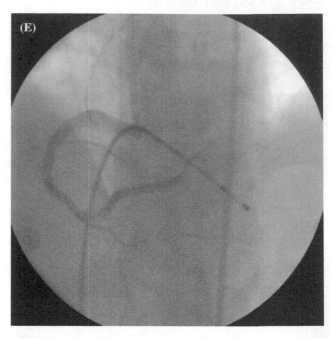

Figure 6.12E After mechanical lysis using the angioplasty balloon, there is some evidence of the distal vascular bed.

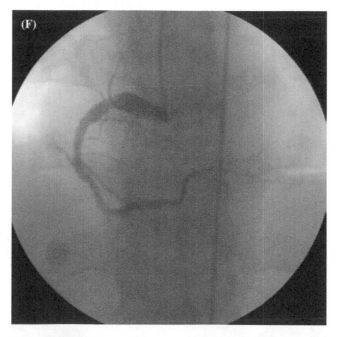

Figure 6.12F At 48 hours, the posterior descending artery remains totally occluded.

CASE 6.13 FOR WANT OF SOMETHING BETTER TO DO

Direct stenting may decrease the risk of embolization. In this case, the tortuosity of the RCA prevented the advancement of the old stiff rheolytic thrombectomy device (AngioJet) to the third tract. Currently the smaller and more trackable rheolytic thrombectomy device may successfully approach such a case.

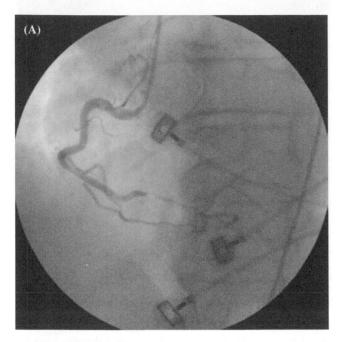

Figure 6.13A Subocclusive thrombosis of the third tract of the RCA.

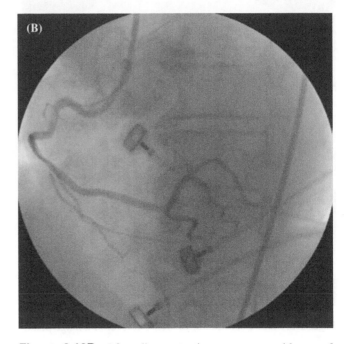

Figure 6.13B After direct stenting no more evidence of thrombosis or embolism.

CASE 6.14 THE NEED FOR STRICTNESS

The need for a stiff wire is very infrequent in the setting of acute myocardial infarction, and the need for stiffness and subsequent high support is limited to transportation of a balloon or a stent through a very tortuous vessel. The straightening of the vessel invariably results in different degrees of pseudonarrowing.

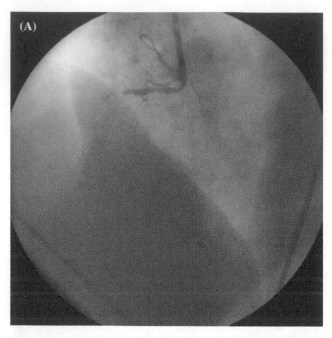

Figure 6.14A Occlusion of the RCA at level of a hinge point.

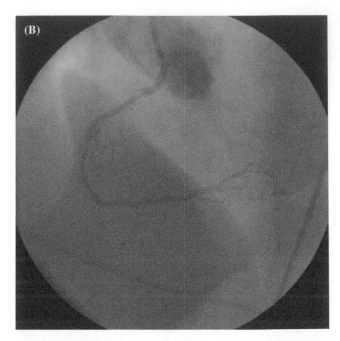

Figure 6.14B The anatomic characteristics of the vessel including two sharp opposite bends prevented the placement of a stent over a normal wire; changing for a stiff wire resulted in the straightening of the vessel, allowing stent placement.

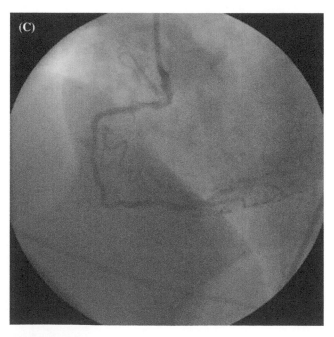

Figure 6.14C After removal of the wire.

CASE 6.15 MUCH SHOW AND BIG SUBSTANCE

In case of massive thrombosis, the aspiration of the thrombus before angioplasty or stenting may be effective in reducing the thrombotic burden, allowing a correct target lesion definition and avoiding the use of multiple stents. In this case multiple stenting was needed to treat a diffuse precrux lesion, and a mild stenosis at the level of occlusion, as revealed by the baseline angiogram.

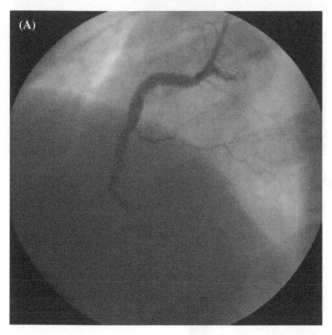

Figure 6.15A Total occlusion of the initial portion of the second tract of the RCA.

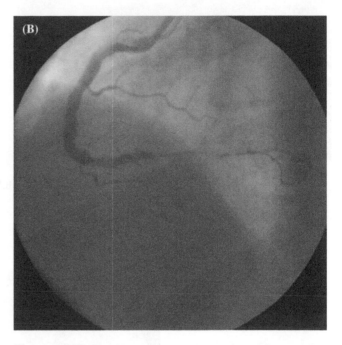

Figure 6.15B Evidence of massive thrombosis after crossing of the wire and placement of an antiembolic occlusive device (GuardWire).

(*Case 6.15 continued on page 106*)

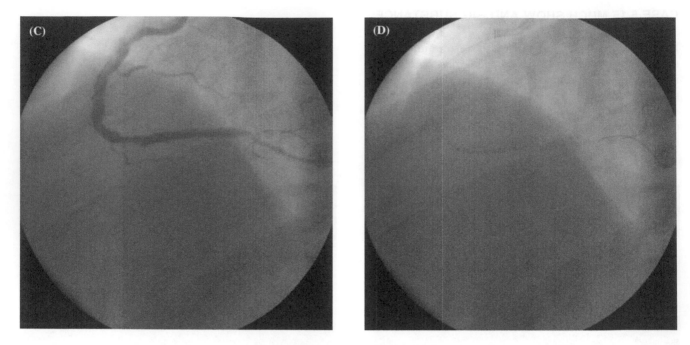

Figure 6.15C,D Multiple direct stenting.

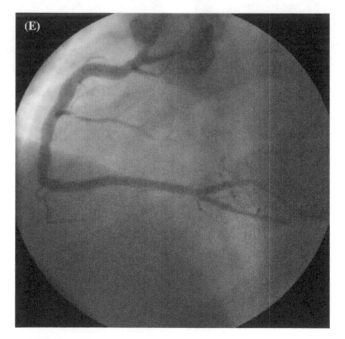

Figure 6.15E Angiographic result after stenting and aspiration using the Export catheter (GuardWire).

CASE 6.16 IT IS ALL SHOW AND NO SUBSTANCE

The disruption of a plaque without significant stenosis or "erosion" may precipitate occlusive thrombosis (see chap. 1). No further intervention is indicated with a normal appearance of the vessel after thrombectomy. Nontarget lesion intervention is indicated for severe stenosis in a major branch.

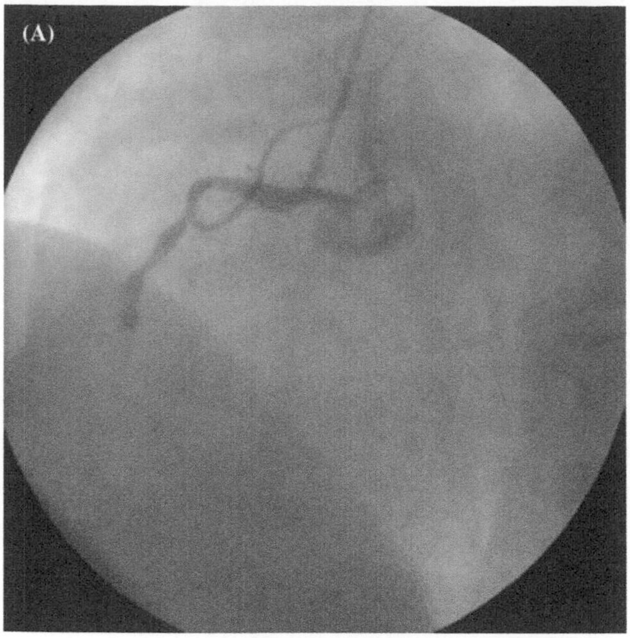

Figure 6.16A Occlusion at the mid-portion of the RCA.

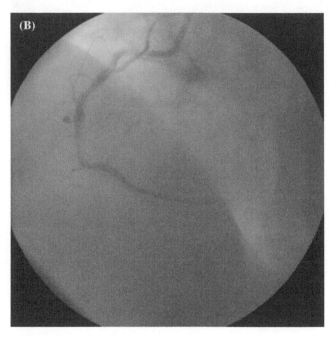

Figure 6.16B Evidence of massive thrombosis after crossing the wire.

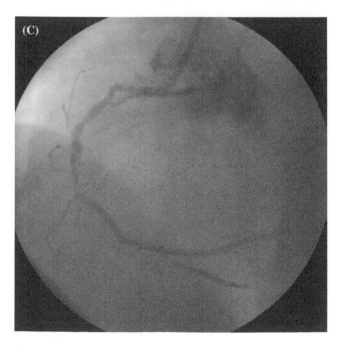

Figure 6.16C After rheolytic thrombectomy (AngioJet), reestablishment of good flow and residual thrombosis; no evidence of significant stenosis at the level of occlusion, and evidence of a severe stenosis of the ostium of a large posterior descending branch.

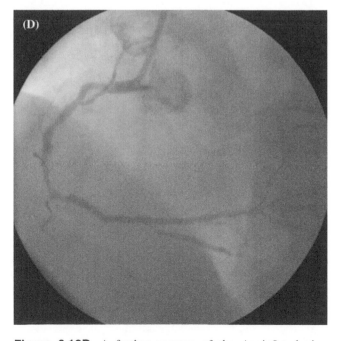

Figure 6.16D A further passage of the AngioJet device decreases the residual thrombosis.

(*Case 6.16 continued on page 108*)

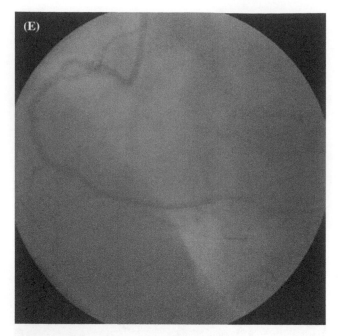

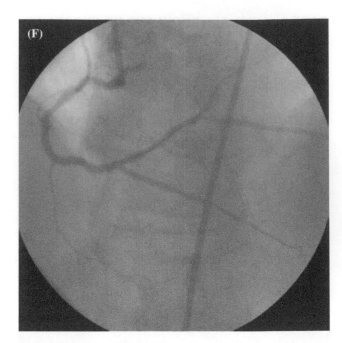

Figure 6.16E After the placement of a second wire in the posterior descending branch, placement of a stent in the proximal portion of the vessel; no further intervention in the midportion of the RCA.

Figure 6.16F Final result.

CASE 6.17 IT IS A VERY STRONG SOAP POWDER

Rheolytic thrombectomy may produce significant regional emolysis resulting in high potassium concentration favoring spasm, and, in dominant RCA, transitory atrioventricular block. The practical implications of these phenomena are the risk of undersizing the stent diameter and the need for temporary pacing. To obviate these problems consider the reference diameter at the baseline angiogram, or wait for the resolution of the vessel spasm. An effective alternative to temporary pacing may be intermittent short-duration thrombectomy.

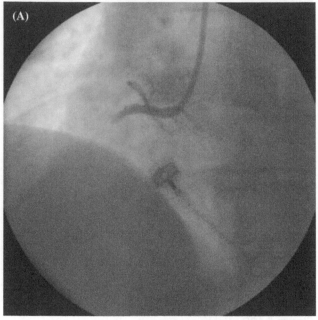

Figure 6.17A Occlusion of the proximal portion of the RCA.

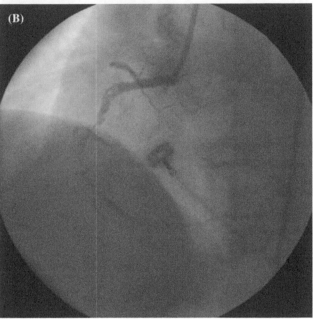

Figure 6.17B After crossing of the wire evidence of diffuse thrombosis.

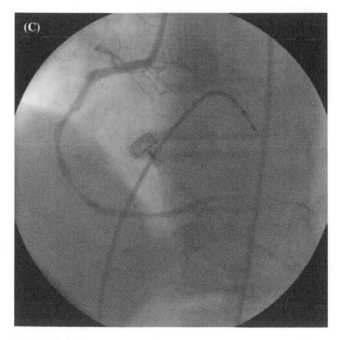

Figure 6.17C After effective rheolytic thrombectomy (Angio-Jet) angiographic evidence of a disrupted plaque in the proximal part of the RCA producing mild stenosis and diffuse spasm of the target vessel.

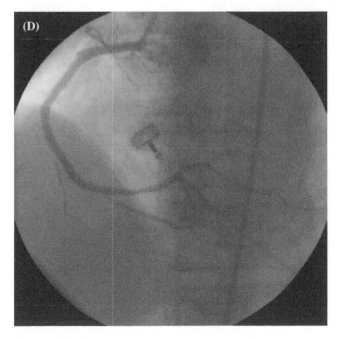

Figure 6.17D After direct stenting of the target lesion and resolution of diffuse spasm.

CASE 6.18 DO NOT BE A STUPID-3

Massive acute thrombotic in-stent reocclusion after successful thrombectomy and direct stenting may be a complication of undersized stenting.

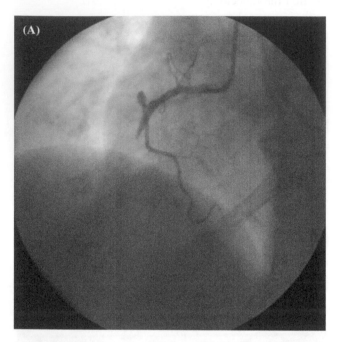

Figure 6.18A Occlusion at the second segment of the RCA.

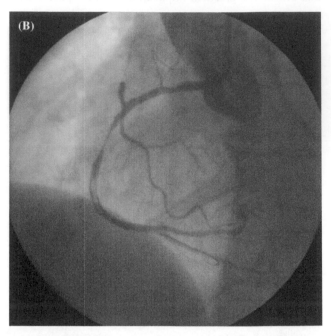

Figure 6.18B Evidence of massive thrombosis after crossing the wire.

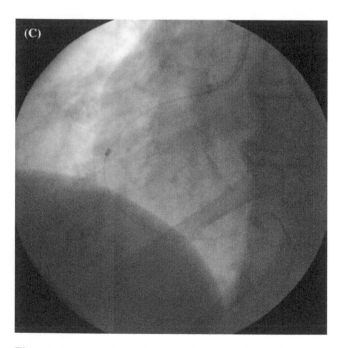

Figure 6.18C Rheolytic thrombectomy (AngioJet, first model) of the vessel.

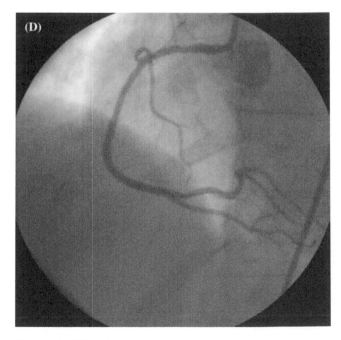

Figure 6.18D Final result after direct stenting at the second tract of RCA; the stent is undersized.

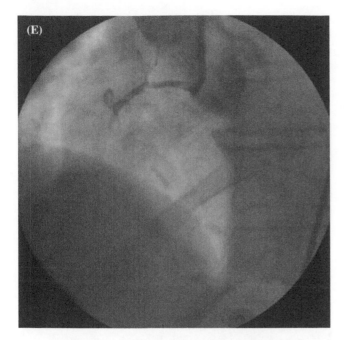

Figure 6.18E Subacute in-stent thrombotic reocclusion.

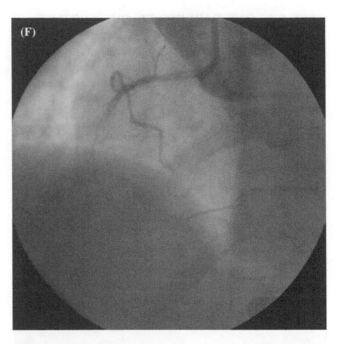

Figure 6.18F Crossing the wire through the thrombotic in-stent reocclusion.

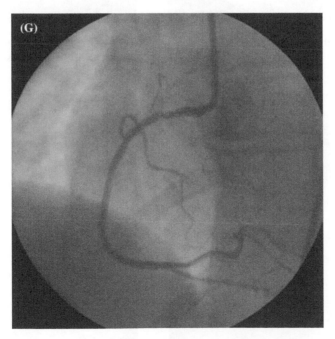

Figure 6.18G Repeat rheolytic thrombectomy and expansion of the stent with a right-sized balloon.

CASE 6.19 ONE PAIN DRIVES OUT ANOTHER

Antiplatelet treatments have dramatically decreased stent thrombosis also in the setting of acute myocardial infarction. A nonoptimal result, such as poststent nonocclusive dissection, may disturb the flow and promote thrombosis. Keep in mind that the strongest antithrombotic factor is a normal no-disturbed flow.

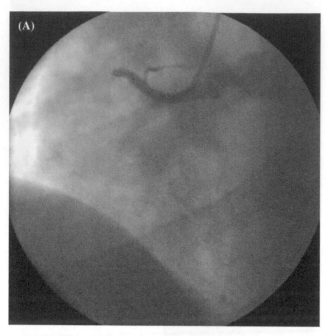

Figure 6.19A Occlusion of the proximal RCA.

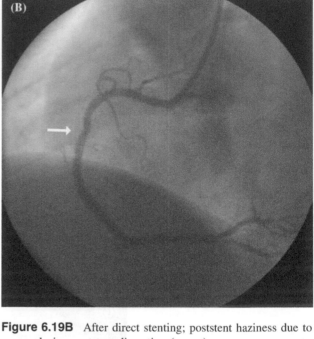

Figure 6.19B After direct stenting; poststent haziness due to non occlusive poststent dissection (*arrow*).

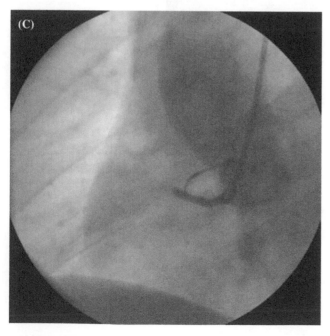

Figure 6.19C Thrombotic reocclusion of the RCA.

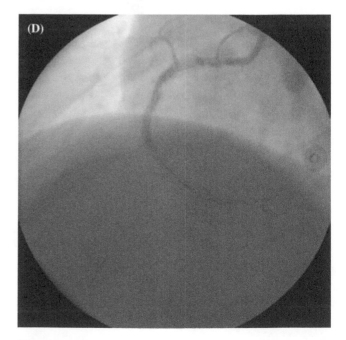

Figure 6.19D Placement of an antiembolic occlusive protection device (GuardWire); contrast injection shows massive thrombosis and the poststent dissection.

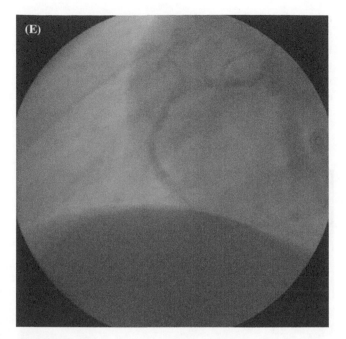

Figure 6.19E Additional stenting.

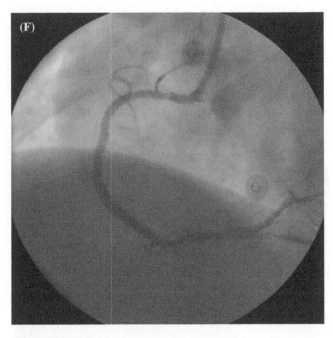

Figure 6.19F After removal of the antiembolic protection device.

CASE 6.20 THE JAIL-2

In aneurysmatical coronary artery disease, the disturbed flow by the ectatic vessel plays a major role in the formation of thrombotic occlusion, or reocclusion after successful recanalization. Thus, besides the reestablishment of the flow by thrombectomy or angioplasty, there is indication for the correction of the aneurysm. This may be achieved with the use of covered stents (see case 7.14); however, the potential disadvantage of covered stents is the need of high pressure for the complete expansion of the stent. An alternative approach may be the use of a mesh stent that dramatically decreases the flow in the extrastent portion of the aneurysm, resulting in complete thrombotic obliteration.

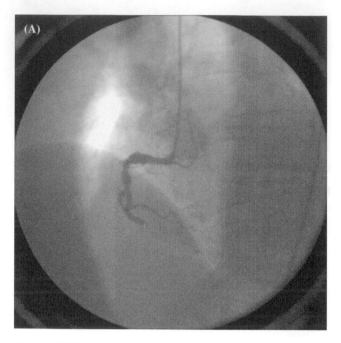

Figure 6.20A Thrombotic occlusion of an aneurysmatic RCA.

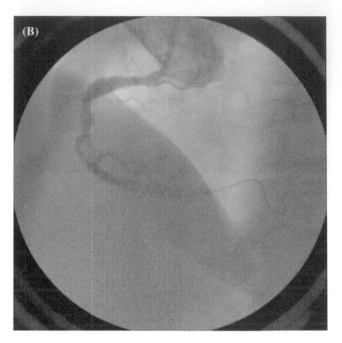

Figure 6.20B After crossing the wire, evidence of the distal aneurysmatic segment with obliterating massive thrombus.

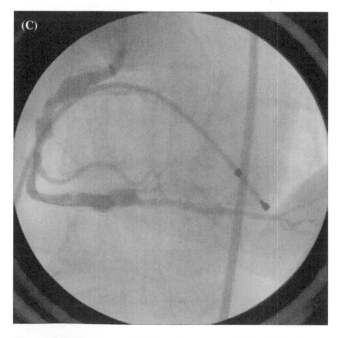

Figure 6.20C Recanalization after successful rheolytic thrombectomy (AngioJet).

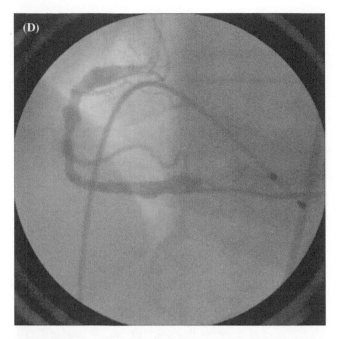

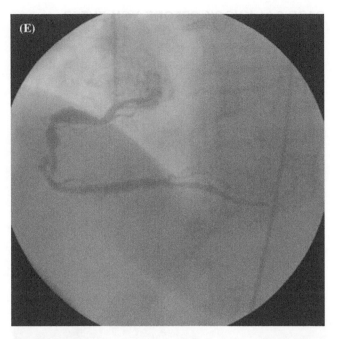

Figure 6.20D Direct stenting with a mesh autoexpandable stent at the distal aneurysmatic segment.

Figure 6.20E The one-month follow-up angiography shows the persistence of RCA patency and the complete obliteration of the aneurysm.

CASE 6.21 KNOCK BEFORE YOU ENTER

Acute occlusion of a venous graft is invariably associated with massive thrombosis; moreover, frequently there is also a diffuse degenerative process of the graft. These two characteristics are associated with a prohibitive risk of embolization and no-flow using a conventional approach. It is likely that the best approach is a combination of thrombectomy to decrease the thrombotic burden and antiembolic protection during stent implantation.

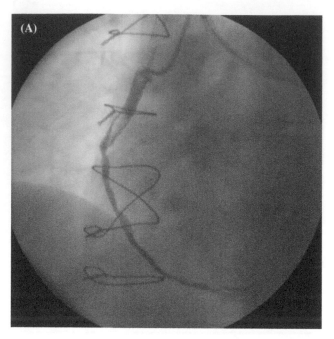

Figure 6.21A Venous graft to RCA with diffuse massive thrombosis.

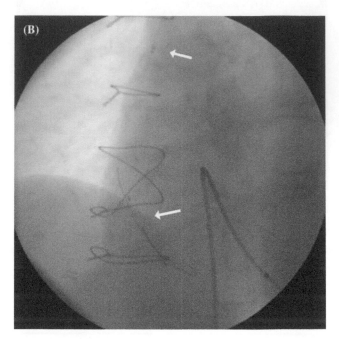

Figure 6.21B Positioning of a distal filter protection device (AngioGuard) at the distal part of the graft and rheolytic thrombectomy (*arrows*).

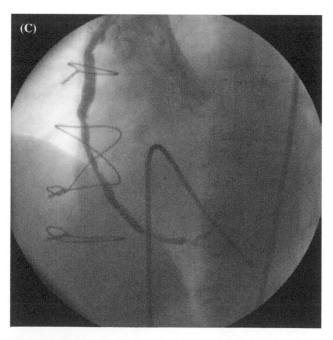

Figure 6.21C Final result after thrombectomy, stenting and removal of the filter device.

CASE 6.22 DO NOT KNOCK BEFORE YOU ENTER

In venous grafts, crossing of the wire or other devices may promote the embolization of thrombus or atherosclerotic debris before thrombectomy or dilation. Thus, the place-

ment of an antiembolic device should be done very carefully. The routine use of abciximab should be considered mandatory.

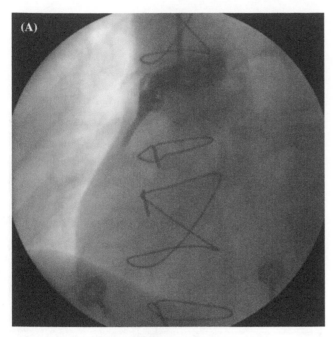

Figure 6.22A Occlusion at the proximal portion of a venous graft to RCA.

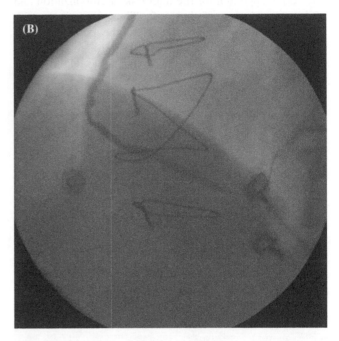

Figure 6.22B After rheolytic thrombectomy persisting thrombotic occlusion at the distal segment of the graft suggesting a possible macroembolization, the mid-portion of the graft shows a long ulcerated plaque.

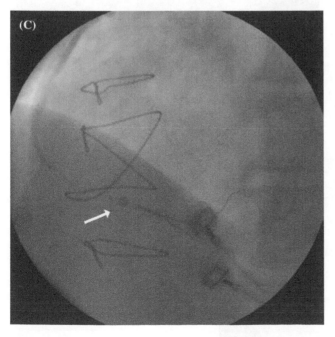

Figure 6.22C Placement of an occlusive antiembolic device (GuardWire) (*arrow*) and stenting of the mid-portion of the graft.

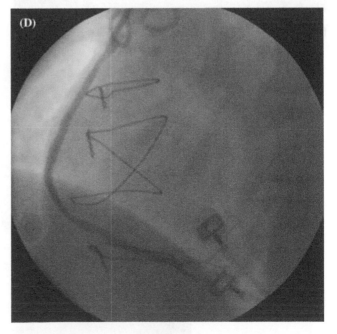

Figure 6.22D After stenting and retrieving by the Export catheter, there is evidence of residual nonocclusive thrombosis in the distal portion of the graft, and no more evidence of the ulcerated plaque.

CASE 6.23 THE OLD WAY MAY BE BETTER THAN THE NEW ONE

The treatment of the native vessel in patients with acute occlusion of a venous graft should be considered as an alternative approach for the high risk of embolization and of late reocclusion of the graft. Thus, in patients with acute myocardial infarction due to the occlusion of a venous graft, a careful evaluation of the feasibility of the revascularization procedure in the native vessel should always be considered.

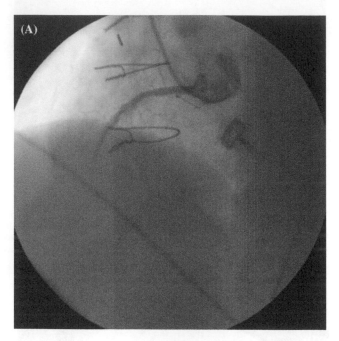

Figure 6.23A Chronic occlusion of the RCA.

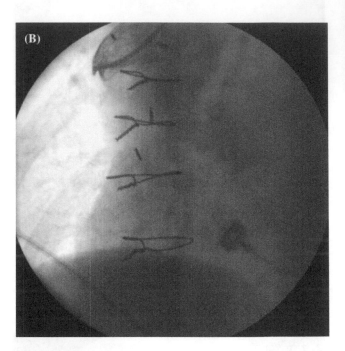

Figure 6.23B Acute proximal occlusion of a graft to the RCA.

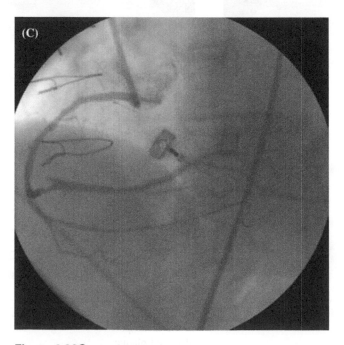

Figure 6.23C Angioplasty and stenting of the native RCA.

CASE 6.24 THE PROBLEM WAS A SOFT NUT TO CRACK

Vessel perforation is a very uncommon complication of percutaneous intervention. If the rupture is not related to an operator mistake (traumatic advancement of the wire, oversized balloon), the rupture may be strongly favored by the anelastic structure of the vessel wall, typically an old degenerated venous graft.

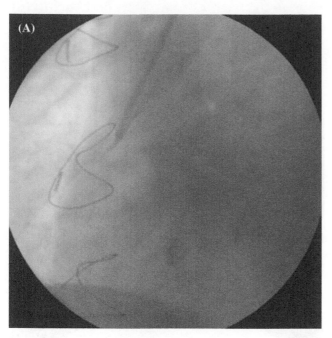

Figure 6.24A Acute occlusion of a venous graft to the RCA.

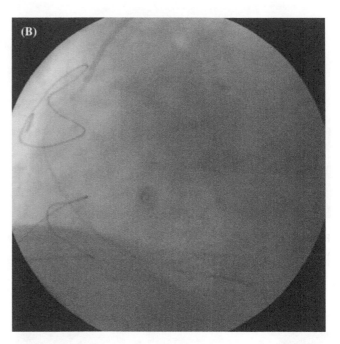

Figure 6.24B Dye injection beyond the occlusion by a dual lumen catheter (Multifunctional Probing) shows massive thrombosis. Failure to advance an antiembolic protection device.

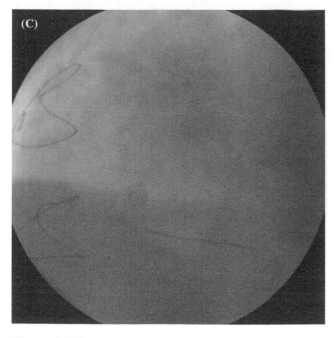

Figure 6.24C After angioplasty with a long undersized balloon; evidence of severe stenosis at the level of the crux.

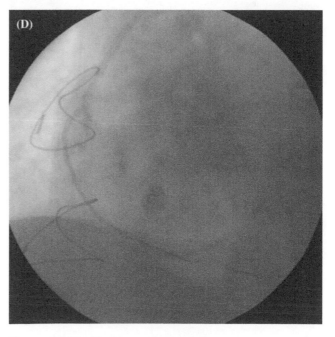

Figure 6.24D Placement of two wires.

(Case 6.24 continued on page 120)

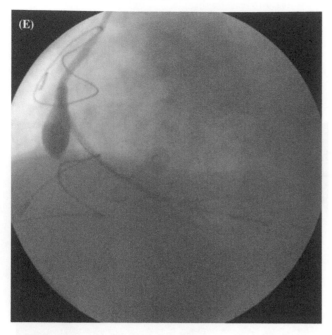

Figure 6.24E After repeat angioplasty, rupture of the graft with temporary containment of dye loss.

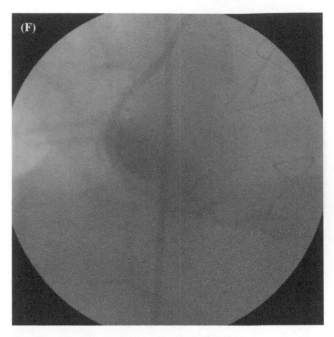

Figure 6.24F Spreading of dye into the pericardial space.

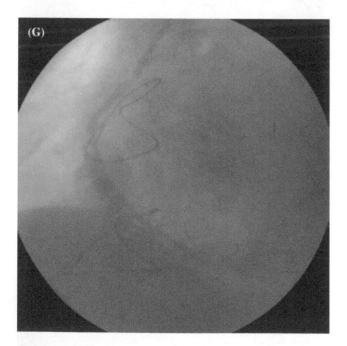

Figure 6.24G Placement of two covered stents (Jostent, Jomed).

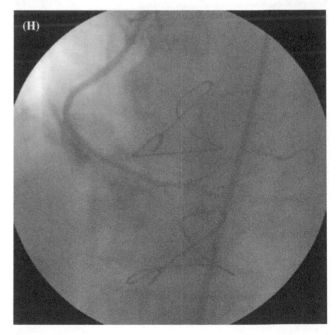

Figure 6.24H No more evidence of the rupture; staining of dye into the pericardial space.

CASE 6.25 DO NOT DO MORE THAN NECESSARY

A minimal approach should be considered in diffuse disease associated with a small reference diameter in the distal portion of the infarct artery if an acceptable result is achieved by angioplasty.

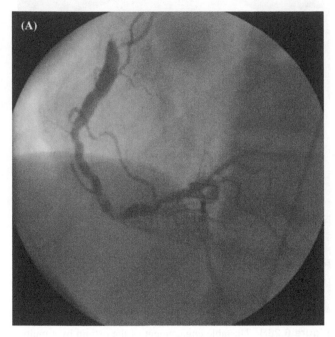

Figure 6.25A Subocclusion of the ostium of the RCA, and diffuse disease of the mid- and distal portion of the vessel.

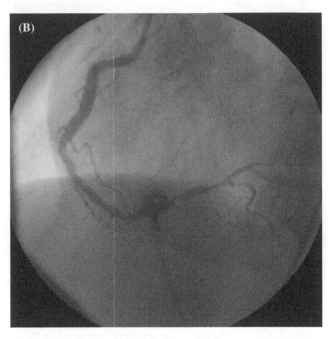

Figure 6.25B Stenting of the ostium and first segment of RCA and conventional angioplasty of the mid- and distal portion of the vessel.

CASE 6.26 TO DROP TWO ANCHORS

This type of RCA origin and takeoff prevents the successful use of standard RCA guide catheters (Judkins, Amplatz, or hockey stick catheters). The best approach is a multipurpose-type guide catheter, or alternatively, a long left Amplatz catheter. In both cases the guide catheter cannot provide sufficient support, and the placement of two coronary wires may increase the anchorage, favoring a successful procedure.

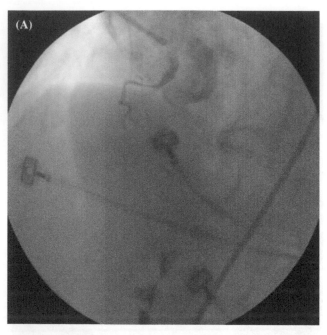

Figure 6.26A Occlusion of the proximal portion of an RCA with a posterosuperior origin from the aorta and caudal takeoff.

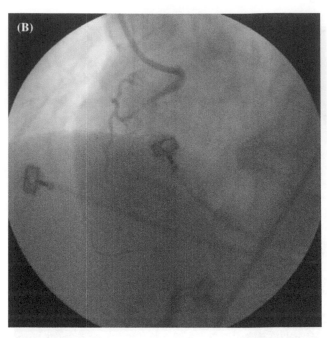

Figure 6.26B Unstable engagement of the ostium by a multipurpose guide catheter.

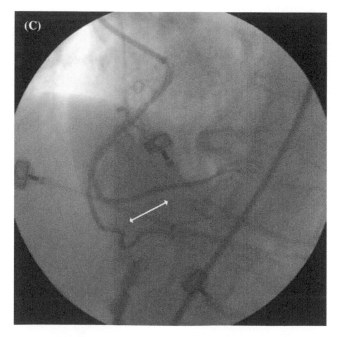

Figure 6.26C Double wire anchorage (*arrows*) and angioplasty.

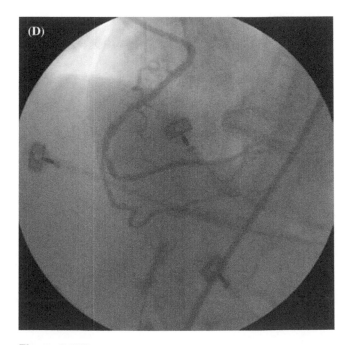

Figure 6.26D After stenting.

CASE 6.27 TO DROP TWO ANCHORS-2

Another example of the utility of the double anchorage technique.

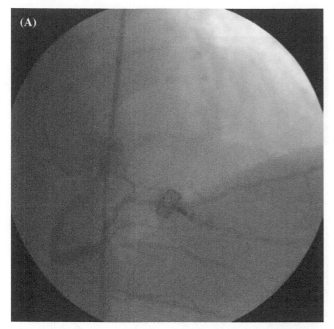

Figure 6.27A Subocclusion of the ostium of the posterior descending artery; the tip of the guide catheter cannot engage the ostium of RCA because of the posterior position of the ostium.

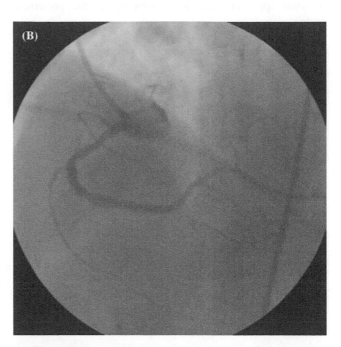

Figure 6.27B Placement of two coronary wires stabilizes the position of the guide catheter.

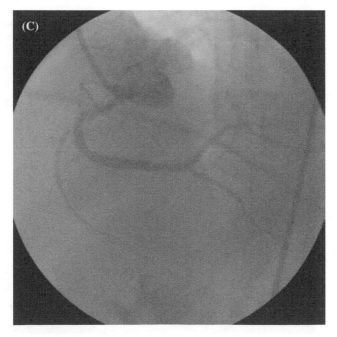

Figure 6.27C After direct stenting of the ostium of posterior descending artery.

CASE 6.28 AT LOWEST RATE

The relative small area at risk as revealed after recanalization of the posterior descending artery may suggest a minimal approach like direct stenting as the preferred strategy.

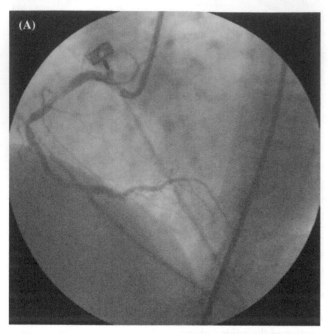

Figure 6.28A Total occlusion of the posterior descending artery.

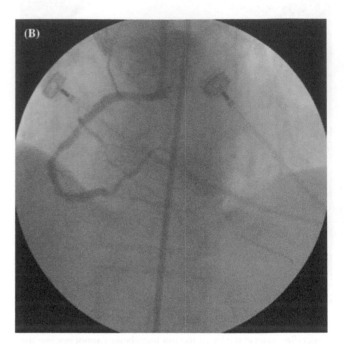

Figure 6.28B Recanalization after crossing the wire; the target lesion is short, and there is evidence of thrombus.

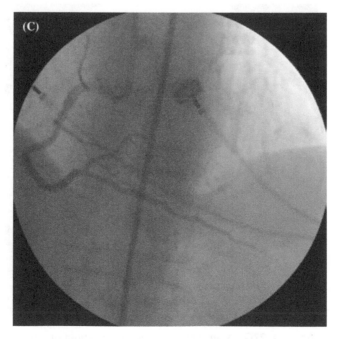

Figure 6.28C After direct stenting of the posterior descending artery.

CASE 6.29 TO GO FAR

Diffuse target vessel disease suggests a large thrombotic burden and, indirectly, a high risk of embolization during intervention. The use of an antiembolic protection device should be considered also in distal coronary occlusion.

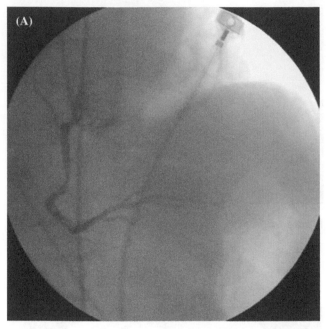

Figure 6.29A Diffuse disease of the RCA and occlusion of the RCA after the origin of the posterior descending artery; moderate stenosis of the proximal posterior descending artery.

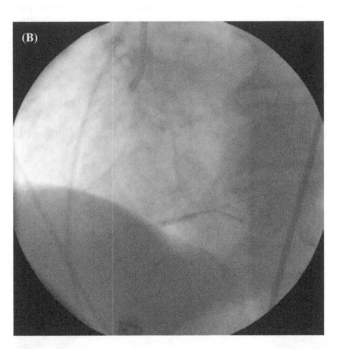

Figure 6.29B Coronary angioplasty and spot stenting of the RCA with distal occlusive antiembolic protection (GuardWire).

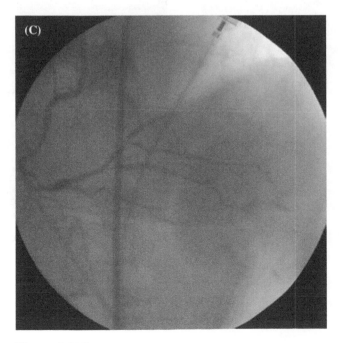

Figure 6.29C Final result.

CASE 6.30 IT IS NOT TOO SMALL TO UNDERSTAND

Isolated right ventricular infarction due to the occlusion of a nondominant RCA is very uncommon and associated with a low-output state or cardiogenic shock unresponsive or poorly responsive to fluid administration or inotropic drugs. Successful recanalization of the vessel is generally associated with a prompt reversal of cardiogenic shock. This quick response may be related to the high resistance of the right ventricular wall to ischemia and subsequent stunning or necrosis. Mortality of a nonreperfused right ventricular infarction is high, and every attempt should be done to restore flow into at least one major right ventricular branch, also in the more frequent association with inferior left ventricular infarction.

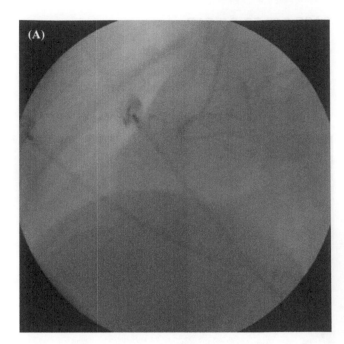

Figure 6.30A Occlusion of a nondominant RCA.

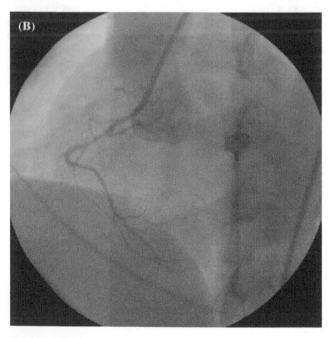

Figure 6.30B Evidence of a large acute marginal branch after crossing the wire.

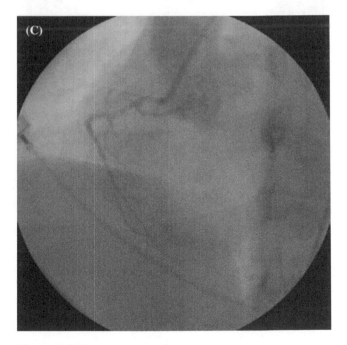

Figure 6.30C After direct stenting.

CASE 6.31 IT IS TOO LARGE TO NOT UNDERSTAND

Cardiogenic shock may complicate an acute occlusion of a hyperdominant RCA. In these cases the low cardiac output state or cardiogenic shock is due to both ventricle failures.

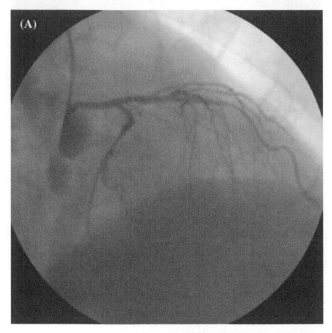

Figure 6.31A Left coronary angiogram showing a hypoplasic circumflex artery.

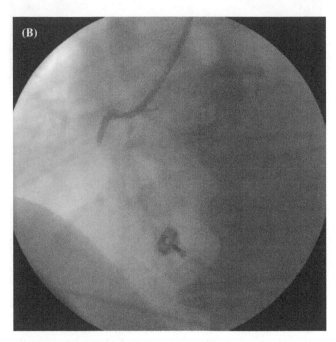

Figure 6.31B Occlusion of the proximal segment of the RCA.

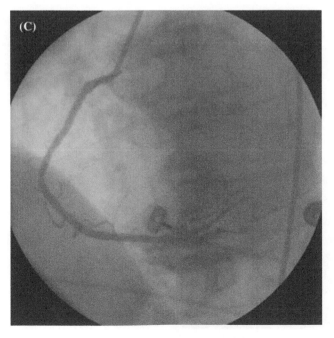

Figure 6.31C After direct stenting of the RCA occlusion.

CASE 6.32 TAKE TWO, PAY ONE

An alternative mechanism of cardiogenic shock due to acute occlusion or subocclusion of the RCA is the contemporary chronic occlusion of the left anterior descending artery if the RCA occlusion compromises the collateral flow to the left anterior descending artery.

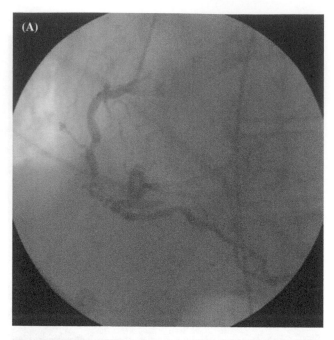

Figure 6.32A Acute occlusion of the third tract of the RCA and evidence of an ulcerated disrupted plaque involving the origin of a large marginal branch.

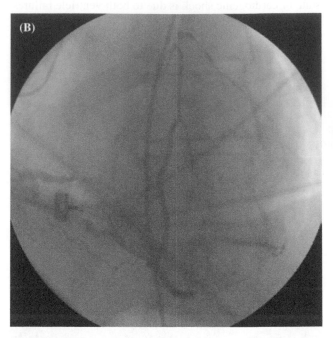

Figure 6.32B The marginal branch provides a collateral flow to the left anterior descending artery.

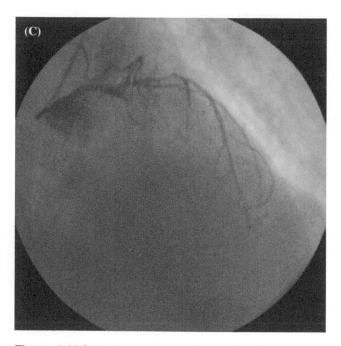

Figure 6.32C Left coronary angiogram showing proximal chronic occlusion of the left anterior descending artery.

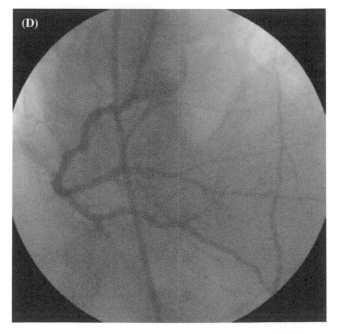

Figure 6.32D After stenting of the occlusion of the third tract of the RCA and of the disrupted plaque at the proximal segment of the third tract.

CASE 6.33 DO NOT GO WRONG FROM THE BEGINNING

True RCA ostium occlusion or subocclusion should be approached very cautiously with the guide catheter and the wire. Both may produce a very proximal false lumen that may prevent the crossing of the lesion due to the absence of any space to try to find the true lumen. Guide catheter should be placed just in front of the ostium, and a soft hydrophilic wire advanced without any resistance.

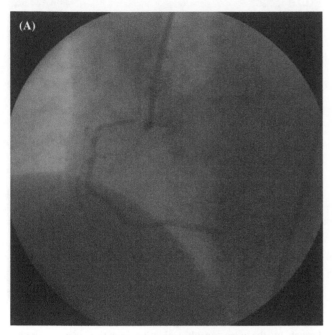

Figure 6.33A True ostial RCA subocclusion; severe stenosis at the end of the first tract of the RCA.

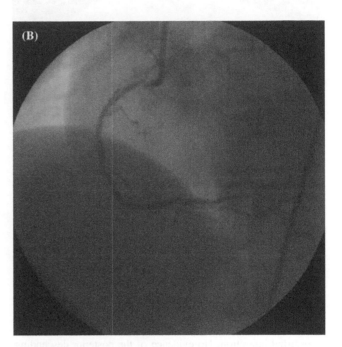

Figure 6.33B Postangioplasty dissection.

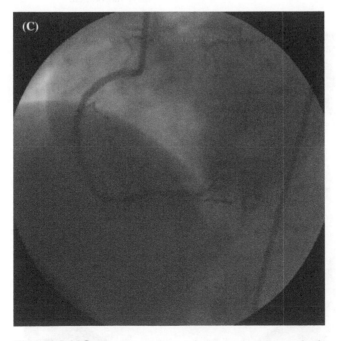

Figure 6.33C Stenting using a long stent to cover both lesions.

CASE 6.34 WHERE ARE YOU?

Vascularization of the inferior wall from a right ventricular marginal branch is an anatomic alternative to the posterior descending artery. The absence of the posterior descending artery on the baseline right coronary angiogram may be due to ostial occlusion of the vessel, or to this anatomic alternative.

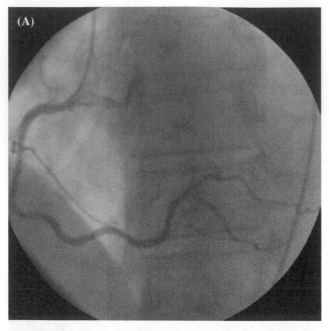

Figure 6.34A RCA angiogram of a patient with acute inferior myocardial infarction. No evidence of the posterior descending artery.

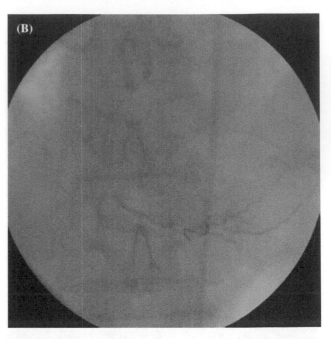

Figure 6.34B After the engagement of an occluded marginal branch by the wire, an ultraselective injection using a double lumen catheter (Multifunctional Probing) allows the correct definition of the vascularization of the inferior wall from the marginal branch.

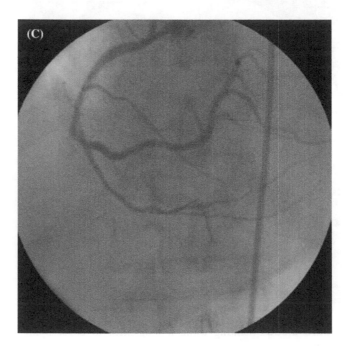

Figure 6.34C After stenting.

CASE 6.35 GET YOU CAUGHT!

Among the coronary anomalies, the origin of RCA from left sinus is the more problematic from the interventional perspective. The engagement of the ostium may be really difficult. The first option guide catheter is multipurpose if the aorta allows wide maneuverability. Otherwise, a short Judkins left-curve catheter may be the best option.

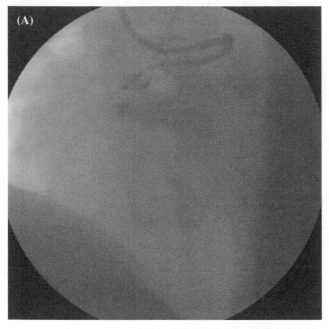

Figure 6.35A Occlusion of an RCA with an anomalous origin from the left coronary sinus.

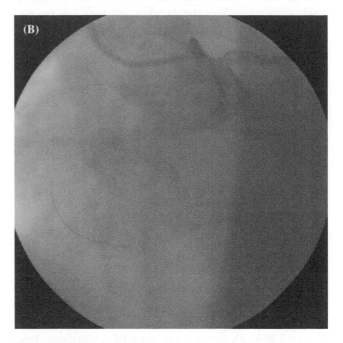

Figure 6.35B Crossing the occlusion and disengagement of the guide catheter from the anomalous ostium.

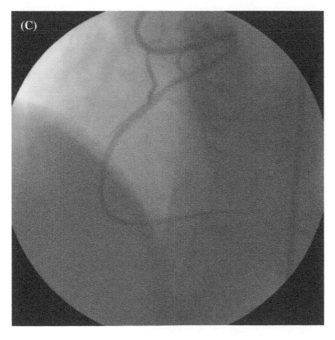

Figure 6.35C Stabilization of the guide catheter with a second wire and direct stenting of the occlusion.

CASE 6.36 A DANGEROUS CURVE

This type of takeoff of the RCA was really a nightmare for stenting when the only available stent was the tubular Palmaz-Schatz stent. Thus, the use of a strong backup guide catheter such as the Amplatz left type was mandatory. Currently, the profile and trackability of the available coronary stents is such that a strong backup from the guide catheter is no more needed, with the advantage of a decreased risk of traumatic dissection of the proximal RCA by a stiff long tip guide catheter. If the vessel curve prevents an easy placement of the stent, deep intubation of the guide catheter over the shaft of the delivery balloon may be the more effective maneuver.

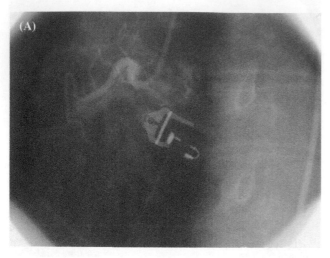

Figure 6.36A Occlusion of a proximal RCA with a sharp bend before the occlusion ("shepherd crook").

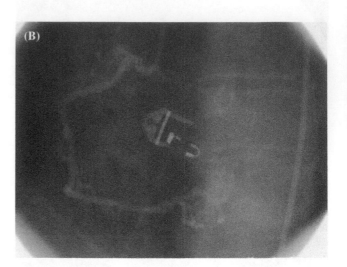

Figure 6.36B After direct stenting.

CASE 6.37 ACT WITH THE GREATEST TACT

A minimal soft approach is required in spontaneous coronary dissection; the goal is the achievement of a normal flow by low-pressure slightly oversized balloon and stenting only for persistent occlusion or subocclusion. A normal flow strongly favors the complete healing of the dissection.

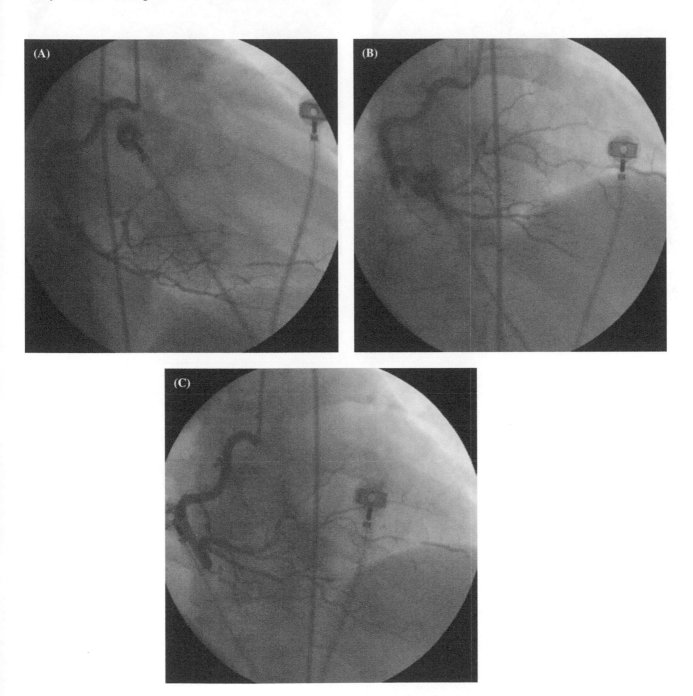

Figure 6.37A–C Long spontaneous dissection of the RCA (see chap. 2). The following features allow the angiographic diagnosis of diffuse dissection: (*i*) unexpected diameter reduction at the beginning of the third tract of the vessel; (*ii*) the very distal dissection involvement of the retroventricular branches that are focally suboccluded or occluded; (*iii*) no angiographic evidence of atherosclerosis.

(*Case 6.37 continued on page 134*)

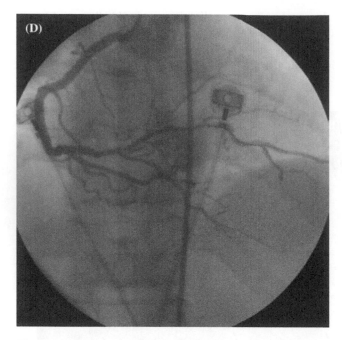

Figure 6.37D After balloon angioplasty partial correction of the dissection with a satisfactory angiographic result.

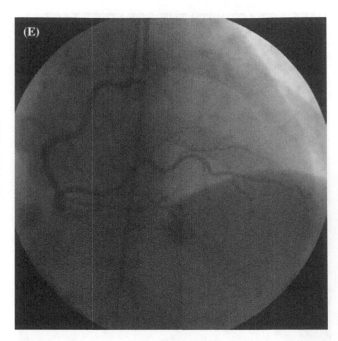

Figure 6.37E The six-month follow-up angiography shows a complete healing of the dissection.

7

Left Anterior Descending Artery (LAD)

RENATO VALENTI AND ANGELA MIGLIORINI
Division of Cardiology, Careggi Hospital, Florence, Italy

CASE 7.1 DO NOT BE A STUPID

The conventional balloon angioplasty is an outdated approach for proximal LAD occlusion. The achievement of an outward "normal" flow in the epicardial branches after macroembolization is generally associated with a poor or absent myocardial salvage due to extensive microvessel disruption.

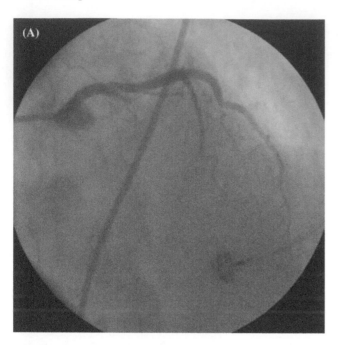

Figure 7.1A Proximal occlusion of the LAD.

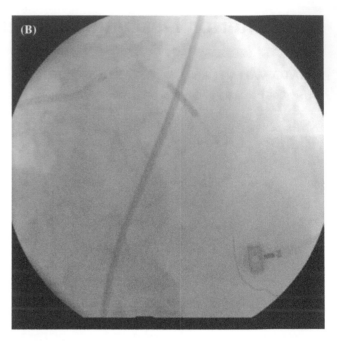

Figure 7.1B Balloon angioplasty.

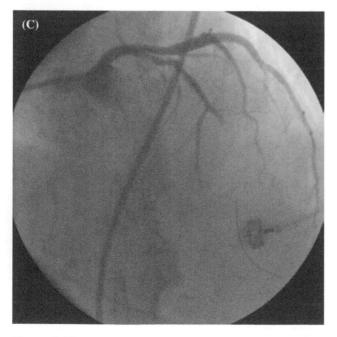

Figure 7.1C Restoration of flow but evidence of macroembolization into the septal and the diagonal branch of a dual LAD.

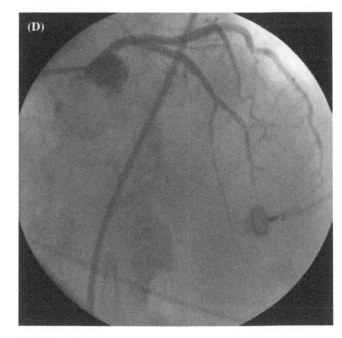

Figure 7.1D After mechanical lysis by balloon angioplasty, residual total occlusion of a first septal branch and restoration of flow in the two principal branches of the LAD.

CASE 7.2 A VERY GOOD SUCTION

A thrombotic component of acute vessel occlusion is invariably present in patients with acute myocardial infarction. Infrequently thrombus may be the only component of the occlusion, as revealed by angiography. In these cases, thrombectomy alone may lead to an optimal angiographic result without the need for further intervention.

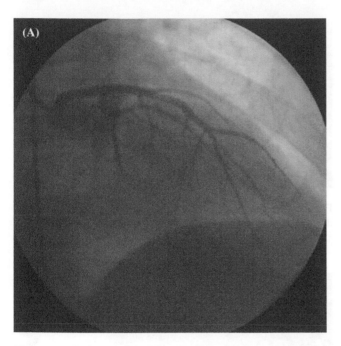
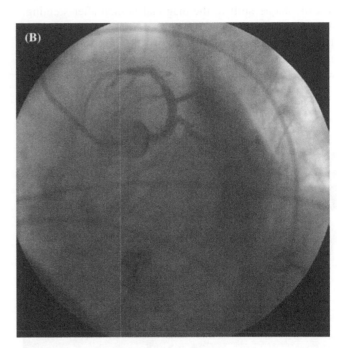

Figure 7.2A, B Subocclusive thrombosis of the mid-portion of the LAD.

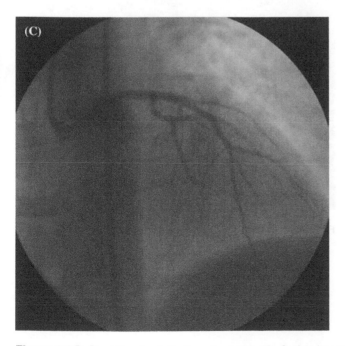
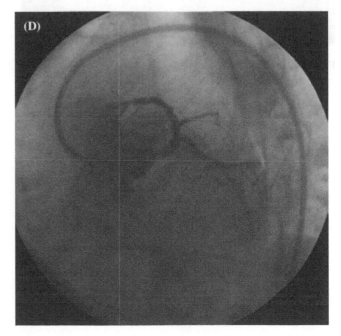

Figure 7.2C, D After rheolytic thrombectomy. No further intervention.

CASE 7.3 AN OPEN JAIL

In LAD occlusion, the involvement of a collateral branch is extremely frequent due to the high number of the branches and the high shear stress at these levels. Thus a correct approach includes a detailed analysis of the anatomy of the vessel. In this case, after thrombectomy there is not a large atherosclerotic burden suggesting a low risk of plaque shift to the diagonal branch after stenting. An open cell design stent is the more indicate stent type. This design allows easy access to the branch if needed, and balloon dilation of the cell is less distorting compared with a closed cell design stent.

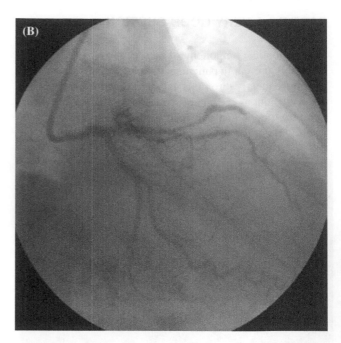

Figure 7.3B Placement of two wires in the LAD and in the diagonal branch.

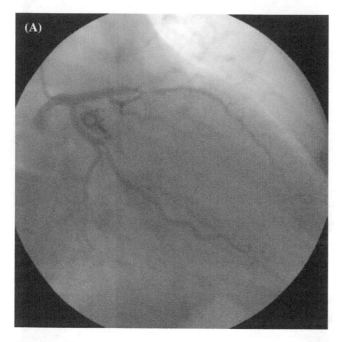

Figure 7.3A Diffuse disease; occlusion of the LAD immediately after the origin of a major diagonal branch.

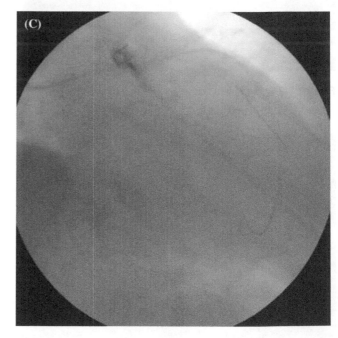

Figure 7.3C Rheolytic thrombectomy (AngioJet).

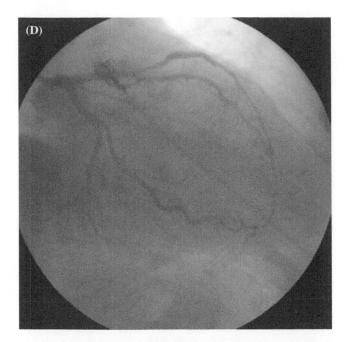

Figure 7.3D After thrombectomy residual severe stenosis of the LAD at the level of the previous occlusion.

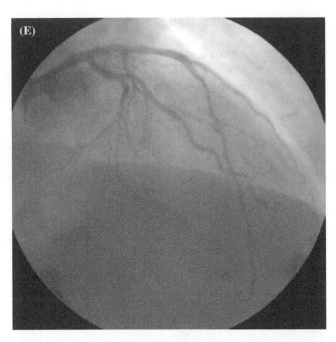

Figure 7.3E After placement of an open cell design tubular stent in the LAD covering the origin of the diagonal branch.

CASE 7.4 AN OPEN JAIL-2

Thrombectomy before stenting of the main vessel in a bifurcation or trifurcation target lesion strongly decreases the risk of atheromatous debris shift to the branches, and generally there is no need for further intervention after direct stenting of the main vessel.

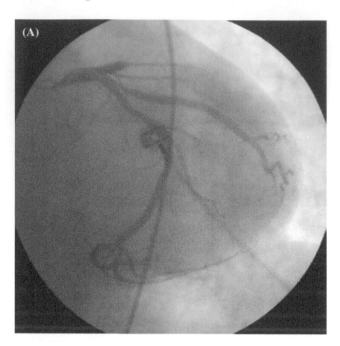

Figure 7.4A Proximal LAD occlusion.

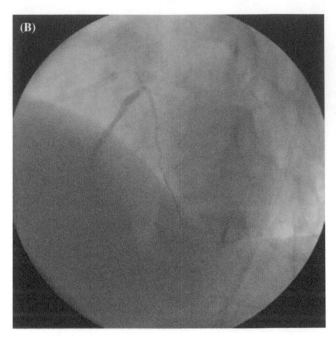

Figure 7.4B After crossing the occlusion, ultraselective dye injection beyond the occlusion shows that the wire is placed first in a large diagonal branch and the target lesion involves also a large septal branch (trifurcation).

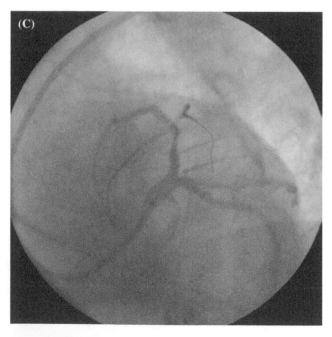

Figure 7.4C Placement of other two wires into the main vessel and in first septal branch and restoring the flow after rheolytic thrombectomy (AngioJet).

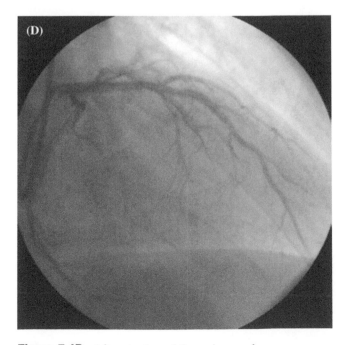

Figure 7.4D After stenting of the main vessel.

CASE 7.5 A DANGEROUS CROSSROADS

The distal migration of the macroembolus from the branch does not contraindicate the use of bailout thrombectomy. Conversely, mechanical lysis by balloon angioplasty of the thrombus is absolutely contraindicated since the fragmentation of the embolus may result in extensive disruption of the microvessel network.

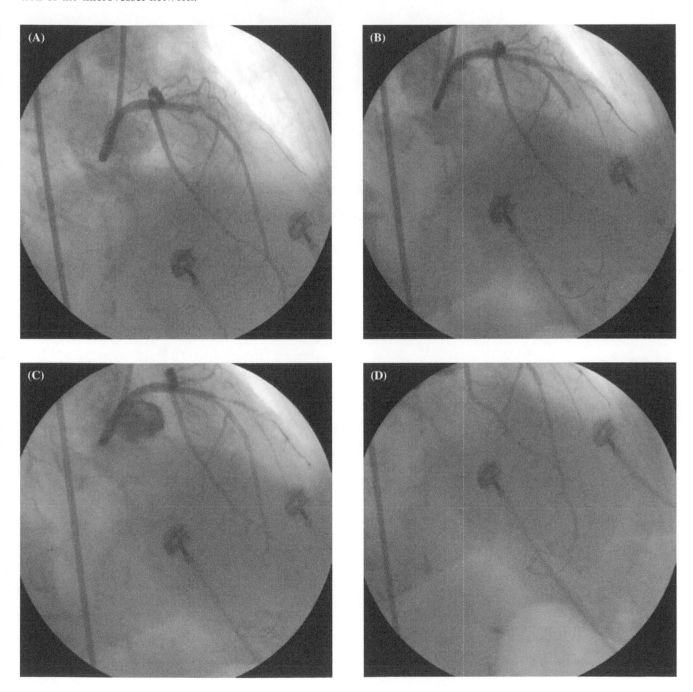

Figure 7.5A–D **(A)** Complex disrupted plaque of the LAD bifurcation with occlusion of the first diagonal branch and decreased dye density of the main vessel. **(B–D)** Balloon angioplasty of the diagonal branch is followed by plaque and thrombus shift to the main vessel and final embolization of the apical segment of the LAD.

(Case 7.5 continued on page 142)

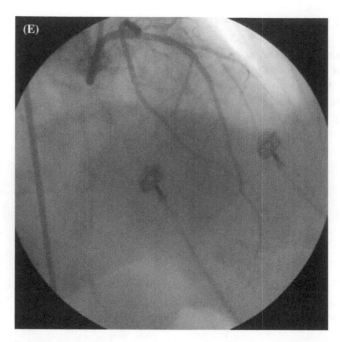

Figure 7.5E   After stenting of the main vessel at the level of
the bifurcation.

CASE 7.6 HAVE A CLEAR VISION OF THE FUTURE

The correct definition of the angiographic anatomy of the vessel by the ultraselective injection of dye beyond the occlusion allowed an easy and uncomplicated procedure.

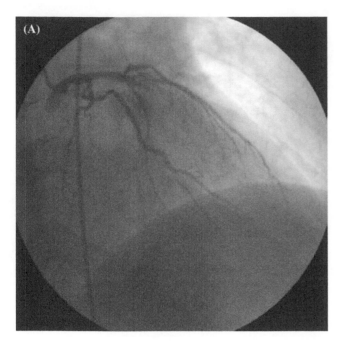

Figure 7.6A LAD occlusion.

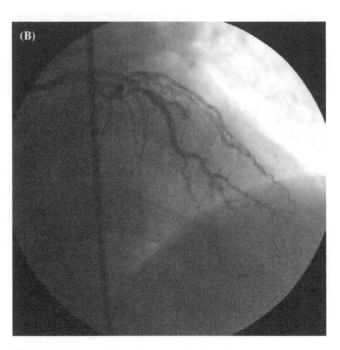

Figure 7.6B No flow after crossing the wire.

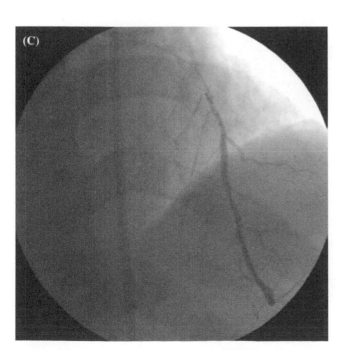

Figure 7.6C Ultraselective dye injection (Multifunctional Probing) beyond the occlusion reveals a relatively short occlusion without massive thrombosis or involvement of major septal or diagonal branches.

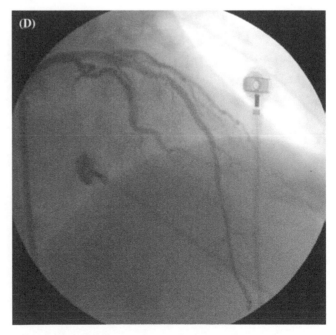

Figure 7.6D After direct stenting of the occlusion.

CASE 7.7 TO GET THE PROBLEM UNDER CONTROL

Simultaneous double injection of dye through the guide catheter and the dual lumen catheter is a simple alternative for more precise assessment of the length of the lesion.

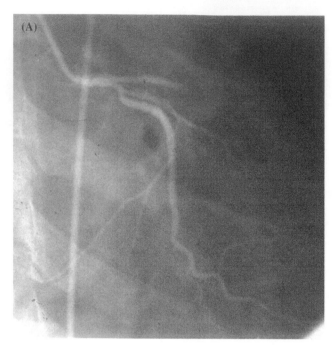

Figure 7.7A Proximal LAD occlusion.

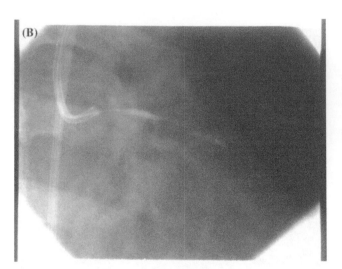

Figure 7.7B Simultaneous dye injections through the guide catheter and the dual lumen catheter (Multifunctional Probing).

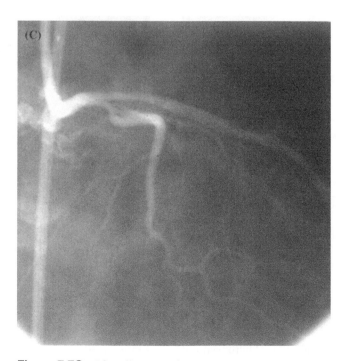

Figure 7.7C After direct stenting.

CASE 7.8 "ELEMENTARY MY DEAR WATSON"

The absence of left coronary system lesions other than the LAD occlusion makes the possibility of a long atherosclerotic plaque remote and suggests the dominance of the thrombotic component of the long occlusion.

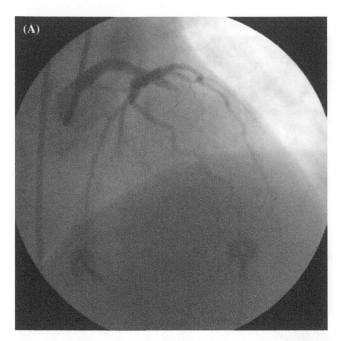

Figure 7.8A Proximal LAD occlusion.

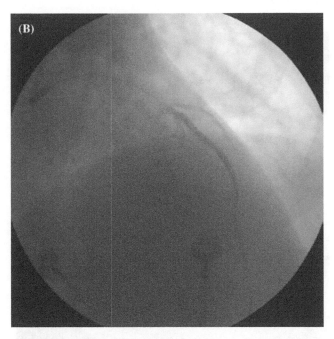

Figure 7.8B Dye injection beyond the occlusion using a dual lumen catheter (Multifunctional Probing) shows a long occlusion, and indirectly a large thrombotic burden.

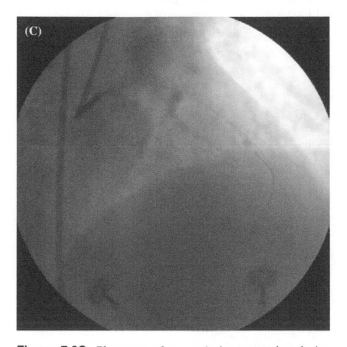

Figure 7.8C Placement of an occlusive protection device (GuardWire).

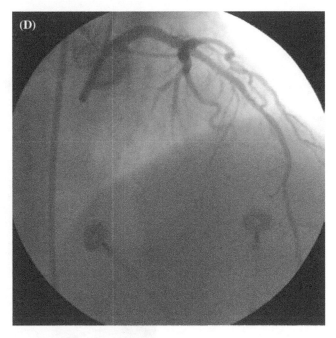

Figure 7.8D After direct stenting and aspiration with the Export catheter.

CASE 7.9 AS THE RIGHT PUTS ON THE RIGHT TRACK

Dual LAD is a frequent anatomic alternative to the normal LAD distribution, and occlusion immediately before the bifurcation of the main vessel is frequent due to the high shear stress.

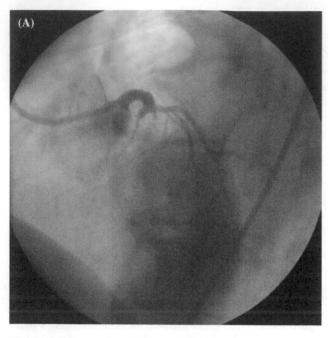

Figure 7.9A Proximal LAD occlusion.

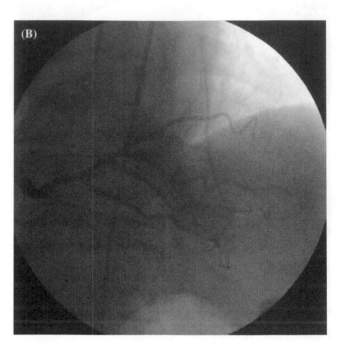

Figure 7.9B Right coronary angiography shows a collateral flow to the LAD and allows the correct anatomic definition of a dual LAD with chronic occlusion of the septal LAD and acute occlusion of the diagonal LAD.

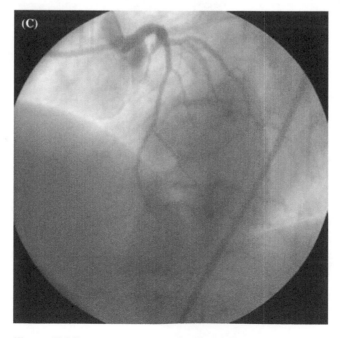

Figure 7.9C After stenting of the diagonal LAD.

CASE 7.10 TAKE ONE, PAY TWO

The need for a bifurcation stenting should be considered only if a satisfactory result cannot be achieved by repeat balloon inflations in a major branch. The favorable remodeling of an acute disrupted plaque is not infrequent, while the risk of restenosis or reocclusion of the branch after bifurcation stenting is high.

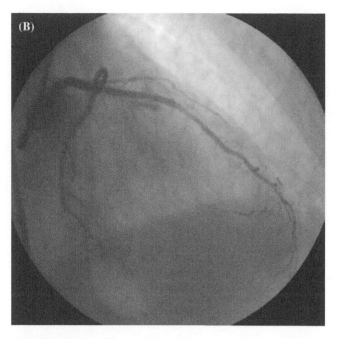

Figure 7.10B After crossing the occlusion, angiography shows that the wire is placed into a large septal branch and that the target lesion involves a true bifurcation with a persistent occlusion of the proximal portion of the second tract of the LAD.

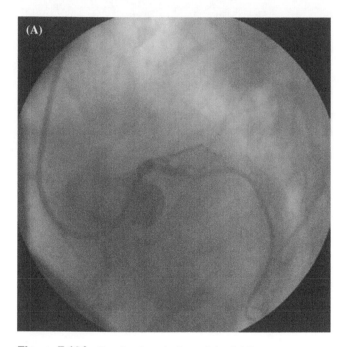

Figure 7.10A Proximal occlusion of the LAD.

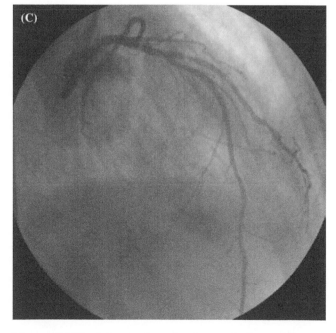

Figure 7.10C Suboptimal results after angioplasty of the two vessels.

(Case 7.10 continued on page 148)

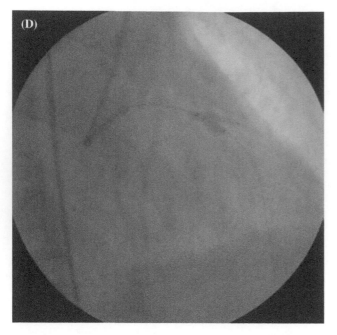

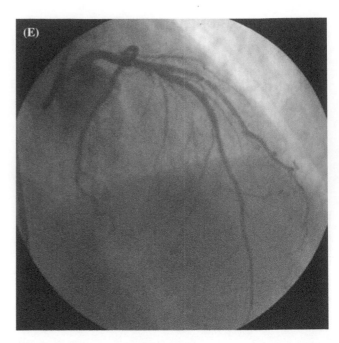

Figure 7.10D Kissing balloon after "T" stenting of the bifurcation.

Figure 7.10E Final result.

CASE 7.11 TAKE ONE, PAY ONE

The optimal angiographic result after angioplasty of the diagonal branch suggests the opportunity to stent only the main vessel.

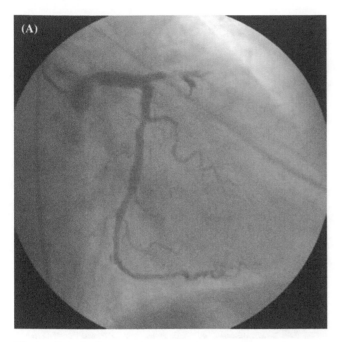

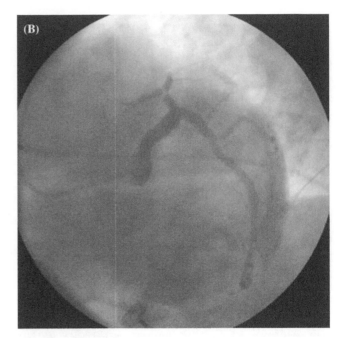

Figure 7.11A, B   True bifurcation LAD occlusion.

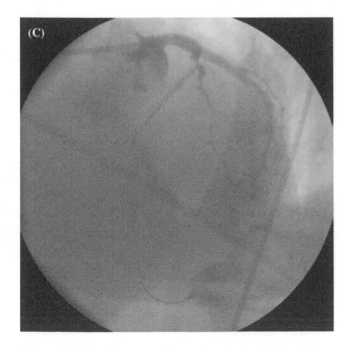

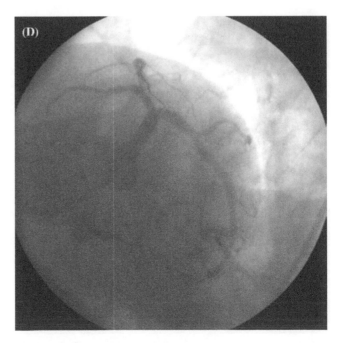

Figure 7.11C   Placement of two wires in the LAD and diagonal branch.

Figure 7.11D   After angioplasty of the two vessels and stenting of the main vessel.

CASE 7.12 A HARD WAY OUT

Crossing the occlusion of an aneurysmal coronary artery may be troublesome due to the absence of flow and the wide space of the aneurysmal sac. Both characteristics make difficult the engagement of the way out of the aneurysm by the wire. The use of a soft, plastic, and nontraumatic wire, with a long distal curve, and of multiple angiographic views may be considered the right approach.

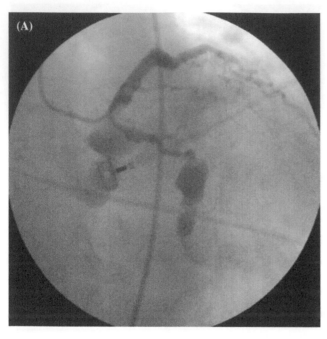

Figure 7.12A Diffuse aneurysmal LAD and circumflex arteries and occlusion at the second tract of the LAD.

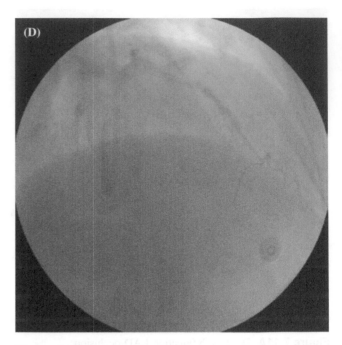

Figure 7.12B Ultraselective injection (Multifunctional Probing) beyond the occlusion shows a diffuse disease of the LAD with a normal vessel diameter.

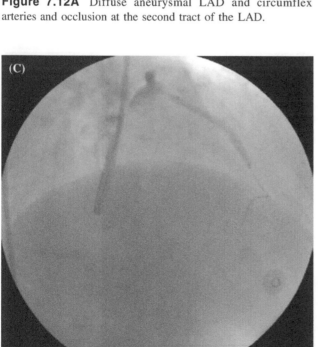

Figure 7.12C Angioplasty with a long balloon and spot stenting.

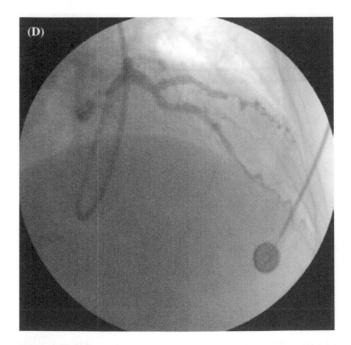

Figure 7.12D Final result.

CASE 7.13 ARMORED OCTOPUS

An aneurysmal bifurcation adds together the technical problems of a bifurcation lesion and an aneurysmal lesion, and the different steps of the procedure include the use of soft wires to twice cross the aneurysm and high support wires to straighten the bifurcation. Straightening allowed successful deployment of two stents.

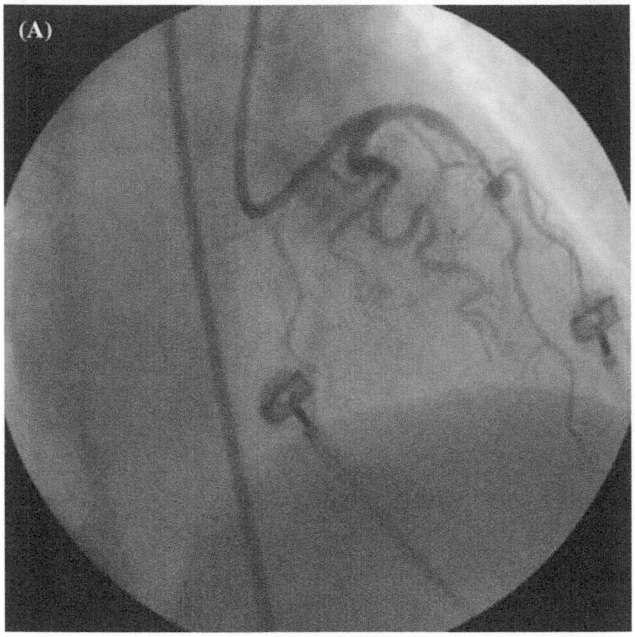

Figure 7.13A A disrupted plaque at the level of an aneurysmal dual LAD bifurcation; placement of two hydrophilic wires in the two branches of the LAD.

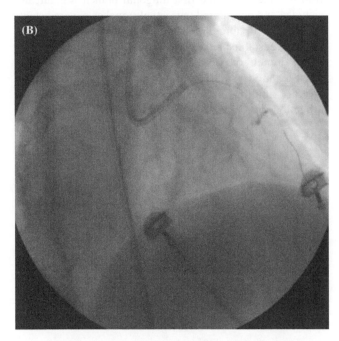

Figure 7.13B Balloon angioplasty of the diagonal branch and evidence of the very sharp takeoff of the branch.

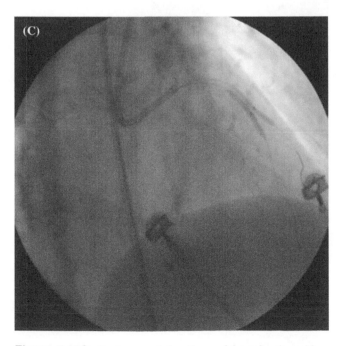

Figure 7.13C Exchange of the diagonal branch wire with a high-support wire to straighten the takeoff of the vessel and kissing balloon angioplasty.

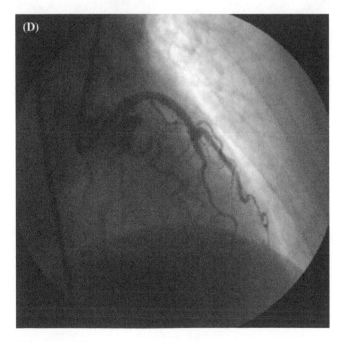

Figure 7.13D After T stenting.

CASE 7.14 MORE AND MORE

This very complex case called for a very complex approach. The absence of open major branches arising from the aneurysm (the first diagonal branch was already occluded and considered untreatable) makes covered stenting the best option. The stent obliterates the aneurysmal sac and reestablishes a normal angiographic appearance of the lumen of vessel. The risk of embolization in massive aneurysmal thrombosis persists also with a covered stenting, and as a consequence the use of a protection antiembolic device is indicated.

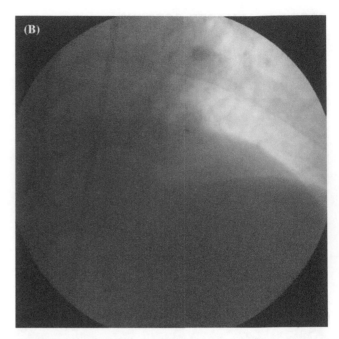

Figure 7.14B Rheolytic thrombectomy (AngioJet).

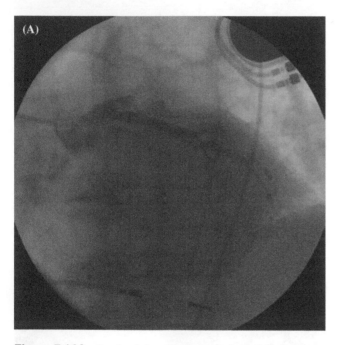

Figure 7.14A Proximal thrombotic occlusion of the LAD.

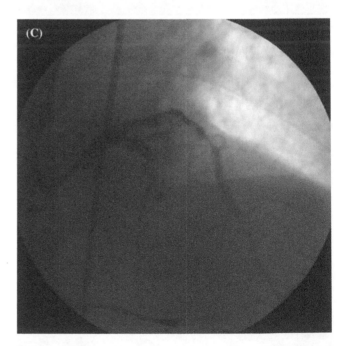

Figure 7.14C After thrombectomy evidence of aneurysmal dilation of the proximal LAD and massive residual thrombosis.

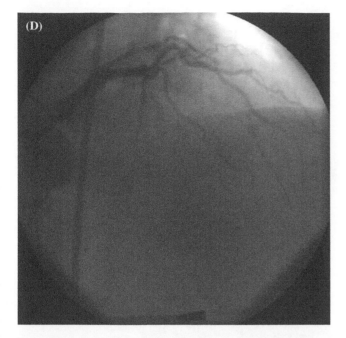

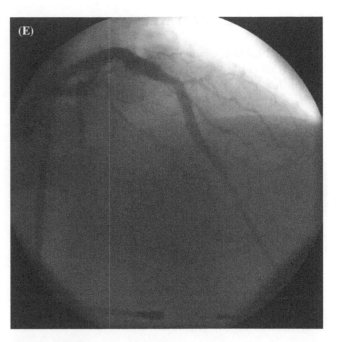

Figure 7.14D Placement of an antiembolic protection device (GuardWire).

Figure 7.14E After placement of a covered stent (Symbiot, Boston Scientific).

CASE 7.15 LOOK AT IT WELL

True ostial LAD occlusion is associated with high risk of shift of atherothrombotic material to the left main or circumflex artery. A right angiographic view can distinguish a true ostial location of the target lesion from a pseudo-ostial lesion.

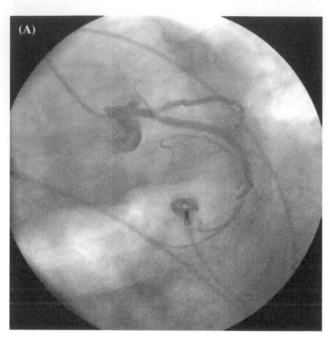

Figure 7.15A Proximal occlusion of the LAD.

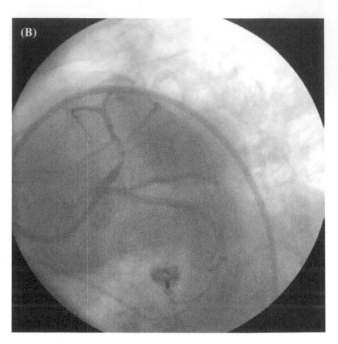

Figure 7.15B The optimized left caudal view of the vessel after crossing the wire; the lesion is far from the ostium and evidence of large thrombus at the level of the target lesion.

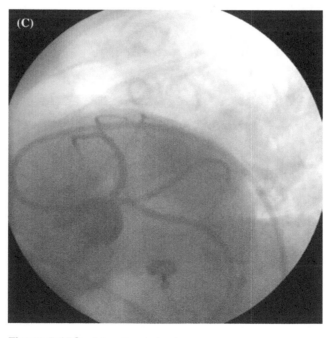

Figure 7.15C After direct stenting.

CASE 7.16 DO NOT BE A STUPID-2

This failed procedure is demonstrative of the limitation of a conventional approach to ostial LAD occlusion. A more complex approach is needed for true ostial LAD occlusion. Thrombectomy should be considered mandatory. A significant residual atheromatous burden after thrombectomy indicates the need for directional atherectomy.

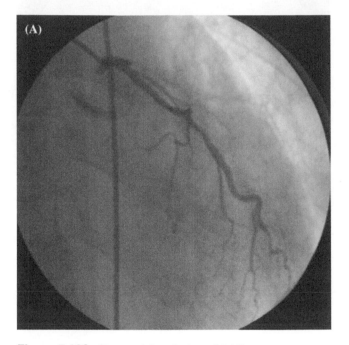

Figure 7.16A True ostial occlusion of LAD.

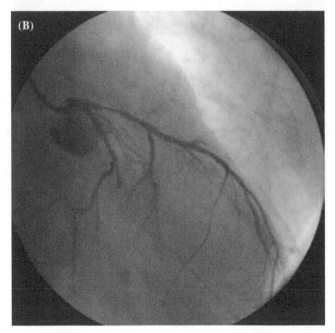

Figure 7.16B After conventional angioplasty significant residual stenosis of LAD and massive embolization to the circumflex artery.

CASE 7.17 NEVER AGAIN

The right approach in such a case should include a correct placement of two wires in the LAD and circumflex artery, thrombectomy of the ostium, and eventually directional atherectomy. However, this strategy could not be used because of the state of profound shock of this patient, the inability to provide mechanical support for severe peripheral vascular disease, and a small brachial artery allowing the use of a small caliper guide catheter (6F) not compatible with the first-generation thrombectomy catheter (5F).

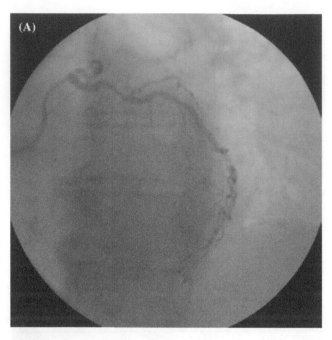

Figure 7.17A Proximal LAD occlusion.

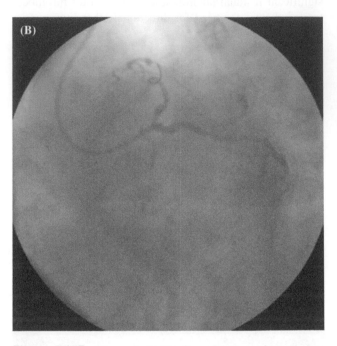

Figure 7.17B The optimized left-caudal view shows a true ostial LAD lesion.

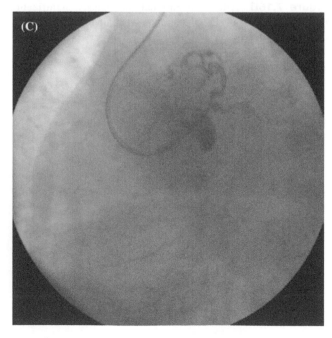

Figure 7.17C A wire crosses the lesion, but the tortuosity of the vessel prevents an easy distal placement of the wire.

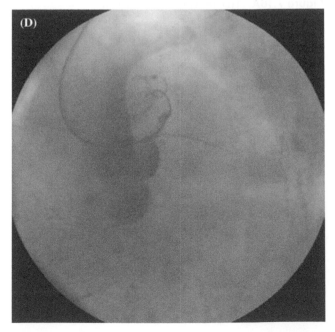

Figure 7.17D Angioplasty of the ostium is followed by embolic occlusion of the circumflex artery and the immediate mechanical cardiac arrest and death.

CASE 7.18 A CRUSHED OPPONENT

The friable nature of the thrombus explains the frequent occurrence of restoring some flow after crossing the wire or the dual lumen catheter for ultraselective dye injection.

The mechanical lysis achieved by the wire movements and the restored flow may result in an apparently insignificant thrombotic burden with a low risk of embolization produced by direct stenting.

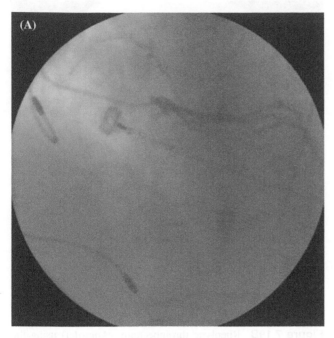

Figure 7.18A Proximal occlusion of the LAD.

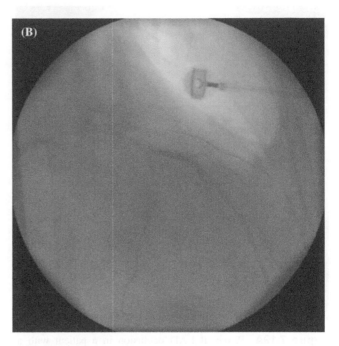

Figure 7.18B Placement of two wires in the LAD and circumflex artery. Ultraselective dye injection beyond the occlusion shows that the distal part of the LAD wire is placed in a major septal branch.

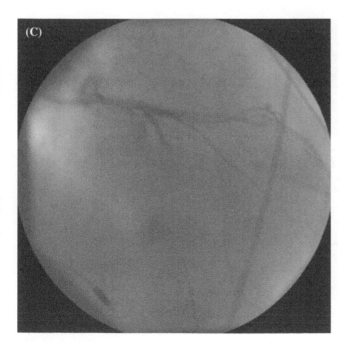

Figure 7.18C After correct repositioning of the LAD wire, some flow is restored and the angiography reveals that the target lesion is far from the ostium. Moreover there is no evidence of large thrombotic burden.

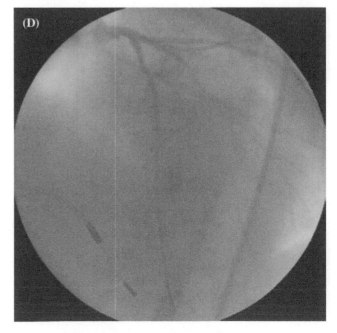

Figure 7.18D After direct stenting.

CASE 7.19 STENT WAS NOT THE REAL CULPRIT

The absence of residual thrombus or large thrombotic burden after thrombectomy allows a safe direct stenting procedure of proximal LAD.

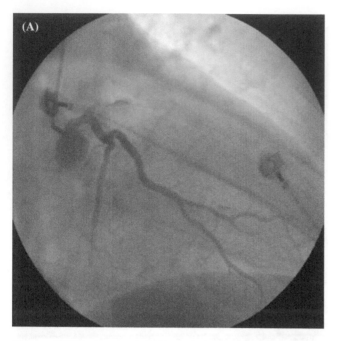

Figure 7.19A Proximal LAD occlusion in a patient with a history of previous stenting of the mid-portion of the LAD.

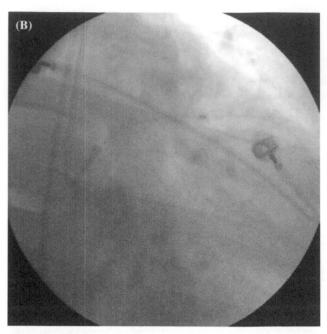

Figure 7.19B Rheolytic thrombectomy (AngioJet) using the first-generation AngioJet catheter.

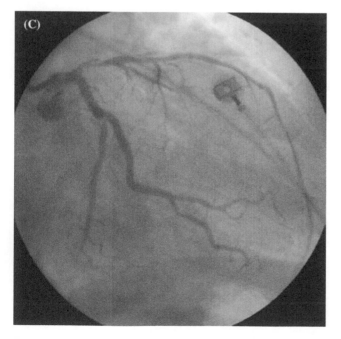

Figure 7.19C After thrombectomy evidence of an ulcerated plaque in the first segment of LAD and residual thrombosis after this new lesion at the level of the middle portion of the vessel.

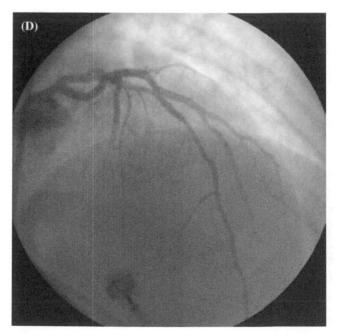

Figure 7.19D After direct stenting of the proximal lesion.

CASE 7.20 AN OCCLUSION WITH A FOREIGN ACCENT

The absence of angiographic signs of atherosclerosis and the angiographic aspect of the occlusion as revealed by ultraselective dye injection suggests an embolic nature of the vessel occlusion.

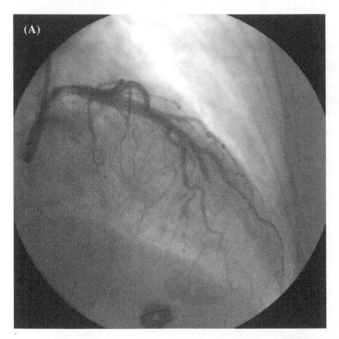

Figure 7.20A Distal occlusion of the LAD in a patient with atrial fibrillation.

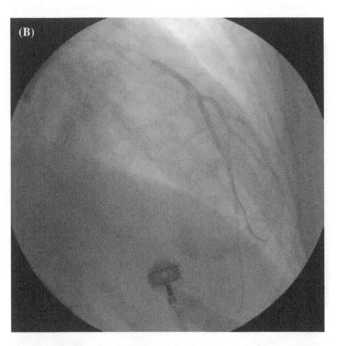

Figure 7.20B Ultraselective dye injection shows large filling defects, while there is no evidence of disrupted plaque.

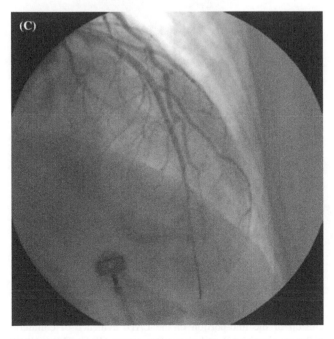

Figure 7.20C Restoration of a normal flow with same residual thrombosis after thrombectomy. No further intervention.

CASE 7.21 WHETHER YOU LIKE IT OR NOT

In elderly patients, as well as in patients under dialysis, the atherosclerotic process is diffuse and may be largely dominant over the thrombotic component of the occlusion. In these extreme cases of old, diffuse, and calcified lesions, the electrocardiographic presentation of the infarction may be with or without ST-segment elevation according to the presence and efficacy of a collateral flow.

The technical issues are the same as in chronic occlusions, and administration of glycoprotein IIb/IIIa inhibitors is absolutely contraindicated, at least before crossing the occlusion. Keep in mind that successfully crossing the occlusion cannot close the multiple prior perforations produced by the wire, and the risk of bleeding into the pericardium is strongly increased and not easily reversed after glycoprotein IIb/IIIa inhibitors administration.

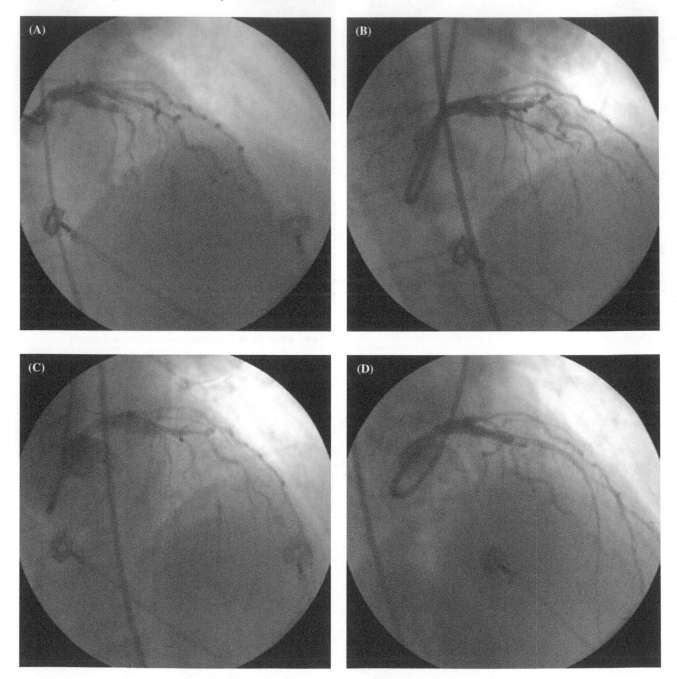

Figure 7.21A–D (A) Long occlusion of the mid-portion of the LAD; evidence of collateral flow to the distal LAD and diffuse atherosclerosis and calcification of the proximal LAD and circumflex artery. (B–C) The occlusion could be crossed with a hydrophilic strong wire and after multiple attempts. The distal part of the wire often went out of the vessel. (D) After rotational atherectomy and adjunctive angioplasty.

CASE 7.22 OLD PLAN BALLOON ANGIOPLASTY AND STENTING FOR OLD LESIONS

Another example of dominance of the atherosclerotic process over the thrombotic component in a patient with severe diffuse disease. No need for thrombectomy or antiembolic protection devices.

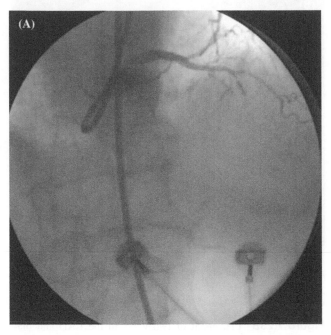

Figure 7.22A Occlusion of the proximal LAD and evidence of diffuse disease.

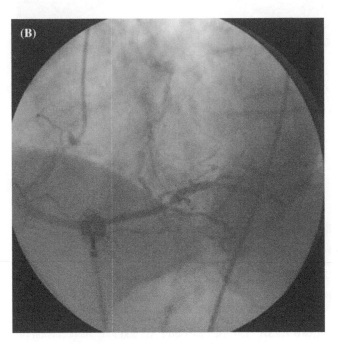

Figure 7.22B Right coronary angiogram shows collateral flow to the LAD.

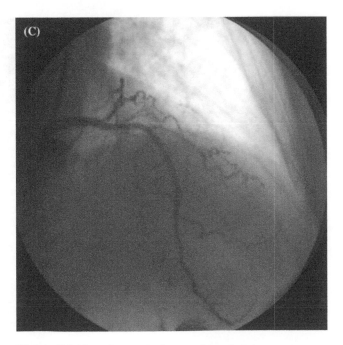

Figure 7.22C After angioplasty and stenting.

CASE 7.23 WHAT SIZE DO YOU TAKE?

Keep in mind that for correct selection of balloon angio-plasty and stent diameters, the baseline angiography in diffuse disease in the setting of acute coronary occlusion or subocclusion invariably underestimates the true vessel reference diameter. The use of undersized devices will negatively affect the procedural result. A suboptimal angiographic result is one of the stronger predictors of early and late target vessel failure.

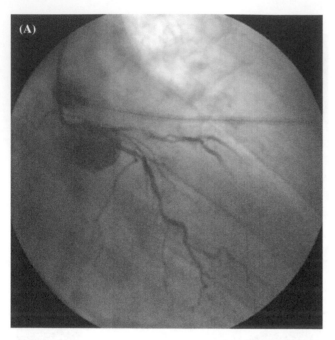

Figure 7.23A Diffuse diseased LAD and long subocclusion of the proximal segment of the LAD involving the origin of the first diagonal branch.

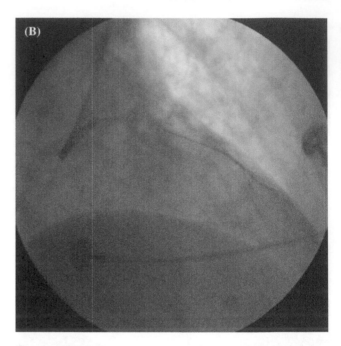

Figure 7.23B Placement of two wires in the LAD and diagonal branch.

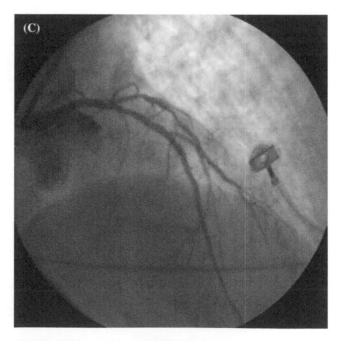

Figure 7.23C After angioplasty and spot stenting of the two branches.

CASE 7.24 IT IS NOT SMALL—IT IS DISEASED

A minimal approach in severe diffuse disease resulting in apparent "small" vessels should be considered the more effective and reliable strategy.

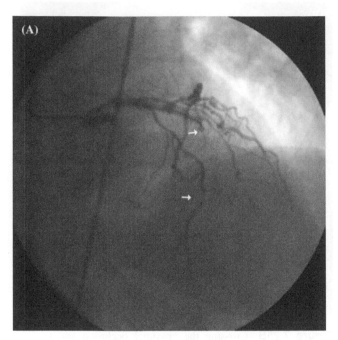

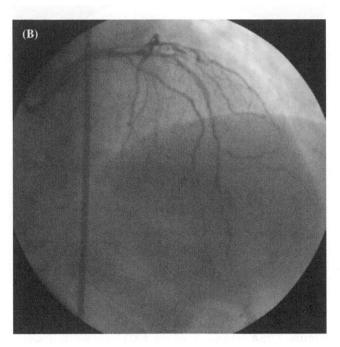

Figure 7.24A Occlusion of the diagonal branch of a dual LAD and subocclusion of the septal branch (*arrows*). Diffuse disease resulting in very small lumen diameters of the entire left coronary system.

Figure 7.24B After angioplasty of the two branches and spot stenting of the diagonal branch.

CASE 7.25 TO OPEN, OR NOT TO OPEN

The indication for the treatment of a chronic occlusion distally to an acute occlusion is questionable because the benefit is unknown, while the procedural risk is increased. A short "soft" attempt may be justified.

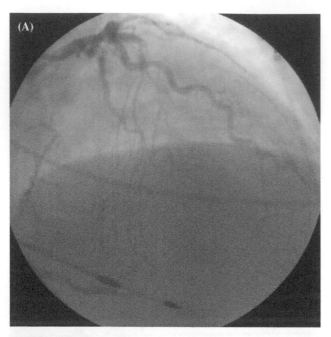

Figure 7.25A Occlusion of the LAD after the first septal branch; diffuse disease of the circumflex artery and collateral flow to the right coronary artery.

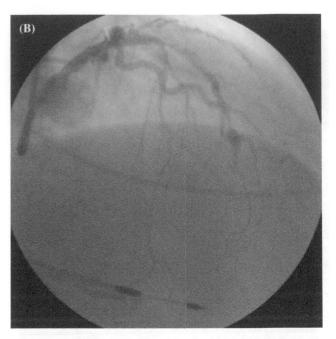

Figure 7.25B Crossing the proximal occlusion and angioplasty; evidence of diffuse disease of the LAD beyond the acute occlusion including a chronic occlusion at the distal segment.

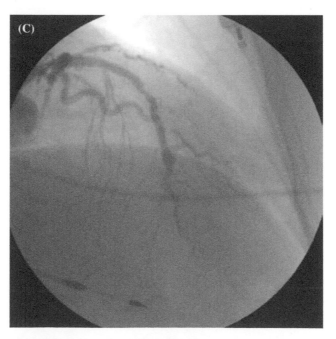

Figure 7.25C After stenting at level of the acute occlusion and angioplasty of the chronic occlusion.

CASE 7.26 HANDLE WITH CARE

Acute occlusion of a venous graft is invariably associated with massive thrombosis. The use of thrombectomy or antiembolic protection devices is mandatory, since extensive embolization complicating a conventional procedure may deteriorate a residual collateral flow and result in further clinical deterioration.

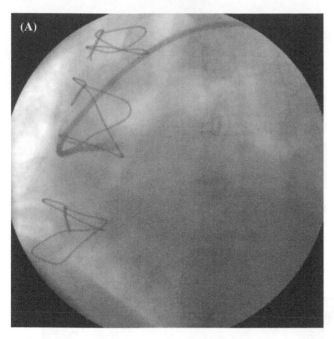

Figure 7.26A Proximal occlusion of a venous graft to LAD; evidence of massive thrombosis.

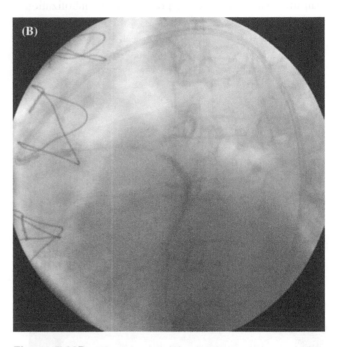

Figure 7.26B Ultraselective injection beyond the occlusion allows the assessment of the length of the occlusion.

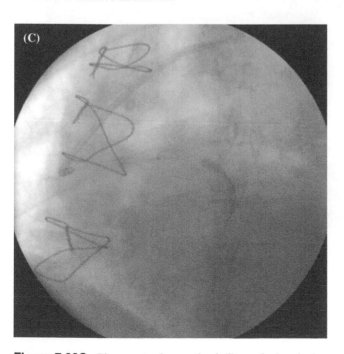

Figure 7.26C Placement of an antiembolic occlusive device and direct stenting.

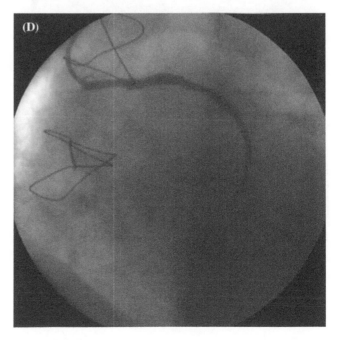

Figure 7.26D After aspiration and removal of the antiembolic protection device.

CASE 7.27 GET IT UNDER THE COVER

Direct stenting using a covered stent may be effective in venous graft occlusion. This approach may be considered in grafts without the angiographic appearance of diffuse disease and degeneration. The covering of the stent jails the atherothrombotic plaque, preventing embolization. Keep in mind that the stent must be abundantly longer than the lesion for effective prevention of embolization.

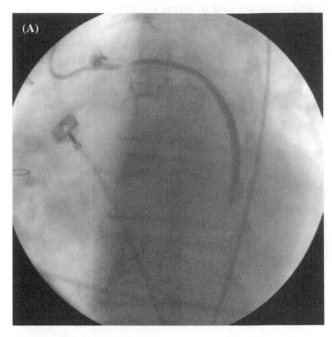

Figure 7.27A Subocclusion coats the proximal segment of a venous graft to LAD.

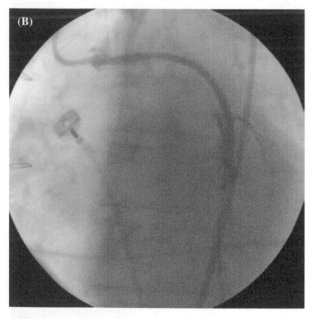

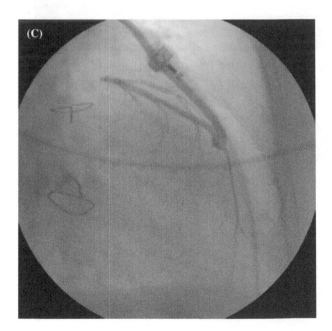

Figure 7.27B, C After direct stenting using a covered stent.

CASE 7.28 A COMPULSORY JAIL

Failure to restore a good flow with conventional angioplasty explains the need for multiple stents of this long dissection.

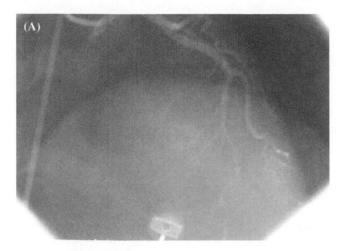

Figure 7.28A Spontaneous subocclusive dissection of the third tract of the LAD.

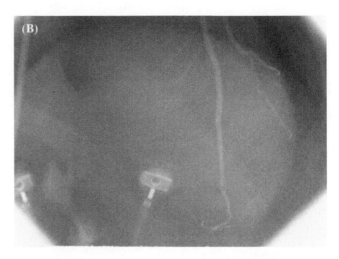

Figure 7.28B Complete coverage of the dissection by multiple stenting.

8

Left Circumflex Artery (LCX)

RENATO VALENTI AND ANGELA MIGLIORINI
Division of Cardiology, Careggi Hospital, Florence, Italy

CASE 8.1 AN INHOSPITABLE VESSEL

As in elective procedures, an unfavorable takeoff of the LCX for intervention is frequent. In this case, the technical approach should include an extra-backup guide catheter and a high support wire.

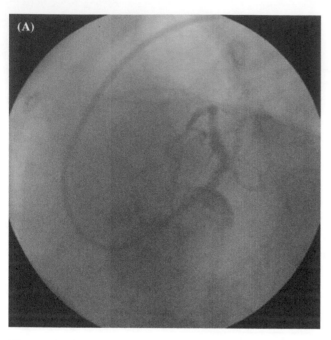

Figure 8.1A Proximal LCX occlusion; the takeoff of the vessel is followed by a sharp bend in the opposite direction of the ostium of the vessel.

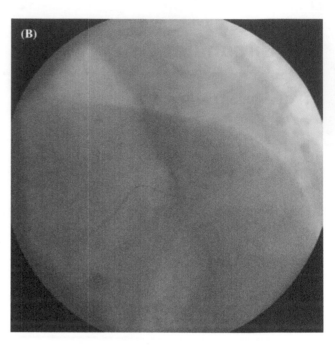

Figure 8.1B Need for a support of the wire, and advancement of an angioplasty balloon to cross the occlusion by the wire.

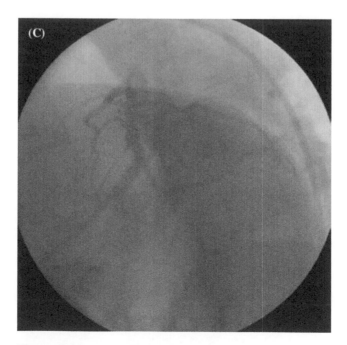

Figure 8.1C After stenting of the entire first tract of LCX.

CASE 8.2 AN INHOSPITABLE VESSEL-2

The procedure was successfully performed using an extra-backup guide catheter and high support wire.

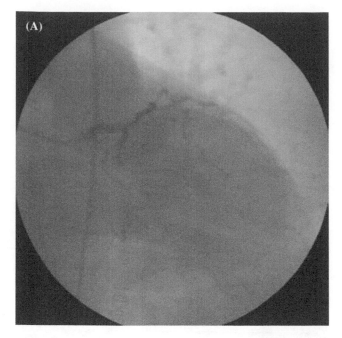

Figure 8.2A Subocclusion of a tortuous first obtuse marginal branch.

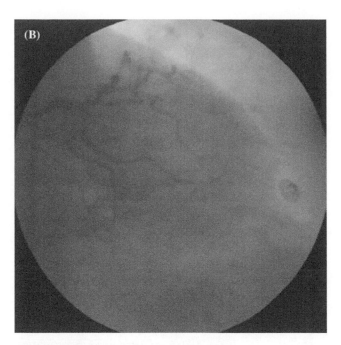

Figure 8.2B After angioplasty and stenting.

CASE 8.3 AN INHOSPITABLE VESSEL-3

An extra-backup guide catheter and high support wire are needed for very distal LCX occlusion, since the stent invariably has to cross at least two opposite bends.

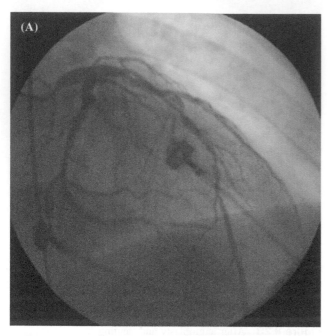

Figure 8.3A Distal occlusion of LCX.

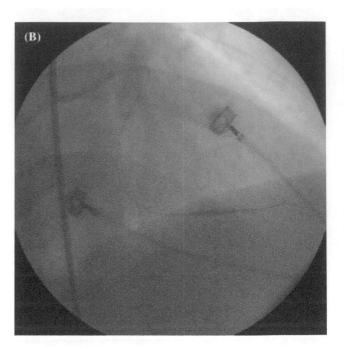

Figure 8.3B Direct stenting.

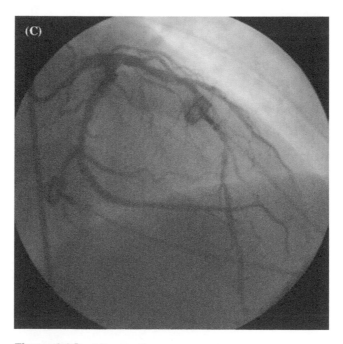

Figure 8.3C After stenting.

CASE 8.4 NOT TOO SMALL

An area at risk larger than expected for the occlusion of a retroventricular branch, or obtuse marginal branch, or diagonal branch is relatively frequent. The potential for this mismatch questions the concept of "small infarction" as a consequence of the occlusion of a small vessel.

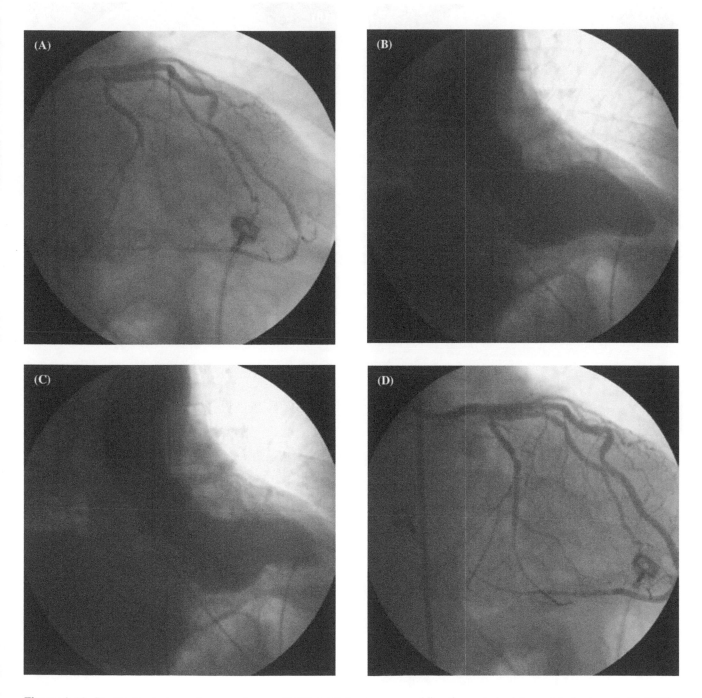

Figure 8.4A–D (A) Occlusion at the second tract of LCX; LAD dominance providing the posterior interventricular branch. (B–C) The occlusion of the distal retroventricular branch is associated with expansion of the posterobasal segment of the left ventricle. (D) After stenting.

CASE 8.5 THE BARE NECESSITIES

Diffuse disease, distal location of the occlusion, and the small lumen of the target vessel suggest the opportunity of a traditional minimal approach.

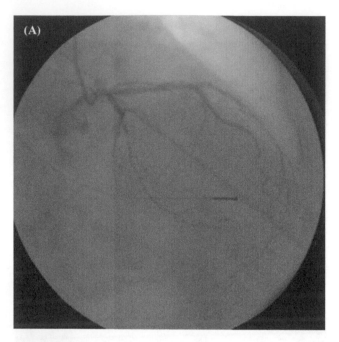

Figure 8.5A Distal occlusion of LCX.

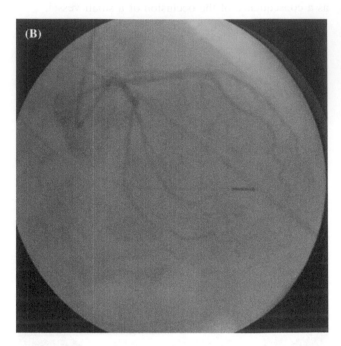

Figure 8.5B After angioplasty and spot stenting.

CASE 8.6 A COMFORTABLE FORK

The diffuse disease of the dominant left main system suggests the opportunity to treat the target lesion alone. The uncommonly favorable takeoff of LAD and LCX from the large left main allows direct stenting of the ostium of the LCX with a relatively low risk of plaque shift.

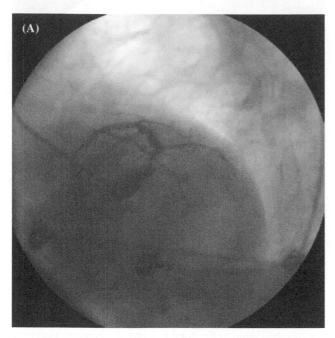

Figure 8.6A Ostial occlusion of LCX and diffuse disease of the LAD.

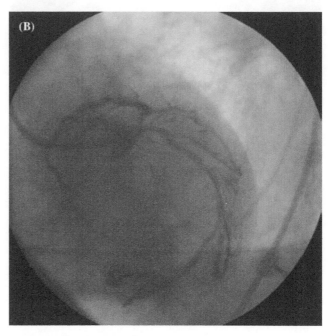

Figure 8.6B The crossing of the wire restores the flow and confirms the diffuse disease extending to a dominant LCX; there is no evidence of thrombus at the level of the target lesion.

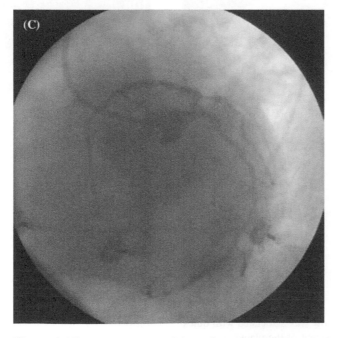

Figure 8.6C Direct stenting of the ostium of the LCX.

CASE 8.7 AUTOTHROMBECTOMY?

The restoring of flow may strongly facilitate the rapid lysis of the thrombotic component of the occlusion allowing the simple approach of direct stenting.

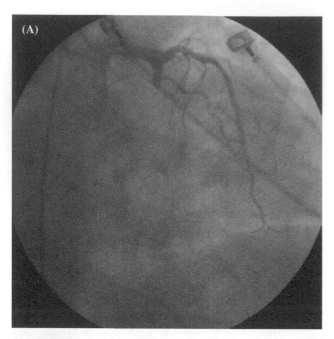

Figure 8.7A Proximal occlusion of a dominant LCX.

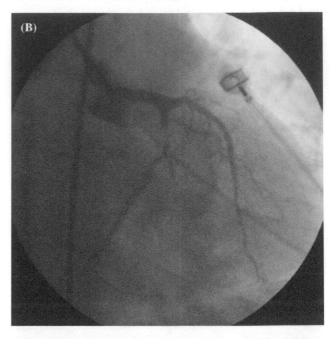

Figure 8.7B After the placement of the wire, evidence of macroembolization to the distal bed and of a complex disrupted plaque involving the first marginal branch.

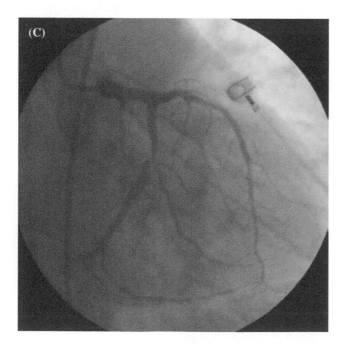

Figure 8.7C Restoring of the flow was associated with quick reduction of the thrombotic component of the plaque.

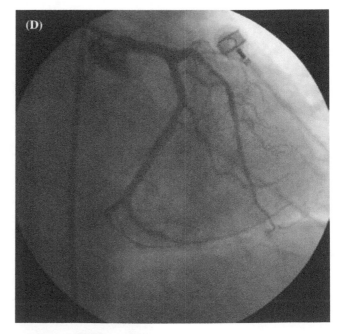

Figure 8.7D Direct stenting.

CASE 8.8 TO CHOOSE THE LESSER OF TWO EVILS

A major disadvantage of antiembolic protection devices (occlusive devices, filters) is that the protection is limited only to the main vessel.

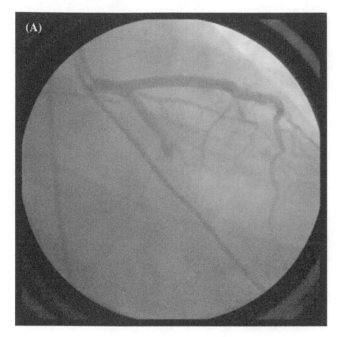

Figure 8.8A Occlusion of the proximal LCX.

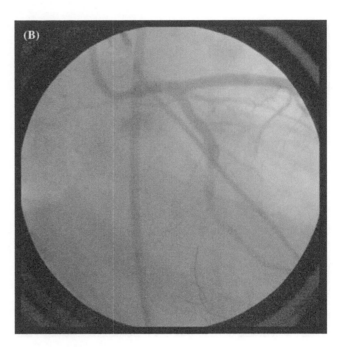

Figure 8.8B After crossing of the wire, evidence of thrombosis immediately before a bifurcation, and placement of an occlusive antiembolic protection (GuardWire) device in one of the two branches of the bifurcation.

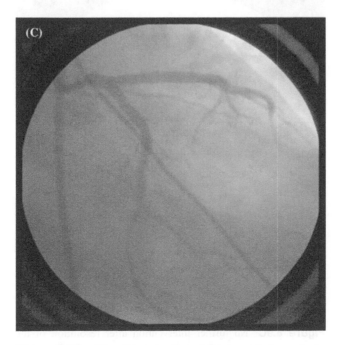

Figure 8.8C After direct stenting of the target lesion.

CASE 8.9 A VERY TOUCHY VESSEL GETS OFFENDED FOR NOTHING

Rheolytic thrombectomy and the straightening of the very tortuous vessel by the wire and the device both may favor intense diffuse spasm of the target vessel.

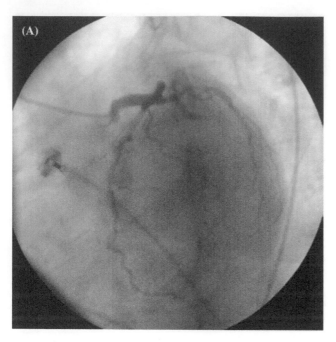

Figure 8.9A Proximal occlusion of the LCX.

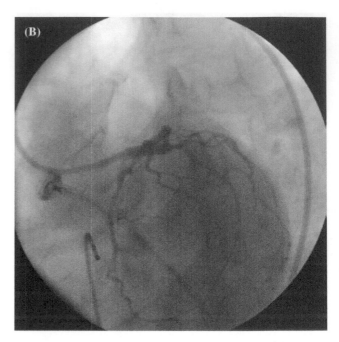

Figure 8.9B After rheolytic thrombectomy diffuse severe spasm of the vessel.

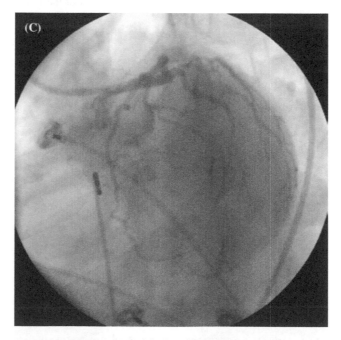

Figure 8.9C No further intervention after resolution of the spasm.

CASE 8.10 A PROVISIONAL JAIL

Thrombectomy is mandatory in the acute occlusion of the last vessel. Residual thrombus after repeat passages of the thrombectomy device suggests that the thrombus is not too friable and that direct stenting may jail it without significant embolization.

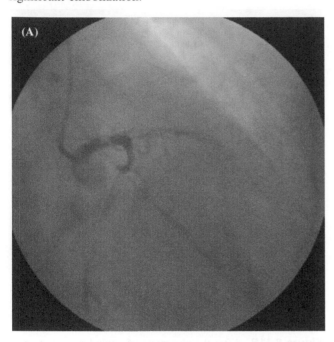
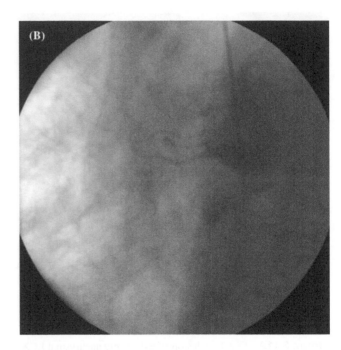

Figure 8.10A,B Acute occlusion of proximal LCX and chronic occlusion of the LAD at the ostium and RCA at the first tract.

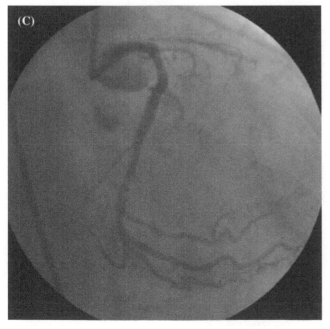
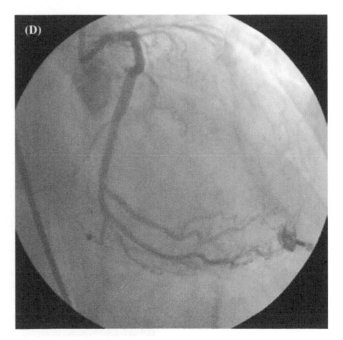

Figure 8.10C Rheolytic thrombectomy (AngioJet) restores a good flow; residual large thrombus in the distal portion of the LCX despite repeat passages of the device.

Figure 8.10D Direct stenting.

CASE 8.11 AN OPEN JAIL

The mesh stent was the first choice device to treat this large aneurysm. The length of the aneurysm and the large marginal branch arising from the aneurysm prevented the use of a single, covered stent.

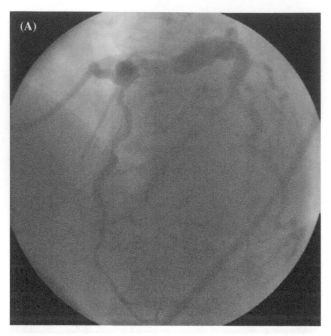

Figure 8.11A   Distal occlusion of a diffusely aneurysmal LCX.

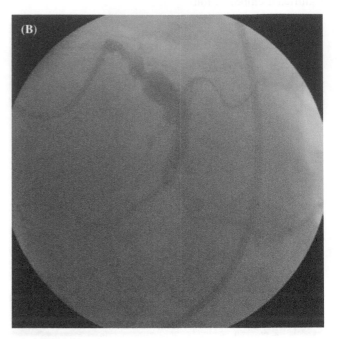

Figure 8.11B   After the placement of a tubular short stent of the distal LCX occlusion.

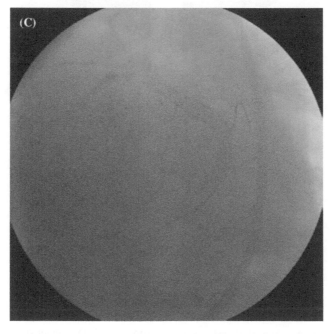

Figure 8.11C   Placement of a wire protection in the large marginal branch arising from the aneurysm and of a long mesh stent to cover all the aneurismal tract.

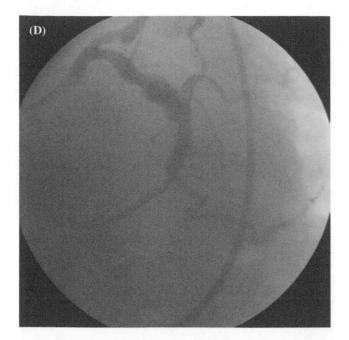

Figure 8.11D Acute angiographic result.

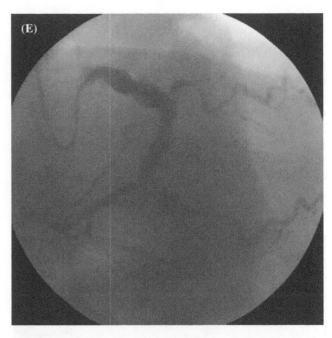

Figure 8.11E The angiographic control after 24 hours shows a nearly completed obliteration of the extrastent aneurysmal sac.

CASE 8.12 A SLIGHT IMPERFECTION

The origin of the LCX from RCA or from the right
coronary sinus is the more frequent coronary anomaly.
Generally, the technical approach is easy using a multipurpose guide catheter for the engagement of the LCX
ostium. Alternative guide catheters are the right Amplatz
2 or the left Amplatz 1. The more difficult step of the
procedure may be the crossing of the stent through the
sharp bend of the proximal vessel. Multipurpose catheter
allows the deep intubation of the vessel, while the
Amplatz curve catheters may provide a strong backup.

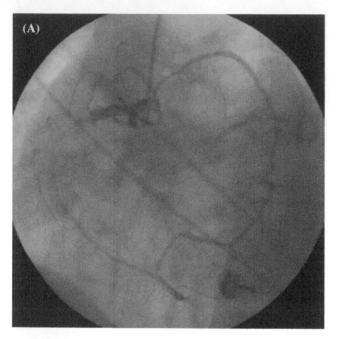

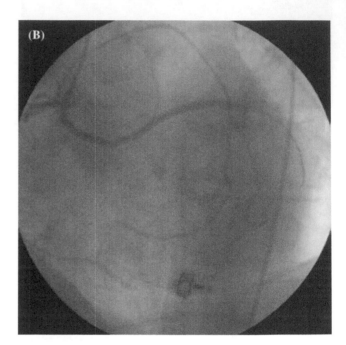

Figure 8.12A Acute proximal occlusion of the LCX arising
from the RCA; chronic occlusion of the RCA; collateral flow to
RCA by a large atrial branch communicating directly with the
retroventricular branch of the RCA.

Figure 8.12B After angioplasty and stenting.

CASE 8.13 A GOOD FISHING

This case directly shows the embolus entrapment ability
of the AngioGuard device.

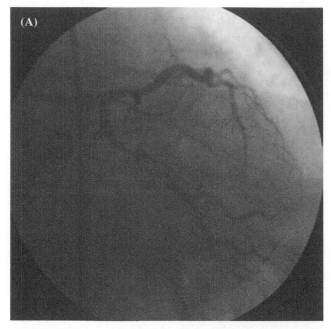

Figure 8.13A Large thrombus distal to severe stenosis of the
proximal LCX.

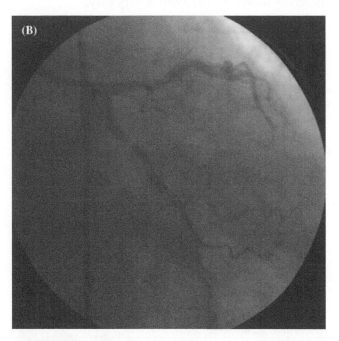

Figure 8.13B Migration and entrapment of the thrombus into
the basket of a filter (AngioGuard).

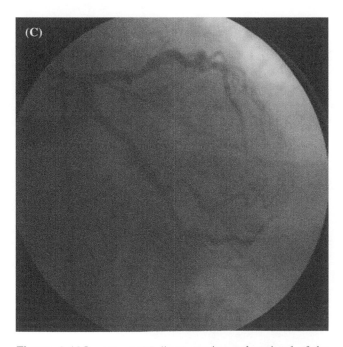

Figure 8.13C After LCX direct stenting and retrieval of the
AngioGuard.

CASE 8.14 A HOSPITABLE VESSEL

The intermediate branch may arise independently from the
left main or as the more proximal branch of the LCX or
LAD. The independent and straight origin of the vessel
generally makes the intervention very easy.

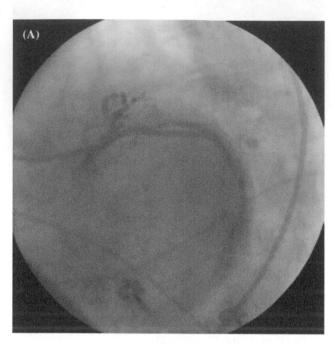

Figure 8.14A Proximal occlusion of the intermediate branch
arising independently from the left main.

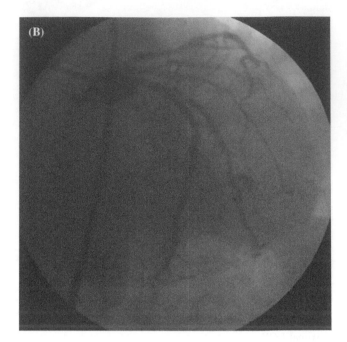

Figure 8.14B After angioplasty and stenting.

9

Left Main Trunk (LMT)

RENATO VALENTI AND ANGELA MIGLIORINI
Division of Cardiology, Careggi Hospital, Florence, Italy

CASE 9.1 TO MAKE SOMEONE'S LIFE DIFFICULT

Despite the dramatic clinical scenario of acute left main occlusion, this case could be treated easily by direct

stenting. The intervention was strongly facilitated by the restoring of a normal flow after crossing of the wires and prompt reversal of cardiogenic shock, and the nondirect involvement of the three ostia of the trifurcation in the very focal distal lesion of the LMT.

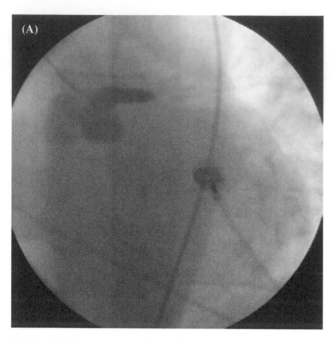

Figure 9.1A   Occlusion of the LMT.

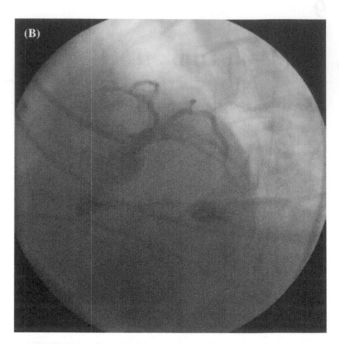

Figure 9.1B   After the placement of two wires in the LCX and LAD, restoring of the flow and evidence of a distal target lesion apparently involving a trifurcation (LAD, intermediate, and LCX).

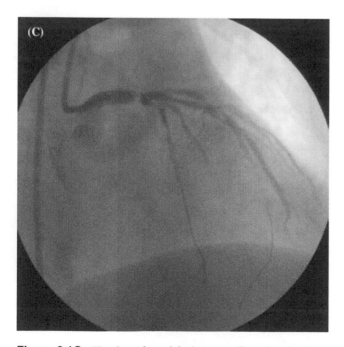

Figure 9.1C   The frontal-caudal view revealing that the three ostia are not directly involved in the left main lesion.

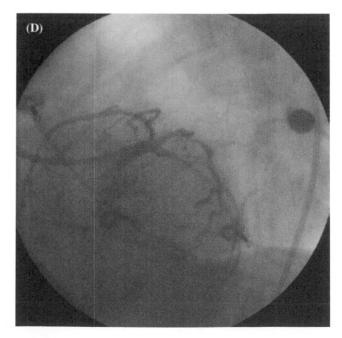

Figure 9.1D   Placement of a third wire into the intermediate branch and direct stenting of the distal LMT.

CASE 9.2 TO HURRY UP

The "V" stenting technique in the setting of acute LMT bifurcation occlusion and subsequent profound shock has some major advantages such as the ease and rapidity of the procedure. This technique provides a new carina and cannot be used in small or short left main, and in the presence of a large intermediate branch arising from LMT.

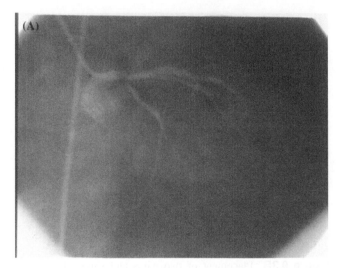

Figure 9.2A   Distal occlusion of the LMT involving the ostia of LAD and LCX.

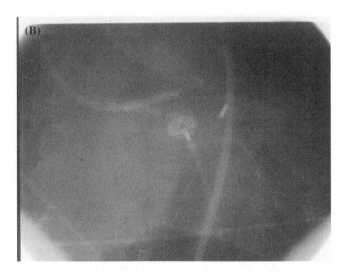

Figure 9.2B   Kissing balloon of the bifurcation.

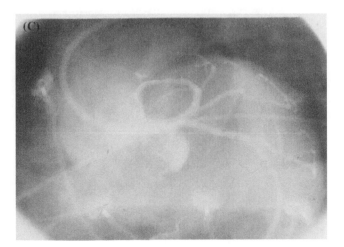

Figure 9.2C   After "V" stenting of the bifurcation.

CASE 9.3 PLAN OLD STENTING

The Gianturco–Roubin stent is no longer available due to
the low mechanical performance of stent (high elastic
acute recoil, high rate of plaque prolapsing, and high late
restenosis rate). However, the ease and quickness of Y
stenting technique for bifurcation lesions using this type
of stent remains unsurpassed.

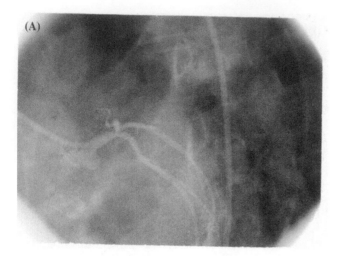

Figure 9.3A Proximal occlusion of the LAD and severe
stenosis of the distal LMT.

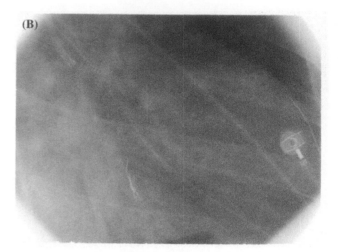

Figure 9.3B Placement of two wires and single stenting of
LAD occlusion and Y stenting of LMT-LCX-LAD using two
coil stents (Gianturco–Roubin stent).

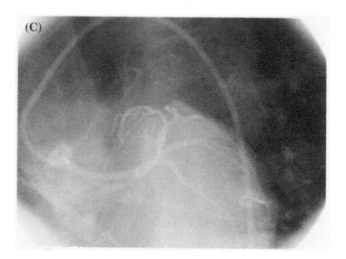

Figure 9.3C After stenting.

CASE 9.4 BE PREPARED FOR EVERY EVENTUALITY

The anomalous origin of LMT from the right coronary sinus is exceptionally uncommon. A large first septal branch before the true bifurcation provides flow to the upper portion of interventricular septum. The engagement of the ostium by the guide catheter may be really troublesome due to the origin of the ostium from the upper part of the right sinus. In this case, the engagement of the ostium was made possible by a right Amplatz curve catheter.

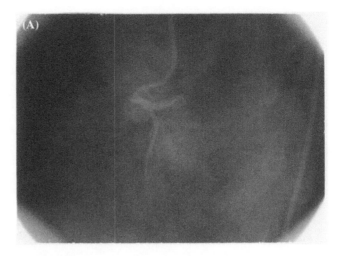

Figure 9.4A Acute occlusion of an LMT arising from the right coronary sinus. A large septal branch arises proximally to the LMT bifurcation.

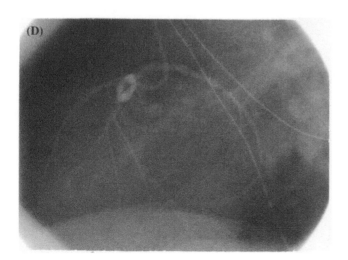

Figure 9.4B A second dye injection revealing some flow in the long LMT allows the recognition of a mild stenosis before the bifurcation as the target lesion and diffuse disease of the LCX.

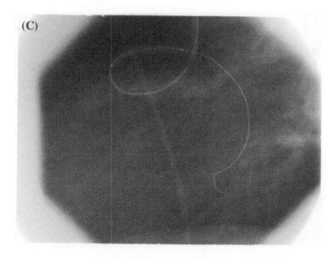

Figure 9.4C Placement of a stent in the proximal LCX.

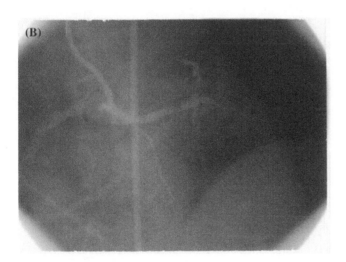

Figure 9.4D After LCX stenting.

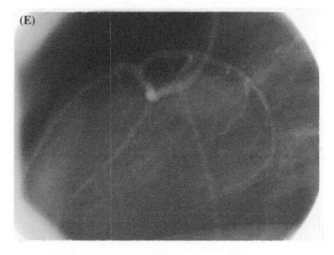

Figure 9.4E After direct stenting of the LMT.

10

Multivessel Coronary Intervention

RENATO VALENTI AND ANGELA MIGLIORINI
Division of Cardiology, Careggi Hospital, Florence, Italy

CASE 10.1 TEA FOR TWO

Multiple vessel intervention in the setting of acute myocardial infarction is indicated in patients with severe left
ventricular dysfunction. Particularly in patients with
cardiogenic shock, severe stenosis of vessels other than
the infarct artery may be flow limiting, producing ischemia of remote ventricular regions resulting in further
deterioration of the hemodynamic status.

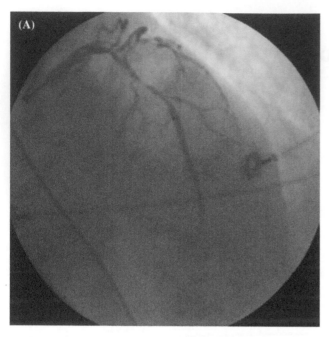

Figure 10.1A Occlusion of the distal LAD and severe stenosis
of the middle portion of the vessel.

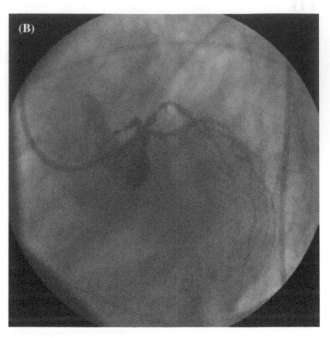

Figure 10.1B The left-caudal view shows severe stenosis of
the intermediate branch.

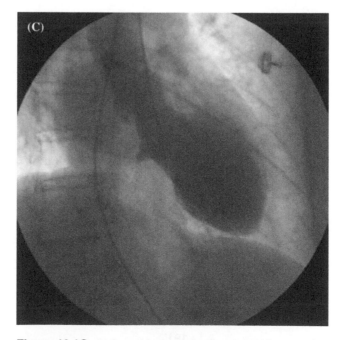

Figure 10.1C Left ventriculography showing wide expansion
of the area at risk.

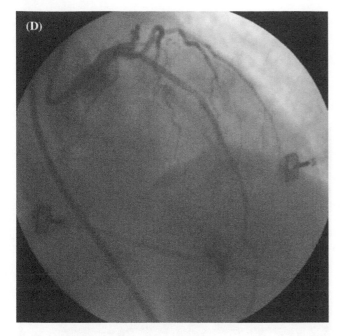

Figure 10.1D After LAD stenting.

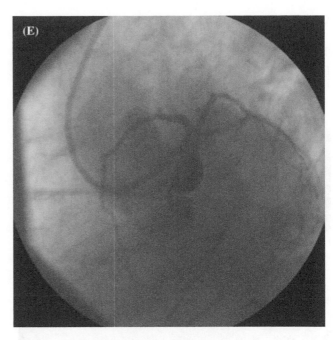

Figure 10.1E After stenting of the intermediate branch.

CASE 10.2 TEA FOR TWO-2

The two-vessel occlusion was associated with a state of profound cardiogenic shock. The treatment of both vessels is mandatory.

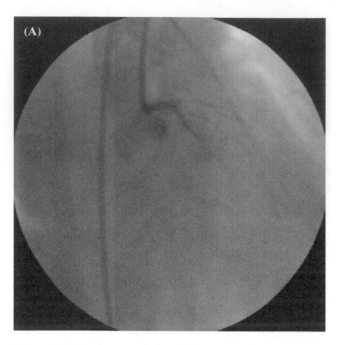 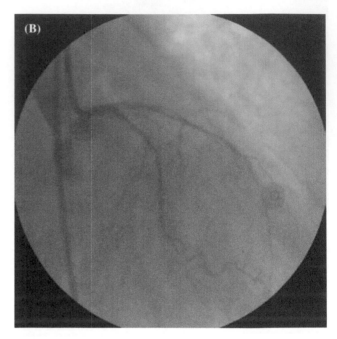

Figure 10.2A Acute occlusion of the LAD and LCX.

Figure 10.2B After stenting of LCX and angioplasty of the LAD.

CASE 10.3 TEA FOR TWO-3

The indication for double vessel intervention was supported by a state of cardiogenic shock.

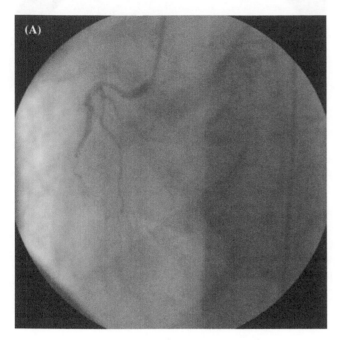

Figure 10.3A Acute mid-portion RCA occlusion.

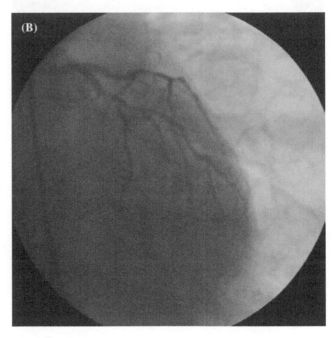

Figure 10.3B Severe, long stenosis of the LCX.

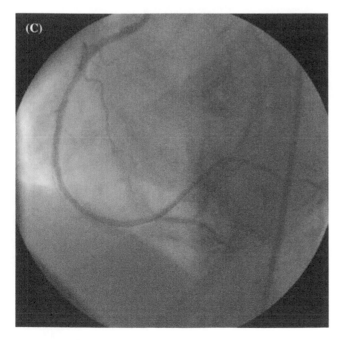

Figure 10.3C After RCA intervention (angioplasty and spot stenting).

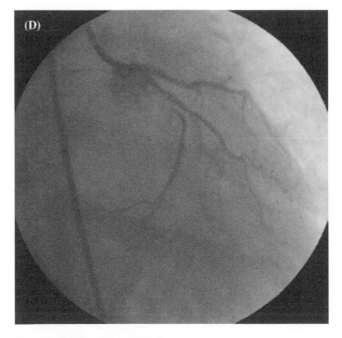

Figure 10.3D After LCX direct stenting.

CASE 10.4 TEA FOR TWO-4

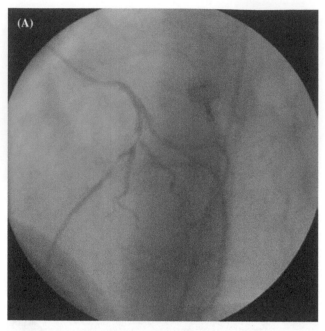

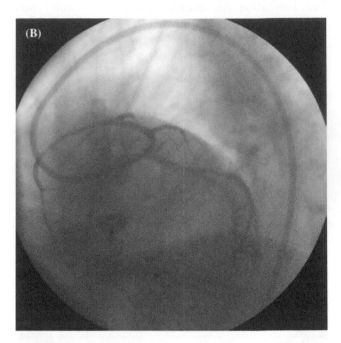

Figure 10.4A Two subocclusive lesions of the LAD and subocclusion of the proximal portion of the LCX.

Figure 10.4B After stenting of both vessels.

CASE 10.5 TEA FOR TWO-5

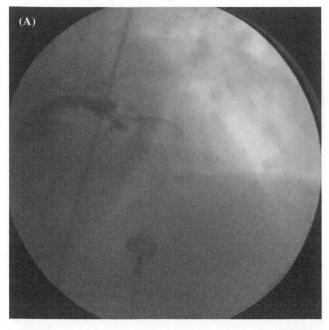

Figure 10.5A Acute occlusion of proximal LAD and LCX.

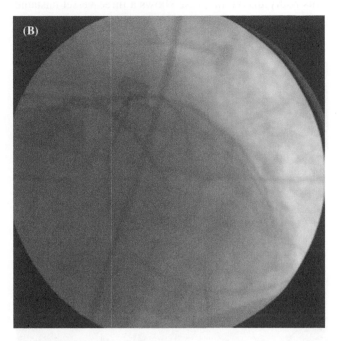

Figure 10.5B Placement of two wires in the LCX and LAD.

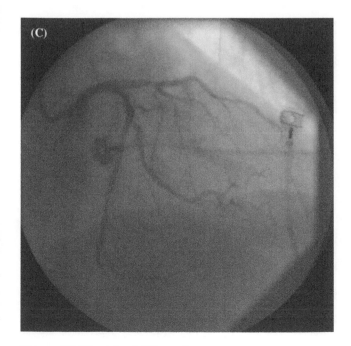

Figure 10.5C After LCX stenting.

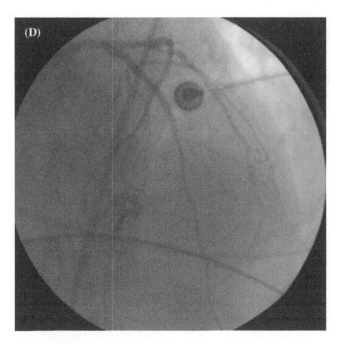

Figure 10.5D After LAD stenting.

CASE 10.6 TEA FOR THREE

This really uncommon case shows a three-vessel unstable plaque with occlusive thrombosis of the LAD and subocclusive thrombosis of the LCX and RCA. The dominant thrombotic component of the multivessel disease indicates thrombectomy as the best initial interventional approach.

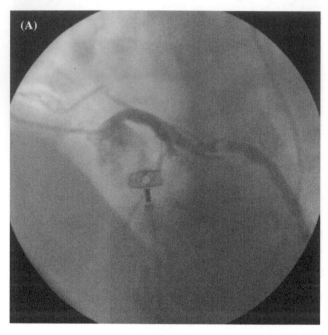

Figure 10.6A Left cranial view showing acute occlusion of the LAD and severe stenosis followed by a large thrombus in the proximal LCX.

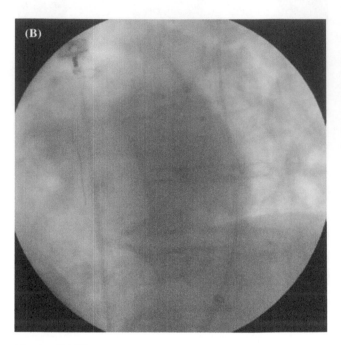

Figure 10.6B Placement of two wires in the LAD and CX; rheolytic thrombectomy (AngioJet) of the two vessels.

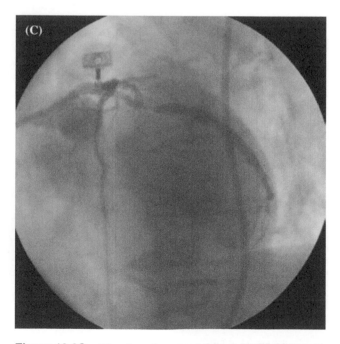

Figure 10.6C After thrombectomy of the LAD and LCX.

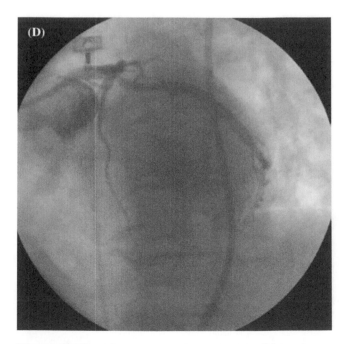

Figure 10.6D After stenting of both vessels.

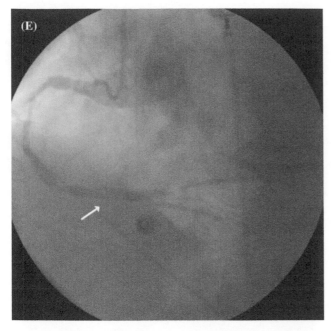

Figure 10.6E Long stenosis of the middle portion of the RCA and angiographic evidence of a large thrombus in the distal RCA (*arrow*).

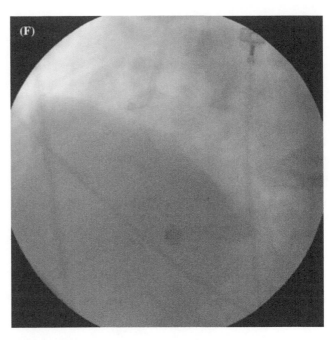

Figure 10.6F Rheolytic thrombectomy (AngioJet).

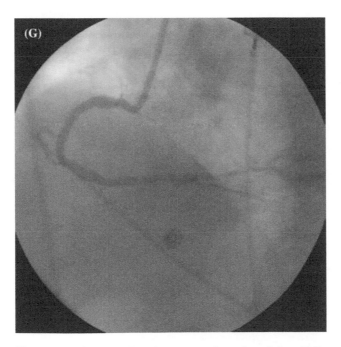

Figure 10.6G After thrombectomy and stenting of the middle portion of the RCA.

Section 4

The Efficacy Perspective

11

Primary Percutaneous Coronary Intervention for Acute Myocardial Infarction in the "Real World"

RENATO VALENTI AND EMILIO VINCENZO DOVELLINI

Division of Cardiology, Careggi Hospital, Florence, Italy

GIOVANNI MARIA SANTORO

Division of Cardiology, San Giovanni di Dio Hospital, Florence, Italy

THE EFFECTIVENESS OF PERCUTANEOUS MECHANICAL INTERVENTION FOR ACUTE MYOCARDIAL INFARCTION

The efficacy of fibrinolytic therapy for patients with acute myocardial infarction (AMI) is not strictly dependent on logistic models, and the results of the treatment are easily foreseen in large populations and in community hospitals and tertiary referral centers. On the contrary, the efficacy of primary mechanical interventions for AMI is quite changeable and dependent on many variables related to the logistic model used for the application of the primary angioplasty program.

Most randomized trials comparing primary percutaneous coronary intervention (PCI) with fibrinolysis have shown that primary PCI provides a better outcome, and this may be easily explained mainly by the achievement of infarct artery recanalization and restoration of a brisk flow in the large majority of patients and subsequent improved myocardial salvage and survival. However, the GUSTO (Global Utilization of STreptokinase and t-PA for Occluded coronary arteries)-IIb trial and survey studies from the United States and France, based on thousands of patients,

have shown no difference in mortality between the two modalities of treatment (1–6). When the strategy of primary PCI is adopted in the "real world," its effectiveness may be lower than the one achieved in high-volume centers. A prospective observational study of the National Registry of Myocardial Infarction (NRMI) investigators, based on outcome analysis of a cohort of 27,080 consecutive patients with AMI who were treated with primary PCI in 661 community and tertiary care hospitals in the United States, showed a strong relationship between increased mortality and delay in door-to-balloon time longer than two hours (3,4). The adjusted odds of in-hospital mortality did not increase significantly with increasing delay from AMI symptom onset to first balloon inflation, while the adjusted odds of mortality were significantly increased by 41% to 62% for patients with door-to-balloon times longer than two hours. The importance of the door-to-balloon time has been established also by GUSTO-IIb investigators who demonstrated that in the GUSTO-IIb patient cohort, patients treated within one hour of hospital arrival had a mortality rate of 1%, whereas those delayed for 61 to 75 minutes, 76 to 90 minutes, and >91 minutes had a mortality rate of 3.7%, 4.0%, and 6.4%, respectively ($p = 0.001$) (7).

Thus, door-to-balloon time may be considered a valid quality-of-care indicator, and should be minimized as much as possible to achieve good clinical results.

The U.S. real world in reperfusive treatment for AMI has changed dramatically in the last 15 years. Data collected in the NRMI from 1994 to 2005 that include 938,675 patients with ST-segment elevation myocardial infarction have shown impressive changes in the administration of reperfusive therapy and subsequent clinical outcome. The percentage of patients not receiving reperfusive therapy decreased from 45.3% in 1994 to 37.0% in 2005. The use of PCI increased from 6.9% to 38.8%, while fibrinolysis decreased from 47.0% to 22.7%. The median delay from symptom onset to hospital admission decreased from 2 to 1.6 hours, and the delay from hospital admission to PCI (door-to-balloon time) decreased from 125 to 98 minutes, with an increase of patients with a door-to-balloon time <90 minutes from 29.8% to 44.8%. Also the median time for transfer from hospital without PCI facilities to hospital with PCI facilities decreased from 2.8 to 1.8 hours. These changes in logistics were associated with a dramatic decrease in in-hospital mortality, from 8.6% in 1994 to 3.8% in 2005 (Williams DO, unpublished data).

The U.S. real world is not the only mirror of current clinical practice. Studies from Germany, Czech Republic, and Denmark have shown that nationwide high standards of care may be achieved.

In two German registries, MITRA (Maximal Individual Therapy in Acute Myocardial Infarction) and MIR (Myocardial Infraction Registry) (8), based on the outcome analysis of 9906 fibrinolysis-eligible patients with AMI, the mean time from admission to treatment was 30 minutes for fibrinolytic treatment and 70 minutes for PCI, nearly half of previous randomized and survey studies. The in-hospital mortality rate in 1327 patients undergoing primary PCI was 6.4%, while the mortality rate of patients receiving fibrinolytic treatment was 11.3% (OR 0.54; 95% CI, 0.43–0.67; $p < 0.001$).

The DANAMI-2 (Danish Multicenter Randomized Study on Thrombolytic Therapy vs. Acute Coronary Angioplasty in Acute Myocardial Infarction) trial compared primary PCI with fibrinolysis in 1572 patients with AMI (9). The trial was conducted in Denmark at 5 tertiary centers and 22 referral centers. The average transport distance from referral centers to invasive centers for patients randomized to PCI was 35 miles, and patients eligible for randomization to mechanical intervention should have a transfer time less than three hours from randomization. The trial was stopped prematurely since an interim analysis already showed a clear advantage of primary mechanical intervention: the primary end point of death, reinfarction, or disabling stroke occurred in 8% of the primary mechanical intervention group and in 13.7% of the fibrinolysis group (40% reduction in relative risk favoring mechanical intervention). The small number of enrolled patients, and the relatively low-risk population (eligible patients should be suitable for fibrinolysis, and patients with cardiogenic shock were excluded from enrolment) prevented the recognition of a significant difference in mortality between groups (7.8% in the fibrinolysis group, and 6.6% in the PCI group, $p = 0.35$), while the component of the composite primary end point that drove the difference between groups was reinfarction (6.3% in the fibrinolysis group, and 1.6% in the PCI group, $p < 0.001$).

The PRAGUE-2 (PRimary Angioplasty in patients transferred from General community hospitals to specialized PTCA Units with or without Emergency thrombolysis) trial compared primary PCI for patients with AMI transferred from community hospitals to tertiary referral centers with emergency fibrinolysis (10). The study was based on a sample of 850 patients with AMI, and excluded from enrolment patients with contraindication to fibrinolytic treatment, advanced cardiogenic shock, and patients with absence of femoral pulsation due to obstructive vascular atherosclerotic disease. The one-month mortality rate was 6.8% for the transfer PCI group, and 10% for the fibrinolysis group ($p = 0.12$). For patients who had the treatment from 3 to 12 hours from AMI onset, PCI provided a significant reduction in one-month mortality compared with fibrinolysis (6.0% vs. 15.3%, respectively; $p < 0.02$), while the mortality rates were nearly identical for patients who had the treatment within three hours from AMI onset (7.3% and 7.4%). It is important to highlight that in this real world nationwide study, the used logistic model allowed a very short delay from randomization to the administration of fibrinolytic treatment (12 minutes) and from admission to the tertiary center to the first balloon inflation (20 minutes). The results of the PRAGUE-2 trial suggest that PCI provides a great benefit compared with fibrinolysis for patients admitted to hospital with a delay from AMI onset of at least three hours, while for patients with very early hospital admission (within 3 hours from AMI onset), the two treatments are equally effective. This hypothesis is consistent with the results of previous studies that show fibrinolysis efficacy inversely related to time to treatment, while the relation for PCI and time to treatment is maintained only for the first two hours from symptom onset, and mortality does not increase with PCI accomplished between 2 and 12 hours from AMI onset.

However, the relationship between time to treatment and mortality in PCI-treated patients is very complex and deserves a specific comparative analysis with fibrinolysis-treated patients to avoid the risk of oversimplification of the issues related to the logistic models and organizative scenarios in PCI for AMI.

THE IMPACT OF TIME TO TREATMENT ON OUTCOME OF PATIENTS TREATED BY PCI FOR ACUTE MYOCARDIAL INFARCTION

It has been shown that the link between a successful reperfusion treatment and improved survival is myocardial salvage and improved ventricular function (11), and fibrinolysis trials have shown that the benefit is strongly dependent on the time delay from symptom onset until treatment (11–15).

The analysis of the Fibrinolytic Therapy Trialists' Group showed that about two lives could be saved per 1000 patients for every hour earlier the treatment began (13). The TIMI-2 (Thrombolysis in Myocardial Infarction) trial investigators showed that 10 lives could be saved for each hour saved when t-PA was given in less than four hours from symptom onset (15). Finally, the GUSTO-IIb trial investigators showed that about 5 lives out of 1000 were saved for each hour earlier that treatment began (7). Several reasons may explain why these studies could easily demonstrate the relationship between time to treatment and mortality despite the relatively low-risk populations enrolled. The most important reasons are the high statistical power provided by thousands of patients enrolled in these trials and the relatively constant and predictable efficacy provided by thrombolytic therapy over time.

On the contrary, studies on the relationship between time to treatment and mortality for patients who undergo primary PCI have produced conflicting results. Several primary PCI trials and survey studies revealed that in-hospital mortality is fairly constant from 2 to 12 hours after symptom onset, while an increased benefit of an early intervention could be revealed only in the small subset of patients who were treated within two hours from symptom onset (4,8,16,17). If these data could be applicable to the generality of patients with AMI, the need for urgent transportation to the catheterization laboratory might be limited only to a minority of patients, just those admitted within two hours from AMI onset, while for the majority of patients, including those who present to hospitals without interventional facilities, the delay to treatment due to the patient transfer to an interventional facility could have no impact on the benefit of primary PCI, overcoming the most important logistic problem of a primary PCI strategy, that is, the delay in referral of patients to a center with a primary PCI program.

In a series of 1352 patients reported by Brodie et al. (16), early mortality was significantly lower in the small group of patients treated within two hours from symptom onset, while it was higher and fairly constant in the later reperfusion groups (4.3%, and 9.0% to 9.5%, respectively, $p = 0.04$).

The Primary Angioplasty in Acute Myocardial Infarction (PAMI) investigators obtained similar results by the analysis of the Stent-PAMI patient cohort (17). In this trial, which included 849 patients, a very low-risk population was enrolled, and the one-month mortality was very low and relatively constant with increasing time to reperfusion (1.8–2.7%).

A relationship between mortality and time to treatment has not been observed also in NRMI-2, which collected data of 27,080 consecutive patients with AMI who were treated with primary PCI from 1994 to 1998 (4). In this registry, the median time from symptom onset to hospital arrival was 1.6 hours, and the median time from symptom onset to treatment was 3.9 hours. Thus, the registry revealed that in this period the door-to-balloon time was longer than the delay from symptom onset to hospital admission. Although unadjusted mortality was higher in the patients treated later, the multivariate-adjusted odds of in-hospital mortality did not increase over the 24-hour period. A following study, including 29,222 patients enrolled in NRMI-3 and NRMI-4 confirmed the key role of door-to-balloon time on mortality in patients receiving PCI. The in-hospital mortality progressively increased with increase in door-to-balloon time: 3.0%, 4.2%, 5.7%, and 7.4% with a door-to-balloon time <90 minutes, from 91 to 120 minutes, from 121 to 150 minutes, >150 minutes, respectively (p for trend <0.01). After adjustment for baseline characteristics a door-to-balloon time >90 minutes was associated with an OR for mortality of 1.42 (95% CI, 1.24–1.62), and the subgroup analysis showed that the effect on mortality was present regardless of time from symptom onset to hospital admission and the baseline risk factors of mortality (18).

The lack of evidence of a relationship between mortality and time to treatment for PCI-treated AMI patients may be explained in several ways. It has been hypothesized that differently from thrombolytic treatment, primary PCI allows successful infarct artery flow restoration also in late-presenting patients, and the efficacy of PCI in opening an occluded infarct artery is not dependent on time to treatment. Another hypothesis asserts that an open artery independently from myocardial salvage may provide a survival benefit by preventing ventricular remodeling and electrical instability (19). Another explanation may be based on a survivor-cohort effect since late-presenting patients have already survived the first high-risk hours from AMI onset. Moreover, the assessment of the time to treatment is not a precise measure since it depends on the subjective patient recall. Finally, an open infarct artery, even if open beyond 12 hours from symptom onset, may provide significant myocardial salvage as shown by the BRAVE-2 trial.

The Beyond 12 hours Reperfusion AlternatiVe Evaluation (BRAVE-2) trial enrolled 365 asymptomatic patients with AMI presenting between 12 and 48 hours from the symptom onset; patients were randomized to an invasive (PCI) or a conservative treatment strategy (20). The primary end point of the study was infarct size as assessed by sestamibi scintigraphy performed between 5 and 10 days after randomization. The median time from symptom onset to hospital admission was 22 hours. In the invasive group, 98.6% of patients had mechanical revascularization. The final infarct size was smaller in the invasive group compared with the conservative group (median 8% vs. 13%, p < 0.001). The scintigraphic substudy that included 261 patients who had paired scintigraphies (before randomization and 5 to 10 days after randomization) showed that the final smaller infarct size in the invasive strategy group compared with the conservative strategy group was due to increased myocardial salvage in the former (21). Beyond these hypotheses, several issues should be addressed to put the results of previous studies on primary PCI into a proper perspective. The large cohort of patients of the NRMI-2 may be considered at "low-risk" (4). Overall, according to the TIMI criteria, slightly more patients receiving fibrinolysis were judged to be "not low-risk" than were those receiving PCI (54% vs. 46%). The incidence of cardiogenic shock was very low (3.7%) and the overall mortality was 6.1%. Mortality was not independently related to time to treatment, while it was to the door-to-balloon time, and it is likely that the impact on mortality of the abnormally long door-to-balloon time in the NRMI-2 patient cohort prevailed that of the symptom onset to treatment.

The issue of the relationship of time to treatment and mortality was addressed with a different approach by the Florence investigators, who analyzed this relationship after stratification of patients by the risk on admission according to the TIMI criteria (22). Patients aged 70 years or older, or with anterior AMI, or a heart rate ≥100 minutes on admission, were considered at not low-risk, while patients younger than 70 years, with non-anterior AMI, or a heart rate on admission <100/min were considered at low-risk (23). Out of the 1336 patients with a successful procedure, 942 (71%) were at not low-risk, and 394 (29%) were at low-risk. Beyond the age, location of AMI, and heart rate on admission, the two groups differed in several ways with a greater incidence in women and diabetes, multivessel disease, chronic occlusion, and cardiogenic shock in the group at not low risk. Patients were not uniformly distributed with respect to the different intervals from symptom onset to treatment. Most patients (70%) were treated between two and six hours, and the higher patient concentration was between two and four hours. Moreover, among not low-risk patients, significant differences in risk profile were associated with increasing time to treatment. Patients with longer time to treatment were older and had a greater incidence of cardiogenic shock, while patients with a history of previous myocardial infarction had shorter time to treatment. The delay from admission to the

catheterization laboratory was very short and similar for the two groups (21 ± 15 minutes and 20 ± 17 minutes, respectively; p = 0.695), while the procedural time (from the arrival to the catheterization laboratory to the end of the procedure) was longer in the not low-risk group (35 ± 17 minutes vs. 32 ± 18 minutes, respectively; p < 0.001). Overall, the time to reperfusion was longer for the not low-risk group compared with the low-risk group (3.9 ± 2.1 hours vs. 3.3 ± 1.7 hours, respectively; p < 0.001). There were no differences in the incidence of stenting procedures, while more low-risk patients had abciximab administration. As expected, peak CK values were higher in the not low-risk group (2741 ± 2400 U/L vs. 1812 ± 1342 U/L, respectively; p < 0.001). The six-month survival rate was 89% ± 1% for the not low-risk group and 99% ± 1% for the low-risk group (p < 0.001).

Unadjusted mortality of the not low-risk patients rose from 4.8% to 12.9% with increasing time to reperfusion up to six hours and did not further increase beyond six hours, while mortality of the low-risk group was very low and constant with increasing time to reperfusion. For the not low-risk group, the univariate analysis revealed a relation between time to treatment and mortality (OR 1.35; 95% CI, 1.06–1.73; p = 0.017). However, time to reperfusion was not an independent predictor of mortality at the multivariate analysis, the only independent variables being age (OR 1.05; 95% CI, 1.03–1.07, p < 0.001), diabetes (OR 1.84; 95% CI, 1.15–2.94, p = 0.011), and cardiogenic shock (OR 8.10; 95% CI, 5.29–12.39, p < 0.001).

Thus, in this study the relationship of time to treatment with mortality was evident for not low-risk patients, while it was lacking for the low-risk patient subset. This figure may be easily explained, considering that the benefit of a treatment is strongly related to the patient risk, and it is very difficult or even impossible to show a benefit of a reperfusive treatment for patients with a very low-risk of death. For not low-risk patients, mortality increased with longer time to treatment, and univariate analysis showed that time to treatment was related to mortality. However, at multivariate analysis, time to treatment did not remain as an independent predictor of death. A potential explanation of these results is the worse patient-risk profiles that were associated with a longer delay to treatment. Late-presenting patients were older and had a higher likelihood to be on cardiogenic shock compared with early-presenting patients. Age and cardiogenic shock are the strongest predictors of mortality and may obscure the incremental prognostic value provided by time-to-treatment variable. Thus, the nonuniform distribution of the patient-risk profile by different intervals from symptom onset to treatment, as revealed in this series of patients, and the relatively small sample population may explain why time to treatment did not emerge as an independent predictor of mortality (22). In this study, most of the confounding effects on mortality revealed in the NRMI-2 and the GUSTO-IIb trial were avoided. This single-center experience included all consecutive unselected patients treated by PCI without any restriction based on age or clinical status on presentation. The direct admission from home to the catheterization laboratory, and the bypass of the emergency room or the coronary care unit for most patients, allowed a very short door-to-balloon time (24,25). All patients were treated with the same standards of care. Moreover, this type of analysis, based on patient stratification by risk on admission, could show an increased mortality by times categories in patients at not low-risk. Nevertheless, stratification by time categories of not low-risk patients showed that late-presenting patients had a worse risk profile that prevented time to reperfusion to be an independent predictor of mortality in this relatively small sample of patients.

Similar results were revealed in a study of the Zwolle group. In a series of 1791 patients treated by primary angioplasty, the one-year mortality rate was 5.8%. Symptom onset to PCI time was associated with one-year mortality, and a strong linear association between symptom onset to balloon time was revealed in not low-risk patients ($p = 0.006$). A symptom-onset-to-balloon time more than four hours was an independent predictor of mortality ($p < 0.05$) (26). In a subsequent analysis, the authors could state that each 30 minutes of delay was associated with a relative risk of one-year mortality of 1.075 (95% CI, 1.008–1.15; $p = 0.041$) (27).

Consistent with the results of these studies, the EMERALD (Enhanced Myocardial Efficacy and Removal by Aspiration of Liberated Debris) investigators in a sample of 501 patients who underwent predischarge sestamibi scintigraphy could reveal a relation between time to treatment and infarct size and a trend toward a low-mortality rate in patients with shorter delay to treatment. Median infarct size was 2%, 9%, 12%, and 11% with time to treatment <2 hours versus 2 to 3 hours, versus 3 to 4 hours, versus >4 hours, respectively ($p = 0.026$), while the mortality rates were 0%, 0%, 2.4%, and 5.3%, respectively ($p = 0.06$) (28).

The first clinical implication of the results of a critical analysis of the complex issue of relationship of time to treatment and mortality is that in not low-risk patients who undergo primary PCI the more rapidly reperfusion is achieved the better the survival. Thus, similar to the results of thrombolytic trials, the traditional paradigm of the early open artery hypothesis is confirmed for not low-risk patients who undergo primary PCI. The second clinical implication is that a fast track to PCI should not be considered unrealistic at a practice level; rather it should be a primary goal for the hospitals with a primary PCI program. Differently from thrombolytic trials that enrolled thousand of patients, it may be very difficult to assess reliably the impact of time delay on mortality in relatively small low-risk patient populations since the potential benefit of an early reperfusion is minimal in low-risk patients, and it would require thousands of patients to be evaluated.

THE INSTITUTIONAL VOLUME OF PRIMARY PCI

Also the institutional volume of primary PCI cases appears to independently influence mortality, with higher volume associated with better outcomes, similar to observations made in elective PCI in other studies (6–8,29).

The NRMI investigators could demonstrate in a study based on 446 hospitals with PCI facilities that primary PCI does not provide a significant reduction in mortality compared with fibrinolytic treatment in centers with a low volume of primary PCI (≤ 16 primary PCI/yr): the mortality rate was 5.9% in fibrinolysis-treated patients and 6.2% in PCI-treated patients. A slight reduction in mortality was evident in intermediate volume centers (17–48 primary PCI/yr) and increased in high-volume centers (≥ 49 primary PCI/yr): 5.9% versus 4.5% ($p < 0.001$) and 5.4% and 3.4% ($p < 0.001$), respectively (6). It is important to highlight that in this study the stratification of the hospitals by procedure volume was subsequent to the categorization in tertiles of the number of procedures per year performed in the hospitals included in the registry. This means that the number of 49 primary PCI per year should not be considered as the optimal quantitative standard for a PCI program. On the contrary, the progressive increased benefit revealed from intermediate volume center tertile to the highest-volume center tertile suggests that the benefit of primary PCI in terms of reduced mortality may progressively increase beyond the number of 49 procedure per year, and that a really high-volume center (>200 procedure/yr) has the potential for the better patient outcome and the most attractive cost/effectiveness ratio.

An analysis of the NRMI-4 investigators shows that the level of specialization with primary PCI has an impact on the clinical outcome. The authors divided 463 hospitals into quartiles of primary PCI specialization based on the relative proportion of patients admitted with a diagnosis of AMI and who underwent primary PCI ($\leq 34\%$, >34–62.5%, >62.5–88.5%, >88.5%). Hospitals in the highest interquartile had a lower in-hospital mortality and shorter door-to-balloon time compared with lower levels of specialization. The adjusted risk reduction in in-hospital mortality comparing the highest and the lowest interquartile was 0.64 ($p = 0.006$) (30). Similar results were demonstrated in a large French registry. The Greater Paris Area Registry investigators performed a case-control analysis to compare in-hospital mortality in low (<400 PCI/yr) and high (>400 PCI/yr) centers. From a total of 37,848 PCI procedures performed from 2001 to

2002, 22.4% were emergent procedures for AMI, cardiogenic shock, and out-of-hospital cardiac arrest. The in-hospital mortality was 6.75% in high-volume centers and 8.54% in low-volume centers ($p = 0.028$) (31).

LOGISTIC MODELS AND ORGANIZATIVE SCENARIOS

The ideal organizative scenario includes a network of mobile coronary care units that allow the diagnosis of AMI at home, and simultaneously alerting the invasive cardiology team. Patients should be directly admitted to the catheterization laboratory, bypassing the emergency room or coronary care unit, resulting in a zero door-to-balloon time. In this ideal scenario all patients with AMI can be treated by primary mechanical intervention. Out of this ideal scenario, all possible logistic models should consider the need for a functional network of community hospitals and referral centers to minimize the delay in reperfusive treatment and optimize therapy. Communities should identify a qualified and experienced center where intervention for AMI could be performed.

The fact that in metropolitan areas the majority of patients with AMI reach the hospital on their own should favor a short time from admission to treatment. Paradoxically, in the real world, the delay in the emergency room seems to be the first reason of the abnormal delay to treatment, and this fact highlights the need for the optimization of in-hospital diagnostic courses. In the DANAMI-2 trial, the time needed for patient transportation from the referral hospitals to the tertiary centers was shorter compared with the time needed for the indication to reperfusive treatment, or the administration of treatment after the decision was adopted (9).

According to the geographic and technical capabilities, an invasive strategy could be considered for all patients with AMI or for the subsets of patients at higher risk or with contraindication to fibrinolytic treatment.

THE ROLE OF CARDIAC SURGERY BACKUP

The role of cardiac surgery in patients with AMI admitted to a center with a program of primary PCI was studied by PAMI investigators (32). In a retrospective analysis of the 1100 patients enrolled in the PAMI-2 trial, cardiac surgery was performed before hospital discharge in a substantial minority of patients (10.9%). Cardiac surgery was performed on an elective basis in 42.6% of cases and on urgent or emergent basis in 57.4%. As expected, patients who underwent coronary surgery were older and had a greater incidence of multivessel disease and diabetes than those managed by percutaneous intervention or medically. The authors conclude that the appropriate use of elective and emergent coronary surgery should be considered an integral component of the primary PCI approach to treat patients at high risk and poorly suitable for a complete revascularization by a percutaneous approach. The emergency surgical treatment may be of great value to patients with cardiogenic shock due to predominant left ventricular failure and, obviously, to patients with cardiogenic shock due to mechanical complications. These data support a logistic model including surgical backup in the centers with a program of primary PCI, or, alternatively, the hospitals without operative facilities should provide expeditious transfer to a nearby tertiary center when necessary.

EDITOR'S COMMENT

It must be emphasized that all the analyses of the results from randomized controlled trial and survey studies could demonstrate that there is strong relationship between the quality of the procedures and survival, and that the potential for the great benefit of mechanical revascularization may be frustrated by low standards of care. Thus, every effort should be done to reach high standards of care by all the hospitals with a program of primary PCI for AMI.

REFERENCES

1. The Global Use of Strategies to Open Occluded Coronary Arteries in Acute Coronary Syndromes (GUSTO IIb) Angioplasty Substudy Investigators. A clinical trial comparing primary coronary angioplasty with tissue plasminogen activator for acute myocardial infarction. N Engl J Med 1997; 336:1621–1628.
2. Every NR, Parsons LS, Hlatky M, et al. A comparison of thrombolytic therapy with primary coronary angioplasty for acute myocardial infarction. N Engl J Med 1996; 335:1253–1260.
3. Tiefenbrunn AJ, Chandra NC, French WJ, et al. Clinical experience with primary percutaneous transluminal coronary angioplasty compared with alteplase (recombinant tissue-type plasminogen activator) in patients with acute myocardial infarction: a report from the Second National Registry of Myocardial Infarction (NRMI-2). J Am Coll Cardiol 1998; 31:1240–1245.
4. Cannon CP, Gibson CM, Lambrew CT, et al. Relationship of symptom-onset-to balloon time and door-to-balloon time with mortality in patients undergoing angioplasty for acute myocardial infarction. JAMA 2000; 283:2941–2947.
5. Danchin N, Vaur L, Genes N, et al. Treatment of acute myocardial infarction in the "real world": one-year results from a nationwide French survey. Circulation 1999; 99:2639–2644.
6. Magid DJ, Calonge BN, Rumsfeld JS, et al. Relation between primary angioplasty volume and mortality for patients with acute myocardial infarction treated with

primary angioplasty vs. thrombolytic therapy. JAMA 2000; 284:3131–3138.

7. Berger PB, Ellis SG, Holmes DR, et al. Relationship between delay in performing direct coronary angioplasty and early clinical outcome in patients with acute myocardial infarction: results from the Global Use of Strategies to Open Occluded Arteries in acute coronary syndromes (GUSTO-IIb) trial. Circulation 1999; 100:14–20.

8. Zahn R, Schiele R, Schneider S, et al. Primary angioplasty versus thrombolysis in acute myocardial infarction: can we define subgroups of patients benefiting most of primary angioplasty? Results from the pooled data of the Maximal Individual Therapy in Acute Myocardial Infarction Registry and the Myocardial Infarction Registry. J Am Coll Cardiol 2001; 37:1827–1835.

9. Andersen HR, Nielsen TT, Rasmussen K, et al. A comparison of coronary angioplasty with fibrinolytic therapy in acute myocardial infarction. N Engl J Med 2003; 349:733–742.

10. Widimsky P, Budesinsky T, Vorac D, et al. Long distance transport for primary angioplasty vs. immediate thrombolysis in acute myocardial infarction. Final results of the randomized national multicentre trial-PRAGUE-2. Eur Heart J 2003; 24:94–104.

11. Simes RJ, Topol EJ, Holmes DR, et al. Link between the angiographic substudy and mortality outcomes in a large randomized trial of myocardial reperfusion. Importance of early and complete infarct artery reperfusion. Circulation 1995; 91:1923–1928.

12. Newby LK, Rutsch WR, Califf RM, et al. Time from symptom onset to treatment and outcomes after thrombolytic therapy. J Am Coll Cardiol 1996; 27:1646–1655.

13. Fibrinolytic Therapy Trialists' (FTT) Collaborative Group. Indications for fibrinolytic therapy and suspected acute myocardial infarction: collaborative overview of early mortality and major morbidity results from all randomized trials of more than 1000 patients. Lancet 1994; 343:311–312.

14. Goldberg RJ, Mooradd M, Gurwitz JH, et al. Impact of time to treatment with tissue plasminogen activator on morbidity and mortality following acute myocardial infarction (the Second National Registry of Myocardial Infarction). Am J Cardiol 1998; 82:259–264.

15. Cannon CP, Antman EM, Walls R, et al. Time as an adjunctive agent to thrombolytic therapy. J Thromb Thrombolysis 1994; 1:27–34.

16. Brodie BR, Stuckey TD, Wall TC, et al. Importance of time to reperfusion for 30-day and late survival and recovery of left ventricular function after primary angioplasty for acute myocardial infarction. J Am Coll Cardiol 1998; 32:1312–1319.

17. Brodie BR, Stone GW, Morice MC, et al. Importance of time to reperfusion on outcomes after primary PTCA for acute myocardial infarction: results from stent PAMI. J Am Coll Cardiol 1999; 33(suppl A):353A.

18. McNamara RL, Wang Y, Herrin J, et al. Effect of door to balloon time on mortality in patients with ST-segment elevation myocardial infarction. J Am Coll Cardiol 2006; 47:2180–2186.

19. Braunwald E. Myocardial reperfusion, limitation of infarct size, reduction of left ventricular dysfunction, and improved survival: should the paradigm be expanded? Circulation 1989; 79:441–444.

20. Schömig A, Mehilli J, Antoniucci D, et al. Mechanical reperfusion in patients with acute myocardial infarction presenting more than 12 hours from symptom onset. JAMA 2005; 293:2865–2872.

21. Parodi G, Ndrepepa G, Conti A, et al. Ability of mechanical reperfusion to salvage myocardium in patients with acute myocardial infarction presenting beyond 12 hours after onset of symptoms. Am Heart J 2006; 152:1133–1139.

22. Antoniucci D, Valenti R, Migliorini A, et al. Relation of time to treatment and mortality in patients with acute myocardial infarction undergoing primary coronary angioplasty. Am J Cardiol 2002; 89:1248–1252.

23. The TIMI Study Group. Comparison of invasive and conservative strategies after treatment with intravenous tissue plasminogen activator in acute myocardial infarction: results of the Thrombolysis in Myocardial Infarction (TIMI) Phase II Trial. N Engl J Med 1989; 320:618–627.

24. Antoniucci D, Valenti R, Santoro GM, et al. Systematic direct angioplasty and stent-supported direct angioplasty therapy for cardiogenic shock complicating acute myocardial infarction: in-hospital and long-term survival. J Am Coll Cardiol 1998; 31:294–300.

25. Antoniucci D, Valenti R, Santoro GM, et al. Primary coronary infarct artery stenting in acute myocardial infarction. Am J Cardiol 1999; 84:505–510.

26. De Luca G, Suryapranata H, Zijlstra F, et al. Symptom-onset-to-balloon time and mortality in patients with acute myocardial infarction treated by primary angioplasty. J Am Coll Cardiol 2003; 42:991–997.

27. De Luca G, Suryapranata H, Ottervanger JP, et al. Time delay to treatment and mortality in primary angioplasty for acute myocardial infarction. Every minute of delay counts. Circulation 2004; 109:1223–1225.

28. Brodie BB, Webb J, Cox DA, et al. Impact of time to treatment on myocardial perfusion and infarct size with primary percutaneous coronary intervention for acute myocardial infarction (from the EMERALD trial). Am J Cardiol 2007; 99:1680–1686.

29. Vakilli BA, Kaplan R, Brown DL. Volume-outcome relation for physician and hospitals performing angioplasty for acute myocardial infarction in New York State. Circulation 2001; 104:2171–2176.

30. Nallamothu BK, Wang Y, Magid DJ, et al. Relation between hospital specialization with primary percutaneous coronary intervention and clinical outcome in ST-segment elevation myocardial infarction. National Registry of Myocardial Infarction-4 analysis. Circulation 2006; 113:222–229.

31. Spaulding C, Morice M-C, Lancelin B, et al. Is the volume-outcome relation still an issue in the era of PCI with systematic stenting? Results of the greater Paris area PCI registry. Eur Heart J 2006; 27(9):1054–1060.

32. Stone GW, Brodie BR, Griffin JJ, et al. Role of cardiac surgery in the hospital phase management of patients treated with primary angioplasty for acute myocardial infarction. Am J Cardiol 2000; 85:1292–1296.

12

Rescue and Facilitated Percutaneous Coronary Interventions

GUIDO PARODI

Division of Cardiology, Careggi Hospital, Florence, Italy

INTRODUCTION

The use of thrombolytic therapy has revolutionized the medical management of patients with acute myocardial infarction (AMI), increasing survival and preserving left ventricular function. Despite these beneficial effects of fibrinolytic therapy, many limitations exist, such as high rates of persistent occluded vessel, recurrent ischemia, intracranial bleeding, and contraindications preventing its use. To improve these deficiencies, several strategies of myocardial reperfusion have emerged. The efficacy of primary angioplasty (mechanical reperfusion without prior thrombolysis) has been widely evaluated, and in the last years other strategies, such as early rescue angioplasty (angioplasty for failed thrombolysis) and facilitated primary angioplasty (pharmacological reperfusion before angioplasty) have became an area of intense investigation.

RESCUE ANGIOPLASTY

Pharmacological reperfusion with full-dose fibrinolysis is not uniformly successful in restoring antegrade flow in the infarct artery. Rescue percutaneous coronary intervention (PCI) is defined as PCI performed on a coronary artery that remains occluded despite fibrinolytic therapy (1). Although this procedure is common, in current clinical practice the diagnosis of failed thrombolysis is frequently delayed, affecting negatively the outcome after PCI. Patients with persistently impaired flow [Thrombolysis In Myocardial Infarction (TIMI) $\leq$ 2] after thrombolysis have worse left ventricular function, more mechanical defects, and higher mortality. Limited and outdated past experiences suggest a trend toward clinical benefit if the infarct-related artery can be recanalized by angioplasty (2). Old studies of rescue angioplasty reported an acute patency in 71% to 100% of occluded coronary arteries after failed thrombolysis (2). However, the infarct-related artery reocclusion occurred in 18% (range 3–29%, twofold higher than primary angioplasty), in-hospital mortality in 10.6% (range 0–17%), and there was no significant recovery of left ventricular function (2). Although, in-hospital mortality and late mortality has been reported to be similar in patients with successful thrombolysis or successful rescue angioplasty after failed thrombolysis, failed rescue angioplasty had a mortality rate of 28% to 39% (mortality was significantly higher in patients with cardiogenic shock) (2). It should be pointed out that virtually the majority of the studies of rescue angioplasty were performed in the pre-stent era. With greater understanding of the importance of infarct-artery stenting (3,4), in association with the use of aspirin, heparin, thienopyridines, glycoprotein (GP) IIb/IIIa inhibitors, ACT monitoring, and intra-aortic balloon counterpulsation, the results of rescue angioplasty lead to a greater degree of technical success and clinical outcomes.

Despite these historical differences, recent data support the initial observation that rescue PCI decreases adverse clinical events compared with medical therapy. In the Wijeysundera meta-analysis (5), which included 1177 patients from eight randomized controlled trials, there was a trend toward reduced mortality rates with rescue PCI from 10.4% to 7.3% (RR 0.69; 95% CI, 0.46–1.05; $p = 0.09$), reduced reinfarction rates from 10.7% to 6.1% (RR 0.58; 95% CI, 0.35–0.97; $p = 0.04$), and reduced heart failure rates from 17.8% to 12.7% (RR 0.73; 95% CI, 0.54–1.00; $p = 0.05$). These event rates suggest that high-risk patients were selected for enrollment, so these data do not inform the clinical community about the role of rescue PCI in lower-risk patients. Probably, the benefits of rescue PCI need to be balanced against the risk. There was an excess occurrence of stroke in two trials (10 events vs. 2 events), but the majority of the strokes were thromboembolic rather than hemorrhagic, and the sample size was small, so more data are needed to define this risk. There also was an increase in absolute risk of bleeding of 13%, suggesting that adjustments in antithrombotic medication dosing are needed to improve safety. It should be noted that the majority of patients who underwent rescue PCI received fibrinolytic therapy with streptokinase.

In clinical practice, the most important issue is the early detection of failed epicardial reperfusion after fibrinolytic therapy that is the prerequisite for the prompt referral of the patient for rescue PCI. In fact, some units do not look for evidence of failed reperfusion at all. In general, it is highly likely that patients referred for consideration after failed reperfusion are those perceived to be at higher risk (e.g., those with anterior myocardial infarction or cardiogenic shock) (6). Since angiographic signs of reperfusion are not available, bedside-available clinical signs must be carefully evaluated. Ongoing chest pain, hemodynamic worsening, persistent ST-segment elevation, and slow release of myocardial injury markers are key parameters for identifying patients candidates for rescue PCI (6). The decision to perform emergency angiography should be made promptly. Critical to the success of rescue PCI is the initial clinical identification of patients who are suspected of having failed reperfusion with full-dose fibrinolysis. Because the presence or absence of ischemic discomfort may be unreliable for identifying failed reperfusion, clinicians should search for evidence of inadequate ST-segment resolution on the 12-lead electrocardiogram (ECG). Operationally, the 12-lead ECG should be scrutinized after adequate time has elapsed before it is decided that fibrinolytic therapy has not been effective. Although earlier times have been used in some studies, 90 minutes after initiation of fibrinolysis was the best time point for evaluating the need for rescue PCI; hence, if there is <50% ST resolution in the lead showing the greatest degree of ST-segment elevation at presentation, fibrinolytic therapy has likely failed to produce reperfusion. A <50% ST-segment resolution at 90 minutes after the administration of the lytic agent is well correlated with persistent infarct vessel occlusion and should be considered a reliable marker. Moreover, the use of combination of these noninvasive criteria increases positive predictive values.

FACILITATED PRIMARY ANGIOPLASTY

By restoring high rates of normal anterograde epicardial (TIMI 3) flow, primary angioplasty has been shown to improve survival of patients with AMI. Nonetheless, the delay from hospital arrival to angioplasty, which averages about two hours in the United States, is considered a major drawback of a primary angioplasty strategy and may adversely affect survival. It has therefore been suggested that early pharmacological reperfusion before angioplasty (so-called facilitated primary angioplasty) may further improve outcome in AMI. A number of studies have evaluated the alliance of pharmacological and mechanical reperfusion approaches (7). The complementary use of both approaches lead to a combination of the speed of patency and the improved microvascular function provided by a pharmacological strategy with the speed of flow following more definitive, albeit later, mechanical intervention (8).

Facilitated PCI is defined as planned immediate PCI after the administration of an initial pharmacological regimen to improve the coronary patency before the procedure. The rationales for facilitated primary angioplasty include: enhanced incidence and speed of myocardial reperfusion (i.e., less ischemia time, greater myocardial salvage, and lower infarct size) and greater technical success (higher preintervention patency of the infarct-related artery, improved patient stability in the catheterization laboratory), with ultimately an expected lower mortality. The potential risks and limitations of facilitated PCI are (*i*) increased bleeding complications (especially in older patients), (*ii*) fibrinolytic-induced platelet activation, (*iii*) intramural coronary haemorrhage, (*iv*) myocardial hemorrhage (predisposing to free-wall rupture), and (*v*) increased costs.

Theoretically, the ways to facilitate primary angioplasty are innumerable. Currently, four combinations of treatment options have been investigated: (*i*) low dose of lytic agent before angioplasty, (*ii*) precatheterization laboratory abciximab, (*iii*) low dose of lytic agent plus abciximab before angioplasty, and (*iv*) full dose of thrombolytic agent before angioplasty. All these strategies have the potential for efficacy.

The PACT (Plasminogen-activator Angioplasty Compatibility Trial) study randomized 606 patients with AMI to half-dose t-PA or placebo before angiography, and angioplasty if needed. Patency of the infarct-related artery on catheterization laboratory arrival was 61% with t-PA, and 34% with placebo ($p = 0.001$); no differences were observed in stroke or major bleeding between groups. This study demonstrated that a reduced-dose (half-dose) of t-PA could be safely combined with PCI and lead to more frequent early infarct-related artery recanalization before intervention. This trial reaffirmed the time-dependent nature of the "open vasculature hypothesis": those patients who had TIMI flow grade 3 restored early, before PCI, had improved ejection fractions compared with those who had delayed restoration of TIMI flow grade 3 after PCI (62% vs. 58%, $p = 0.0001$) (9). Thus, thrombolysis, as employed in this trial, and angioplasty may be compatible.

In the ADMIRAL (Abciximab before Direct Angioplasty and Stenting in Myocardial Infarction Regarding Acute and Long-Term Follow-up) trial the early administration of abciximab in patients with AMI-improved coronary patency before stenting, the success rate of the stenting procedure, the rate of coronary patency at six months, the left ventricular function, and the clinical outcomes (a composite of death, reinfarction, or urgent revascularization of the target vessel: 6.0%, vs. 14.6% in the placebo group; $p = 0.01$), with only a 0.7% increase in major bleeding in patients randomized to abciximab (10). Unfortunately, these results were obtained in a small number of patients.

The first large trial exploring the possible benefit of the combination therapy with abciximab and a lytic agent was the GUSTO-V (Global Utilization of Streptokinase and Tissue-Type Plasminogen Activator for Occluded Coronary Arteries) trial (11) based on 16,588 patients enrolled within six hours of evolving ST-segment elevation AMI. Patients were randomly assigned standard-dose reteplase or half-dose reteplase and full-dose abciximab. The primary end point of the study was the 30-day mortality. The trial showed the noninferiority of half-dose reteplase plus abciximab versus standard-dose reteplase (primary end point: 5.6% vs. 5.9%; $p = 0.43$). Although less nonfatal reinfarctions, recurrent ischemia, and total ischemic complications, a significant increase in non-cerebral-bleeding complications in the overall study population, and in intracranial hemorrhage in patients older than 75 years occurred with the combination half-dose reteplase and abciximab. The GUSTO-V trial suggested that the combination therapy may be harmful in elderly patients.

The TIMI-14 trial (12) randomized 888 patients with ST-segment elevation AMI to either 100 mg of accelerated-dose of alteplase or abciximab alone or in combination with reduced doses of alteplase or streptokinase. Abciximab facilitated the rate and extent of thrombolysis, producing marked increases in infarct-related artery TIMI 3 flow at 60 minutes when combined with half the usual dose of alteplase (72% vs. 43% of the alteplase-only group; $p = 0.0009$). The improvement in reperfusion with the association of abciximab and alteplase occurred without an increase in the risk of major bleeding. Moreover, the TIMI-14 trial results suggest that the combination therapy with abciximab and reduced-dose t-PA improves both epicardial flow and microvascular reperfusion (13). Insight into the mechanism of facilitation of thrombolysis when abciximab is combined with alteplase may be gained by considering the multiple effects of abciximab on clot formation and structure. The inhibition of GP IIb/IIIa receptors prevents aggregation of platelets, leading to reductions in both thrombus mass and the platform for further thrombin generation. Moreover, abciximab inhibits the release reaction from activated platelets, leading to decrease in the local concentration of inhibitors of thrombolysis such as PAI-1 and α-2 plasma inhibitor. Finally, abciximab weakens clot structure by its ability to block binding of activated factor XIII to platelets. By diminishing the tendency to thrombus growth and increasing clot porosity, abciximab may promote penetration of thrombolytic agents deeper into the clot, allowing a more rapid and more extensive thrombolysis (12).

The SPEED (Strategies for Patency Enhancement in the Emergency Department) trial (14) studied 323 patients with AMI who underwent PCI after reteplase with or without abciximab. The trial demonstrated that PCI either after reduced-dose r-PA alone or in combination with abciximab is safe and effective. Patients receiving abciximab with reduced-dose reteplase (5 U double bolus) showed an 86% incidence of TIMI grade 3 flow at 90 minutes. Unlike the TIMI-14 trial, which reached a similar conclusion using alteplase, intervention at the time of initial angiography was encouraged in the SPEED trial, resulting in early PCI in 61% of enrolled patients. Although the SPEED trial was a comparison of early PCI versus no PCI and carried out same limitations, its results encouraged the growing body of AMI literature supporting a "union in reperfusion" (14).

The ASSENT-3 (Assessment of the Safety and Efficacy of a New Thrombolytic) PLUS trial compared, in a series of 1639 patients with ST-segment elevation AMI, the efficacy and safety of pre-hospital single-bolus tenecteplase with low-molecular-weight heparin (enoxaparin) for a maximum of seven days or weight-adjusted unfractioned heparin for 48 hours. The median treatment delay was 115 minutes (53% within 2 hours). The combination of 30-day mortality, in-hospital reinfarction or ischemia, showed a trend to significant lower rate of events among patients treated with enoxaparin than among those treated with unfractioned heparin (14.2% vs. 17.4%, $p = 0.08$), with an increase in intracranial hemorrhage in patients older than 75 years (lower doses of low-molecular-weight heparin need to be tested in elderly patients) (15). The results of this study encourage the use of pre-hospital single-bolus tenecteplase with enoxaparin in patients with AMI. Thus the ASSENT-4 trial, one of the most important facilitated PCI study, was designed.

The ASSENT-4 study (16) was an open-label randomized trial in which patients with ST-elevation AMI of less than six hours of duration, scheduled to undergo primary PCI with an anticipated delay of one to three hours, were randomized to standard PCI or PCI preceded by administration of single-bolus full-dose tenecteplase. Four thousand patients were planned, but early cessation of enrollment was recommended by the data and safety monitoring board because of higher in-hospital mortality in the facilitated than in the standard PCI group (6% vs. 3%; $p = 0.0105$). The primary end point (90-day death or congestive heart failure or shock) was reached in 19% and 13% ($p = 0.0045$) of patients randomized to facilitated or standard primary PCI, despite the facilitated strategy allowed the achievement of higher infarct vessel patency before PCI (43% vs. 15% in the PCI-alone group). Strokes as well as ischemic cardiac complications were higher in the facilitated group. Thus, the ASSENT-4 investigators concluded that a strategy of full-dose tenecteplase, preceding PCI by one to three hours, is associated with more major adverse events than primary PCI in ST-elevation myocardial infarction (STEMI) patients. This study had several limitations, in particular regarding the suboptimal co-therapy in the facilitated arm, the long time from symptom onset to lytic therapy, the short time from TNK administration to PCI, and finally the open label design. Nevertheless, the ASSENT-4 trial is still the more important trial on facilitated PCI and significantly weighted in the meta-analysis-based data reported by Keeley and coworkers (7). From this meta-analysis, which included 4500 patients from 17 randomized trials on facilitated versus primary angioplasty, despite more than twofold increase in the number of patients with TIMI grade 3 flow at baseline angiography, facilitated PCI offered no benefit (higher mortality, reinfarction, urgent revascularization, and major bleeding rates!) over primary PCI in STEMI treatment (Fig. 12.1). However, if we divide the 17 included studies according to the type of facilitation regimen used [lytic alone ($n = 9$; 2953 patients), GP IIb/IIIa inhibitors alone ($n = 6$; 1148 patients), and lytic + GP IIb/IIIa inhibitors ($n = 2$; 399 patients)], we can notice that the worse performances were provided by the more numerous group treated by lytic-alone-facilitated strategy, in which mortality, reinfarction, and target vessel revascularization rates were higher than the control group (Fig. 12.1). While the other two facilitated PCI regimens considered, and in particular the pretreatment with only GP IIb/IIIa inhibitors, resulted to be safer and not associated with a significant increase in adverse events (no clear clinical advantage, but at the same time no harm).

Recently, the ACC/AHA 2004 Guidelines for the Management of Patients with STEMI has been updated (17). A

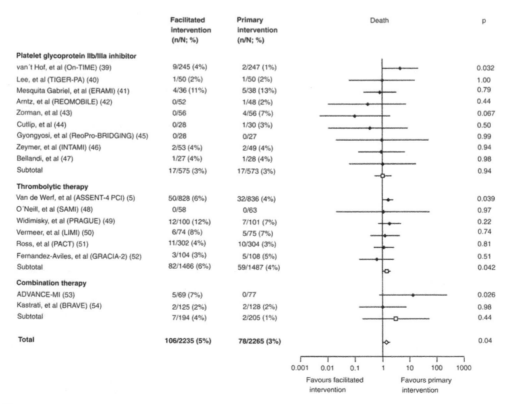

Figure 12.1 Short-term death in patients treated with facilitated or primary PCI. *Source*: From Ref. 17.

focused update has been prepared for facilitated PCI. With a class IIb recommendation (level of evidence C) it is stated that facilitated PCI using regimens other than full-dose fibrinolytic might be considered a reperfusion strategy when all of the following patients' characteristics are present: (*i*) higher-risk patients, (*ii*) low bleeding risk, and (*iii*) PCI not immediately available within 90 minutes. Thus, the use of facilitated PCI is further limited and confined to particular situations. Moreover, an option of facilitation (full-dose fibrinolytic) is no more considered. However, in the last lines of the Guidelines paragraph dedicated to facilitated PCI, a room is left to such a strategy stating that further trials with reduced-dose fibrinolytic therapy, with or without GP IIb/IIIa inhibitors, may yield different efficacy/safety results. Actually, two other important trials have been concluded. These are the Facilitated Intervention With Enhanced Reperfusion Speed to Stop Events (FINESSE) trial and the Combined Abciximab Reteplase Stent Study (CARESS) in AMI trial.

The FINESSE trial (18) enrolled patients with a new STEMI within six hours of pain onset with estimated time to catheterization laboratory of one to four hours. Patients were randomized in a double-blind, double-dummy fashion to either one of three treatment strategies: (*i*) primary PCI, (*ii*) facilitated PCI with abciximab alone, and (*iii*) facilitated PCI with half-dose reteplase plus abciximab. Study enrollment was stopped because of budgetary issues in December 2006 after 2452/3000 patients were entered into the study. TIMI flow 2/3 prior to PCI was achieved in 61% of patients treated with reteplase/abciximab versus 25% in the primary PCI group and 26% in the placebo/abciximab group. Consistently with other facilitated PCI trials, at 90 days, there was no difference in the primary composite end point (all-cause mortality/rehospitalization for congestive heart failure, resuscitated ventricular fibrillation more than 48 hours after randomization, and cardiogenic shock) between the three study groups. However, total amount of TIMI bleeding complications was significantly higher in the facilitated PCI arms. There was also a higher rate of intracranial hemorrhage in the reteplase/abciximab group compared with the other two groups, but the difference was not significant. In this trial, there was no significant improvement in the primary end point or its components in patients treated with either abciximab-facilitated PCI or reteplase/abciximab-facilitated PCI compared with primary PCI with administration of abciximab in the catheterization laboratory. Therefore, primary PCI with in-laboratory abciximab administration still provides better benefit/risk profile than the two facilitated strategies tested in the FINESSE trial in patients with STEMI who can undergo PCI within four hours of first medical contact. The results of this trial lead to the same question evoked by prior studies, namely, why does facilitated PCI, the marriage between two proven reperfusion strategies for the treatment of ST-elevation AMI, enhance early reperfusion and does not improve the clinical outcome? At least four reasons were postulated by the investigators. First, the differences in time to reperfusion may affect myocardial salvage only during the first two hours after the onset of infarction (an interval that is shorter than that in which patients can be treated). After two hours time dependency of PCI-mediated salvage may be attenuated. Second, the importance of the timing of treatment for myocardial salvage may not be as great with PCI as it is with thrombolysis. Third, only high-risk patients are likely to have a major benefit from early reperfusion with PCI (in the FINESSE trial only 67% of the enrolled patients were classified as being at high risk). Fourth, the rates of major complications and events after primary PCI with adjunctive abciximab therapy are quite low and therefore difficult to improve.

Differently, the CARESS in AMI study (19) compared a strategy of early transfer of patients to a PCI center after thrombolysis versus medical treatment continued in the admitting hospital and transfer for rescue PCI only if there was evidence of lack of reperfusion. Higher-risk STEMI patients less than 12 hours from symptom onset admitted to centers without PCI facilities were randomized to either facilitated PCI (lytics and transfer to the nearest PCI center) or medical treatment/rescue PCI (lytic and transfer for rescue PCI if persistent ST-elevation). After protocol amendment, a total of 600 patients were randomized to facilitated PCI ($n = 297$) or to the medical/rescue ($n = 300$) arms of the study. In the immediate PCI group, baseline angiography TIMI 3 flow was observed in 61% of patients prior to PCI, and after the procedure, TIMI 3 flow was achieved in 91% of patients. The combined end point of death/reinfarction/refractory ischemia at 30 days was significantly lower in the facilitated arm compared with the medical/rescue-treated patients (4.1% vs. 11.1%, respectively; $p = 0.001$). Of note, the CARESS in AMI trial did not include a standard primary PCI control arm. Moreover, the difference in the primary end point was mainly driven by a reduced incidence in the relatively soft end point of refractory ischemia (defined as recurrent chest pain with ST-elevation or T-wave inversion occurring >12 hours after randomization persisting for at least 10 minutes and not fulfilling the diagnosis of re-MI). Probably, deleterious effect on the platelet aggregation of fibrinolysis was balanced in this trial by the simultaneous use of abciximab. Safety outcomes showed a significantly higher rate of bleeding complications in the facilitated arm of the study, mainly related to an increased vascular access site bleeding. Conversely, because of the exclusion of patients at high risk of bleeding (including elderly), severe bleeding, transfusion, and stroke rates were similar between the two study groups. The investigators concluded that the strategy of immediate transfer of selected high-risk STEMI patients at low bleeding risk treated with half-dose reteplase and abciximab from non-PCI hospitals to high-volume PCI centers (facilitated PCI) is better than standard lytic therapy with clinically indicated rescue PCI strategy.

On the basis of the results obtained from these studies at present time routine facilitated PCI is not recommended to patients with STEMI. ASSENT-4 and FINESSE failed to show a benefit, and results from ASSENT-4 suggest that the strategy may even yield a harmful effect. However, we cannot ignore the fact that in both studies a significantly higher percentage of patients achieved reperfusion (TIMI 2/3) in the infarct-related artery by the time they arrived to the catheterization laboratory. This is a critical observation when we consider that "time is muscle." However, these findings still leave us questioning why the improved reperfusion rates did not translate to improved clinical outcomes. Possible explanations include an increase in bleeding complications, the lack of adequate antithrombotic/antiplatelet adjunctive therapy, or that perhaps these studies were underpowered to show a clinical benefit in a short period of time (30–90 days). Nevertheless, selective use of the facilitated strategy with regimens other than full-dose fibrinolytic therapy in subgroups of patients (at high risk with low bleeding risk) who present to hospitals without PCI capability might be still considered when significant transfer delays for primary PCI are anticipated.

TRANSFER FOR PRIMARY ANGIOPLASTY/ TOWARD MYOCARDIAL INFARCTION CENTER

As the majority of patients with ST-elevation AMI are presented to hospital without the capability to perform primary angioplasty, interhospital transportation of patients with AMI plays a central role.

Data from a number of studies indicate that transfer to a tertiary-care hospital for rescue or primary PCI can be performed safely. Rapid transfer to an intervention center will enhance the ability to recanalize persistently occluded vessels and preserve left ventricular function (20).

In the DANAMI-2 (Danish Multicenter Randomized Study on Fibrinolytic Therapy vs. Acute Coronary Angioplasty in Acute Myocardial Infarction) trial (21), 1572 patients with AMI were randomly assigned to treatment with angioplasty or alteplase. Of the 1572 patients, 1129 were enrolled in 24 community hospitals without angioplasty facilities. Transfer to the nearest angioplasty center had to be completed within three hours. The primary end point (a composite of death, reinfarction, or disabling stroke at 30 days) was reached in 8.5% of patients in the angioplasty group compared with 14.2% of those in

the on-site fibrinolysis group ($p = 0.002$). The transfer of patients was found to be safe. Almost all patients enrolled in the community hospitals arrived in the catheterization laboratory within two hours after randomization. The DANAMI-2 trial demonstrated the superiority of primary PCI over thrombolysis even when patients are admitted to a local hospital without angioplasty capability and must be transported to an invasive-treatment center with transfer times up to 120 minutes.

The PRAGUE-2 (PRimary Angioplasty in patients transferred from General community hospitals to specialized PTCA Units with or without Emergency thrombolysis) trial (22) randomized 850 patients with ST-segment elevation AMI presenting within 12 hours to the nearest community hospital without a catheterization laboratory to either on-site thrombolysis or immediate transport for primary PCI. The primary end point (30-day mortality) was reached in 10.0% in the thrombolysis group compared with 6.8% in the PCI group ($p = 0.12$, intention-to-treat analysis). In patients who actually underwent PCI, mortality rate was significantly lower (6.0% vs. 10.4% of patients treated with thrombolysis; $p < 0.05$). In patients randomized >3 hours after the onset of symptoms, the mortality rate of the thrombolysis group reached 15.3% compared with 6.0% in the PCI group ($p < 0.02$). The PRAGUE-2 trial (22) showed the safety and feasibility of the strategy of long distance interhospital transportation to perform primary angioplasty, with a significant reduction in 30-day mortality compared with on-site thrombolysis, particularly in patients presenting >three hours after symptom onset. The explanation of this finding is complex because multiple factors may interact with time to treatment. The influence of the time-to-treatment interval on the myocardial salvage in patients with AMI depends on the type of reperfusion therapy (23). Time delay of interhospital transportation for primary angioplasty seems to have lower impact on outcome than delay to treatment for patients undergoing thrombolytic therapy. Certainly, as interventional centers treat large numbers of patients with AMI, these patients benefit from the fact that results of procedures as well as the optimal application of other therapies for AMI are volume dependent (17). The DANAMI-2 (21) and the PRAGUE-2 (22) trials are especially important as they show that mechanical reperfusion for AMI can be applied in large country areas.

Studies (20,24,25) have suggested that PCI for AMI is superior to thrombolysis even if the treatment is delayed by >120 minutes by transferring the patient to an interventional center. Thus patients with ST-elevation AMI should be directly transported to specific emergency departments with catheterization facilities, a sort of "myocardial infarction center," avoiding delays in the small hospitals or emergency departments of the large hospitals.

REFERENCES

1. Ross AM, Lundergan CF, Rohrbeck SC, et al.; for the GUSTO-I Angiographic Investigators. Rescue angioplasty after failed thrombolysis; technical and clinical outcomes in a large thrombolysis trial. J Am Coll Cardiol 1998; 31:1511–1517.

2. Ellis SG, Van de Werf F, DaSilva ER, et al. Present status of rescue coronary angioplasty. Current polarization of opinion and randomised trials. J Am Coll Cardiol 1992; 19:681–686.

3. Garot P, Himbert D, Juliard JM, et al. Incidence, consequences, and risk factors of early reocclusion after primary and/or rescue percutaneous transluminal coronary angioplasty for acute myocardial infarction. Am J Cardiol 1998; 82:554–558.

4. Antoniucci D, Santoro GM, Bolognese L, et al. A clinical trial comparing primary stenting of the infarct-related artery with optimal primary angioplasty for acute myocardial infarction: results from the Florence Randomized Elective Stenting in Acute Coronary Occlusion (FRESCO) trial. J Am Coll Cardiol 1998; 31:1234–1239.

5. Wijeysundera HC, Vijayaraghavan R, Nallamothu BK, et al. Rescue angioplasty or repeat fibrinolysis after failed fibrinolytic therapy for ST-segment myocardial infarction: a meta-analysis of randomized trials. J Am Coll Cardiol 2007; 49:422–430.

6. de Lemos JA, Morrow DA, Gibson CM, et al. Early noninvasive detection of failed epicardial reperfusion after fibrinolytic therapy. Am J Cardiol 2001; 88:353–358.

7. Keeley EC, Boura JA, Grines CL. Comparison of primary and facilitated percutaneous coronary interventions for ST-elevation myocardial infarction: quantitative review of randomised trials. Lancet 2006; 367:579–588.

8. Gibson CM. A union in reperfusion: The concept of facilitated percutaneous coronary intervention. J Am Coll Cardiol 2000; 36:1497–1499.

9. Ross AM, Coyne KS, Reiner JS, et al. A randomized trial comparing primary angioplasty with a strategy of short-acting thrombolysis and immediate planned rescue angioplasty in acute myocardial infarction: The PACT Trial. J Am Coll Cardiol 1999; 34:1954–1962.

10. Montalescot G, Barragan P, Wittenberg O, et al. Platelet glycoprotein IIb/IIIa inibition with coronary stenting for acute myocardial infarction. N Engl J Med 2001; 344:1895–1903.

11. The GUSTO-V Investigators. Reperfusion therapy for acute myocardial infarction with fibrinolytic therapy or combination reduced fibrinolytic therapy and platelet glycoprotein IIb/IIIa inhibition: the GUSTO-V randomized trial. Lancet 2001; 357:1905–1914.

12. Antman EM, Giugliano RP, Gibson CM, et al. Abciximab facilitates the rate and extent of thrombolysis. Results of the Thrombolysis In Myocardial Infarction (TIMI) 14 Trial. Circulation 1999; 99:2720–2732.

13. de Lemos JA, Antman EM, Gibson CM, et al. Abciximab improves both epicardial flow and myocardial reperfusion in ST-elevation myocardial infarction. Observations from the TIMI 14 Trial. Circulation 2000; 101:239–243.

14. Herrmann HC, Moliterno DJ, Ohman EM, et al. Facilitation of early percutaneous coronary intervention after reteplase with or without abciximab in acute myocardial infarction. Results from the SPEED (GUSTO-4 Pilot) Trial. J Am Coll Cardiol 2000; 36:1489–1496.

15. Wallentin L, Goldstein P, Armstrong PW, et al. Efficacy and safety of tenecteplase in combination with the low-molecular-weight-heparin enoxaparin or unfractionated heparin in the prehospital setting: the Assessment of the Safety and Efficacy of a new Thrombolytic Regimen (ASSENT)-3 PLUS randomized trial in acute myocardial infarction. Circulation 2003; 108:135–142.

16. ASSENT-4 PCI Investigators. Primary versus tenecteplase-facilitated percutaneous coronary intervention in patients with SE-segment elevation acute myocardial infarction (ASSENT-4 PCI): randomised trial. Lancet 2006; 367:569–578.

17. Antman EM, Hand M, Armstrong PW, et al. 2007 Focused update of the ACC/AHA guidelines for the management of patients with ST-elevation myocardial infarction. Circulation 2008; 117: 2152–2163.

18. Ellis SG, Tendera M, de Berder MA, et al.; for the FINESSE Investigators. Facilitated PCI in patients with ST-elevation myocardial infarction. N Engl J Med 2008; 358:2205–2217.

19. Di Mario C, Dudek D, Piscione F, et al. Immediate angioplasty versus standard therapy with rescue angioplasty after thrombolysis in the Combined Abciximab Reteplase Stent Study in Acute Myocardial Infarction (CARESS-in-AMI): an open, prospective, randomised milticentre trial. Lancet 2008; 371:559–568.

20. Dalby M, Bouzamondo A, Lechat P, et al. Transfer for primary angioplasty versus immediate thrombolysis in acute myocardial infarction: a meta-analysis. Circulation 2003; 108:1809–1814.

21. Andersen HR, Nielsen TT, Rasmussen K, et al. for the DANAMI-2 Investigators. A comparison of coronary angioplasty with fibrinolytic therapy in acute myocardial infarction. N Engl J Med 2003; 349:733–742.

22. Widimsky P, Budesinsky T, Vorac D, et al. Long distance transport for primary angioplasty vs. immediate thrombolysis in acute myocardial infarction. Final results of the randomized national multicentre trial – PRAGUE-2. Eur Heart J 2003; 24:94–104.

23. Schöming A, Ndrepepa G, Mehilli J, et al. Therapy-dependent influence of time-to-treatment interval on myocardial salvage in patients with acute myocardial infarction treated with coronary stenting or thrombolysis. Circulation 2003; 108:1084–1088.

24. Zijlstra F. Angioplasty vs. thrombolysis for acute myocardial infarction: a quantitative overview of the effects of interhospital transportation. Eur Heart J 2003; 24:21–23.

25. Grines CL, Westerhausen DR, Grines LL, et al. A randomized trial of transfer for primary angioplasty versus on-site thrombolysis in patients with high-risk myocardial infarction. The Air Primary Angioplasty in Myocardial Infarction Study. J Am Coll Cardiol 2002; 39:1713–1719.

13

Myocardial Stem Cell After Acute Myocardial Infarction

NAZARIO CARRABBA

Division of Cardiology, Careggi Hospital, Florence, Italy

Despite the advances made in the management of acute myocardial infarction (AMI), congestive heart failure secondary to ventricular remodeling after AMI continues to be a major problem (1).

In the last few years, the positive results in animal experiments have led to the development of cardiac cell therapy in humans. Different types of regenerating cells (embryonic stem cells, skeletal myoblasts, and bone marrow–derived cells) have recently been investigated for their capacity to proliferate and differentiate into functional cardiomyocytes or cardiac vascular cells, such as endothelial cells (2–6), for their therapeutic potential to improve the myocardial perfusion at microvascular level and left ventricular function. Among them, the use of bone marrow–derived stem cells (BMSCs) seems to be the most promising method.

The bone marrow contains several reconstructing stem cell types, with overlapping phenotypes, including hematopoietic stem cells, endothelial stem progenitor cells, mesenchymal stem cells, and multipotent adult progenitor cells (7–12). Experimental studies show that the cardiac function improvement is exclusive not to one cell type but rather to a certain combination of the progenitors.

Some observations indicate that the presumable beneficial effects of BMSC implantation in humans may be connected in particular with the paracrine effects of the injected cells rather than with their transdifferentiation to the myocytes or endothelial cells (13,14).

The first small clinical trials (15–18) justified the safety and feasibility of the intracoronary application of autologous BMSCs in patients after recent myocardial infarction (MI). Larger randomized, controlled studies have revealed the favorable effects of stem cell therapy on the regional and global left ventricular function and myocardial perfusion in a similar patient cohort. The Transplantation of Progenitor Cells and Regeneration Enhancement in Acute Myocardial Infarction (TOP-CARE) study (19) demonstrated a significant increase in global left ventricular ejection fraction (LVEF) and a significant reduction in infarct size measured by contrast-enhanced magnetic resonance imaging one year after the intracoronary application of either bone marrow–derived or blood-derived progenitor cells into the infarct-related artery (IRA) at 4.9 ± 1.5 days after AMI in 59 patients. In the BOne marrOw transfer to enhance ST-elevation infarct regeneration (BOOST) trial (20), significant improvements in regional wall motion and global LVEF could be observed in 30 treated patients as compared with the control subjects six months after the intracoronary application of bone marrow–derived nucleated cells. A recent update of the BOOST trial proved that the beneficial effect of cardiac cell therapy after AMI is sustained at 18 months, although there was a further improvement of the LVEF in the control group, and the difference between the treated and control groups was therefore no longer significant. In the Reinfusion of

Enriched Progenitor cells and Infarct Remodeling in Acute Myocardial Infarction (REPAIR-AMI) study (21), an improvement in LVEF at ventricular angiography (from 48% to 54%) was observed in 204 post-MI patients after the infusion of BMSCs; intriguingly, BMSC-treated patients exhibited a significantly lower rate of prespecified major cardiovascular events (including death, recurrence of MI, and any revascularization procedure), although the study was not powered to test difference in clinical end points. Conversely, the Autologous Stem-cell Transplantation in AMI (ASTAMI) trial (22) did not show any beneficial effect of the intracoronary stem cell therapy on the left ventricular systolic function assessed by cardiac magnetic resonance, single-photon emission tomography, and echocardiography.

Lack of consistent effects of BMSCs on left ventricular function in these early randomized trials is probably related to their limited statistical power and differences in enrolment criteria, BMSC processing, timing of BMSC injection, and methods to assess cardiac function. It is worth noting that the beneficial effects observed in some of these trials are probably related to paracrine effects of BMSCs favorably influencing neovascularization, whereas a convincing demonstration of therapeutic myocardial regeneration in humans is still lacking (23).

The uncertainty of the consistent effects of BMSCs on left ventricular function remains also when you take into account the results of a recent meta-analysis of 10 controlled clinical trials on intracoronary cell therapy performed in patients with AMI (698 patients, median follow-up 6 months) (24). Patients who received intracoronary cell therapy had a significant improvement in LVEF (3% increase), as well as a reduction in infarct size (−5.6%) and end-systolic volume (−7.4 mL), and a trend toward reduced end-diastolic volume (−4.6 mL). Intracoronary cell therapy was also associated with a nominally significant reduction in recurrent AMI and trends toward reduced death, rehospitalization for heart failure, and repeat revascularization. Meta-regression suggested the existence of a dose-response association between injected cell volume and LVEF changes. This meta-analysis included intracoronary cell therapy derived from both BMSCs and peripheral stem cells. Although this may be argued as a limitation of the study, intracoronary cell therapy after AMI appears to improve LVEF regardless of whether BMSCs or peripheral stem cells are employed. However, despite these encouraging results, the question of whether a small increase in LVEF is of clinical significance remains an important issue. On the other hand, it should be stressed that many of the interventions with an established lifesaving effect during or after AMI also provided only moderate yet clinically meaningful increases in LVEF.

INTRAMYOCARDIAL DELIVERY OF STEM CELL

Only in a few recently published trials, autologous BMSCs have been injected intramyocardially, particularly in patients with severe, chronic ischemic heart disease. Tse et al. (25) reported their results on eight patients who received NOGA electromechanical mapping-guided intramyocardial stem cell injection into the ischemic myocardium. After three months, the authors found a 12% increase in wall thickening as measured by magnetic resonance imaging. Fuchs et al. (26) reported that the Canadian Cardiovascular Society (CCS) angina score and the stress-induced myocardial ischemia were decreased significantly three months after the intramyocardial injection of autologous BMSCs into 14 patients not amenable to conventional revascularization. Perin et al. (27) reported an improvement in LVEF, a reduction in end-systolic volume, and a significant mechanical improvement of the injected segment after stem cell therapy guided by the NOGA electromechanical mapping in patients with end-stage ischemic heart disease. In five heart transplant candidates with severe ischemic heart failure, Silva et al. (28) observed a reduction in the amount of ischemic myocardium and a significant improvement in the exercise test results. Of the five patients, four were no longer eligible for cardiac transplantation.

The combined intramyocardial and intracoronary delivery of autologous BMSCs into the fibrotic myocardium has been proposed recently. The promising preliminary results of the pilot nonrandomized study suggest the feasibility and safety of this combined mode of stem cell application (13,29,30). However, the long-term efficacy of this approach is unknown.

THE RISK OF ACCELERATED ATHEROSCLEROSIS

Two recent studies have raised concern with respect to the safety of BMSCs after AMI. In one study, Kang et al. (17) found in-stent restenosis in five of seven patients treated with granulocyte colony-stimulating factor (G-CSF) for five days, followed by bare-metal stent implantation and intracoronary BMSC infusion; notably, they found a correlation between late loss and improvement in the LVEF at follow-up. In addition, in a nonrandomized study in 38 patients, Mansour et al. (31) found that the infusion of CD133+ enriched BMSCs was associated with increased in-stent proliferation and larger luminal loss in nonstented distal segments of the IRA, which resulted in a significant decrease in coronary flow reserve. The risk of accelerated atherosclerosis associated with intracoronary administration of BMSCs observed in these two studies might be due to the prevalence of proinflammatory stimuli caused by coadministration of cytokines or BMSC manipulation. Interestingly, in a more recent study, Kang et al. (32) found an improvement in the LVEF in the absence of a higher rate of in-stent restenosis in post-AMI patients successfully revascularized by drug-eluting stent (DES) implantation, who received G-CSF, followed by intracoronary BMSC infusion. In this study, the anti-inflammatory effects of DES were probably sufficient to counterbalance the potential proinflammatory action of G-CSF.

Taken together, these findings suggest that the risk of accelerated atherosclerosis has to be taken into account in the cell-based treatment of AMI, but this potential risk is protocol dependent and is not a direct consequence of intracoronary BMSC administration.

FINAL CONSIDERATIONS

After the promising results of initial observational studies and randomized trials with surrogate end points, cell-based treatment of AMI will leave the "gray zone" only if large randomized trials reproducibly and convincingly show that this innovative form of treatment can reduce the rate of major cardiac events in the absence of accelerated atherosclerosis. To fully exploit the potential of cell-based therapy of AMI, two issues are critical: (*i*) inclusion criteria and (*ii*) BMSC function and homing. With regard to the first issue, patients who have the highest probability of beneficial effects are poor mobilizers of BMSCs with a low LVEF, while patients who have the lowest probability of beneficial effects are good mobilizers of BMSCs (33,34). With regard to the second issue, the BMSC function is known to be depressed in patients with coronary risk factors. Yet there are ways to improve it, including coadministration of statins and/or of mobilizing factors (such as erythropoietin or a cytokine with low proinflammatory profile). Finally, BMSCs homing is probably denied by the no-reflow phenomenon, which might be limited by coadministration of microvascular vasodilators.

REFERENCES

1. Caplice NM, Gersh BJ. Stem cell to repair the heart: a clinical perspective. Circ Res 2003; 92:6–8.
2. Taylor DA, Atkins BZ, Hungspreugs P, et al. Regenerating functional myocardium: improved performance after skeletal myoblast transplantation. Nat Med 1998; 4:929–933.
3. Gepstein L. Derivation and potential applications of human embryonic stem cells. Circ Res 2002; 91:866–876.
4. Weissman IL. Stem cells—scientific, medical, and political issues. N Engl J Med 2002; 346:1576–1579.
5. Menasché P, Hagège AA, Vilquin JT, et al. Autologous skeletal myoblast transplantation for severe postinfarction left ventricular dysfunction. J Am Coll Cardiol 2003; 41:1078–1083.
6. Reinecke H, Poppa V, Murry CE. Skeletal muscle stem cells do not transdifferentiate into cardiomyocytes after cardiac grafting. J Mol Cell Cardiol 2002; 34:241–249.
7. Orlic D, Kajstura J, Chimenti S, et al. Bone marrow cells regenerate infarcted myocardium. Nature 2001; 410:701–705.
8. Asahara T, Masuda H, Takahashi T, et al. Bone marrow origin of endothelial progenitor cells responsible for postnatal vasculogenesis in physiological and pathological neovascularization. Circ Res 1999; 85:221–228.
9. Kawamoto A, Gwon HC, Iwaguro H, et al. Therapeutic potential of ex vivo expanded endothelial progenitor cells for myocardial ischemia. Circulation 2001; 103: 634–637.
10. Kocher AA, Schuster MD, Szabolcs MJ, et al. Neovascularization of ischemic myocardium by human bone-marrow-derived angioblasts prevents cardiomyocyte apoptosis, reduces remodeling and improves cardiac function. Nat Med 2001; 7:430–436.
11. Ylä-Herttuala S, Alitalo K. Gene transfer as a tool to induce therapeutic vascular growth. Nat Med 2003; 9:694–701.
12. Tomita S, Li RK, Weisel RD, et al. Autologous transplantation of bone marrow cells improves damaged heart function. Circulation 1999; 100(19 suppl):II247–II256.
13. Nyolczas N, Gyongyosi M, Beran G, et al. Beneficial effect of combined intramyocardial and intracoronary administration of autologous stem cells on global and regional left ventricular function and myocardial perfusion in patients with ischaemic cardiomyopathy. J Am Coll Cardiol 2006; 47(suppl A):304.
14. Thum T, Bauersarchs J, Polle-Wilson PA, et al. The dying stem cell hypothesis. J Am Coll Cardiol 2005; 46: 1799–1802.
15. Strauer BE, Brehm M, Zeus T, et al. Repair of infarcted myocardium by autologous intracoronary mononuclear bone marrow cell transplantation in humans. Circulation 2002; 106:1913–1918.
16. Assmus B, Schächinger V, Teupe C, et al. Transplantation of Progenitor cells and regeneration enhancement in acute myocardial infarction (TOPCARE-AMI). Circulation 2002; 106:3009–3017.
17. Kang HJ, Kim HS, Zhang SY, et al. Effects of intracoronary infusion of peripheral blood stem-cells mobilised with granulocyte-colony stimulating factor on left ventricular systolic function and restenosis after coronary stenting in myocardial infarction: the MAGIC cell randomised clinical trial. Lancet 2004; 363:751–756.
18. Fernández-Avilés F, San Román JA, García-Frade J, et al. Experimental and clinical regenerative capability of human bone marrow cells after myocardial infarction. Circ Res 2004; 95:742–748.
19. Schächinger V, Assmus B, Britten MB, et al. Transplantation of progenitor cells and regeneration enhancement in acute myocardial infarction: final one-year results of the TOPCARE-AMI Trial. J Am Coll Cardiol 2004; 44:1690–1699.
20. Wollert KC, Meyer GP, Lotz J, et al. Intracoronary autologous bone-marrow cell transfer after myocardial infarction:

the BOOST randomised controlled clinical trial. Lancet 2004; 364:141–148.

21. Schächinger V, Erbs S, Elsässer A, et al. Intracoronary bone marrow-derived progenitor cells in acute myocardial infarction. N Engl J Med 2006; 355:1210–1221.

22. Lunde K, Solheim S, Aakhus S, et al. Intracoronary injection of mononuclear bone marrow cells in acute myocardial infarction. N Engl J Med 2006; 355:1199–1209.

23. Anversa P, Leri A, Kajstura J. Cardiac Regeneration. J Am Coll Cardiol 2006; 47:1769–1776.

24. Lipinski MJ, Biondi-Zoccai GG, Abbate A, et al. Impact of intracoronary cell therapy on left ventricular function in the setting of acute myocardial infarction: a collaborative systematic review and meta-analysis of controlled clinical trials. J Am Coll Cardiol 2007; 50:1761–1767.

25. Tse HF, Kwong YL, Chan JK, et al. Angiogenesis in ischemic myocardium by intramyocardial autologous bone marrow mononuclear cell implantation. Lancet 2003; 361:47–49.

26. Fuchs S, Satler LF, Kornowski R, et al. Catheter-based autologous bone marrow myocardial injection in no-option patients with advanced coronary artery disease: a feasibility study. J Am Coll Cardiol 2003; 41:1721–1724.

27. Perin EC, Dohmann HF, Borojevic R, et al. Transendocardial, autologous bone marrow cell transplantation for severe, chronic ischemic heart failure. Circulation 2003; 107:2294–2302.

28. Silva GV, Perin EC, Dohmann HF, et al. Catheter-based transendocardial delivery of autologous bone-marrow-derived mononuclear cells in patients listed for heart transplantation. Tex Heart Inst J 2004; 31(3):214–219.

29. Charwat S, Gyongyosi M, Beran G, et al. Combined intra-myocardial and intracoronary administration of autologous stem cells in patients with ischaemic cardiomiopathy. Am J Cardiol 2005; 96(suppl):12H.

30. Gyongyosi M, Beran G, Long I, et al. Improvement of myocardial perfusion and left ventricular function in patients of ischaemic heart disease after combined (intra-myocardial and intracoronary) bone marrow derived stem cell therapy. Am J Cardiol 2005; 96(suppl):12H.

31. Mansour S, Vanderheyden M, De Bruyne B, et al. Intra-coronary delivery of hematopoietic bone marrow stem cells and luminal loss of the infarct-related artery in patients with recent myocardial infarction. J Am Coll Cardiol 2006; 47:1727–1730.

32. Kang HJ, Lee HY, Na SH, et al. Differential effect of intracoronary infusion of mobilized peripheral blood stem cells by granulocyte colony-stimulating factor on left ventricular function and remodeling in patients with acute myocardial infarction versus old myocardial infarction: the MAGIC Cell-3-DES randomized, controlled trial. Circulation 2006; 114(1 suppl):I145–I151.

33. Leone AM, Rutella S, Bonanno G, et al. Mobilization of bone marrow-derived stem cells after myocardial infarction and left ventricular function. Eur Heart J 2005; 26:1196–1204.

34. Wojakowski W, Tendera M, Zebzda A, et al. Mobilization of CD34(+), CD117(+), CXCR4(+), c-met(+) stem cells is correlated with left ventricular ejection fraction and plasma NT-proBNP levels in patients with acute myocardial infarction. Eur Heart J 2006; 27:283–289.

14

The Assessment of Myocardial Reperfusion and Its Clinical Significance in Acute Myocardial Infarction

GIOVANNI MARIA SANTORO

Division of Cardiology, San Giovanni di Dio Hospital, Florence, Italy

In patients with acute myocardial infarction (AMI) early coronary artery recanalization may induce salvage of reversible damaged ischemic myocardium and limit infarct size. The short-term effect is improvement of left ventricular (LV) function and reduction of mortality in the first few weeks after AMI. The long-term effect is prevention of LV remodeling and dilatation and, consequently, reduction of LV failure and death.

Although patency of the infarct artery is the essential prerequisite, the early restoration of an anterograde flow may not be sufficient to offer a benefit because a discrepancy may exist between epicardial coronary flow and myocardial tissue perfusion and because reperfusion may occur too late to salvage myocardium. Therefore, two conditions are needed to ensure myocardial salvage: restoration of myocardial tissue perfusion and persistence of myocardial viability.

THE NO-REFLOW PHENOMENON

Restoration of blood flow in the epicardial coronary artery by fibrinolytic treatment or percutaneous coronary intervention (PCI) does not necessarily imply complete restoration of myocardial tissue perfusion. Prolonged coronary occlusion and subsequent reperfusion may induce structural changes in the microvasculature, which prevent restoration of blood flow to cardiac myocytes. The phenomenon of no-reflow is defined as inadequate myocardial perfusion without angiographic evidence of mechanical vessel obstruction (1). The occurrence of no-reflow is more frequent with longer periods of coronary occlusion. The distribution is predominant in the subendocardium and its manifestation is progressive since no-reflow starts during the ischemic period and then increases during reperfusion (2).

Although it is clear that no-reflow is secondary to abnormalities in the microvasculature, the mechanisms involved in determining the phenomenon are uncertain and probably a variety of factors contribute to it. However, no-reflow is primarily caused by microvascular compression and obstruction (Table 14.1).

During the ischemic phase, endothelial damage may occur in the form of endothelial swelling and endothelial protrusions, which may reduce or occlude the capillary lumen (1). Myocardial cell swelling and interstitial edema secondary to ischemia may contribute to the development of areas of initial no-reflow. Reperfusion-induced myocardial cell swelling and contracture and increase in interstitial edema may exacerbate mechanical compression of the vascular bed after reopening of the coronary vessel. Intravascular plugging by fibrin, platelets, and

Table 14.1 Mechanisms Involved in the Genesis of No-Reflow

Microvascular compression
—Myocardial cell swelling (ischemia reperfusion)
—Interstitial edema (ischemia reperfusion)
—Myocardial cell contracture (reperfusion)
—Interstitial microhemorrhage (ischemia reperfusion)

Microvascular obstruction
—Endothelial blebs (ischemia reperfusion)
—Endothelial swelling (ischemia reperfusion)
—Platelet plugs (reperfusion)
—Neutrophil plugs (reperfusion)
—Red blood cell plugs (reperfusion)
—Spasm (reperfusion)
—Atheroembolism (spontaneous or during reperfusion treatment)

leukocytes has been recognized as the main cause of microvascular obstruction. Capillary leukocyte plugging has been demonstrated in no-reflow areas (3). The negative effect of leukocytes is probably not limited to mechanical plugging. Leukocytes may release oxygen-free radicals, proteolytic enzymes, and lipoxygenase products, which may induce endothelial dysfunction and vasoconstriction (4). Another potential source of microvascular obstruction, particularly in the setting of acute AMI treated either by fibrinolytic treatment or PCI, is atheroembolism caused by microemboli of atherosclerotic debris, blood clots, and platelet aggregates. Animal studies support the role of platelet-dependent microembolization (5). Necropsy studies have demonstrated the presence of thrombi occluding coronary microvessels in patients who died after AMI (6,7). Functional abnormalities of the microvasculature may contribute to no-reflow. Coronary artery occlusion may trigger a cardio-cardiac sympathetic reflex, which results in α-adrenergic macrovascular and microvascular constriction (8). An increase in the density of angiotensin II receptors in the scar tissue has been shown after experimental AMI (9). Angiotensin II may modulate the sympathetic control of coronary vasomotor tone, contributing to increased coronary constriction.

Recently, the traditional concept of secondary microvascular impairment in the setting of ischemia reperfusion damage has been questioned, and a primary dysfunction of the myocardial microvasculature has been suggested as a potential mechanism contributing to the genesis of AMI (10). According to this hypothesis, preexisting transient or permanent microvascular dysfunction might reduce blood flow in the epicardial coronary vessels, leading to an alteration of shear stress and endothelial function, which in turn might contribute to thrombus formation and AMI pathogenesis.

ASSESSMENT OF MYOCARDIAL REPERFUSION

Several diagnostic strategies have been proposed to evaluate myocardial tissue perfusion. Since numerous fibrinolytic and PCI studies have demonstrated unfavorable outcome in patients with AMI who have no-reflow after reperfusion therapy, the recognition of impaired myocardial perfusion allows the early identification of patients who have an adverse clinical prognosis and consequently deserve special attention.

Coronary Angiography

Thrombolysis in Myocardial Infarction Flow Grade

The quality of flow in the epicardial coronary artery is traditionally classified according to the Thrombolysis in Myocardial Infarction (TIMI) flow grade (Table 14.2) (11). In patients treated with fibrinolytic therapy or PCI, TIMI grade 0 to 1 flow has been traditionally considered to identify failure to achieve an acceptable epicardial coronary flow, while TIMI grade 2 to 3 flow has been associated with successful coronary recanalization. Subsequently, however, the clinical significance of TIMI grade 2 flow was recognized closer to that of TIMI grade 0 to 1 flow than to that of TIMI grade 3 flow. Therefore, TIMI grade flow <3 without evidence of obstruction in the epicardial coronary artery is actually considered the angiographic counterpart of no-reflow, and only TIMI grade 3 flow is considered to indicate normal flow. PCI has been shown to be more effective than fibrinolytic treatment in restoring TIMI grade 3 flow. While only 50% to 60% of the patients treated with fibrinolysis had TIMI grade 3 flow at 90 minutes coronary angiography (12), 92.3% of patients treated with angioplasty had TIMI grade 3 flow after the intervention, a higher rate than that observed in

Table 14.2 TIMI Flow Grade

Grade 0–No perfusion; no antegrade flow beyond the point of occlusion.
Grade 1–Penetration without perfusion; contrast material passes beyond the area of obstruction but fails to opacify the entire coronary bed.
Grade 2–Partial perfusion; contrast material passes across the obstruction and opacifies the coronary artery distal to the obstruction. However, the rate of entry of contrast material into the vessel distal to the obstruction or its rate of clearance from the distal bed (or both) is slower than its flow into or clearance from adjacent vessels.
Grade 3–Complete perfusion; antegrade flow into the bed distal to the obstruction and clearance of contrast material is as rapid as in adjacent vessels.

Abbreviation: TIMI, Thrombolysis in Myocardial Infarction.
Source: From Ref. 11.

patients treated with stent implantation (88.6%) (13). Both fibrinolytic and PCI studies have demonstrated improvement in clinical outcome in patients with AMI who had early restoration of TIMI grade 3 flow in the infarct artery. In a meta-analysis of five fibrinolytic trials (11), overall mortality was 3.7% for TIMI grade 3 flow, 7.0% for TIMI grade 2 flow, and 8.8% for TIMI grade 0 to 1 flow. LV global and regional systolic function was also significantly improved in patients with TIMI grade 3 flow in comparison to those with TIMI grade 2 and TIMI grade 0 to 1 flow. Similarly, a better clinical outcome has been observed in patients treated with PCI, who had restoration of TIMI grade 3 flow. In the PCI group of the GUSTO IIb (14), 30-day mortality rate was 1.6% in patients with TIMI grade 3 flow, 19.9% in patients with TIMI grade 2 flow, and 20.0% in patients with TIMI grade 0 to 1 flow. The same result was found in patients treated with coronary stent implantation. The six-month composite end point of death, reinfarction, or target vessel revascularization was 15.8% in patients with TIMI grade 3 flow and 40% in patients with TIMI grade 0 to 2 flow ($p = 0.02$) (15). TIMI grade 3 flow was the strongest determinant of survival. The results of the Florence registry, including 1894 consecutive patients with AMI treated with primary PCI in the period 1995 to 2002, are similar. The six-month composite end point of death, reinfarction, or target vessel revascularization was 22% in patients with TIMI grade 3 flow, 33% in TIMI grade 2 flow, and 55% in TIMI grade 0 to 1 flow ($p < 0.001$ vs. TIMI grade 3) (Fig. 14.1).

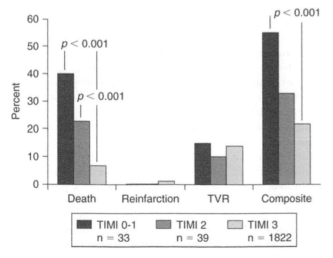

Figure 14.1 TIMI flow grade and six-month composite end point (including death, reinfarction, and target vessel revascularization) rate in 1894 patients treated with primary PCI in the Division of Cardiology, Careggi Hospital, Florence, Italy between January 1995 and December 2002. *Abbreviations*: TIMI, Thrombolysis in Myocardial Infarction; PCI, percutaneous coronary intervention.

Corrected TIMI Frame Count

Although the TIMI flow grade is a valuable and widely used qualitative classification of the epicardial coronary flow, it is limited by its subjective and categorical nature. To standardize the assessment of the epicardial coronary flow and develop a simple continuous index of coronary flow, another method has been proposed, which is based on the number of cineframes required for contrast dye to first reach standard distal coronary landmarks (TIMI frame count) (16). Since in normal coronary arteries the left anterior descending coronary artery TIMI frame count was 1.7 times longer than the mean of the right coronary and circumflex counts, the longer frame count of this vessel was corrected by dividing by 1.7 to obtain the corrected TIMI frame count (CTFC). In contrast to the conventional TIMI flow grade system, the CTFC allows a quantitative rather than a qualitative evaluation; is a continuous rather than a categorical method; and is objective, reproducible, and sensitive to flow changes (16). Despite high rates of TIMI grade 3 flow reported in the literature, a truly normal flow (defined as CTFC < 28) was observed in only one-third of patients with an open artery at 90 minutes after fibrinolysis (16). In a study including 1248 patients of the TIMI 4, 10A, and 10B trials (17), faster flow (lower 90-minute CTFC) was related to improved in-hospital and one-month clinical outcomes after fibrinolytic treatment in both univariate and multivariate models. In a multivariate model that excluded TIMI flow grades, the 90-minute CTFC was an independent predictor of in-hospital mortality (OR 1.21 per 10-frame rise, $p < 0.001$), even when other significant predictors of mortality were considered. The CTFC was found to identify a subgroup of patients with TIMI grade 3 flow, who were at a particularly low risk of adverse outcome. The risk of in-hospital mortality increased from 0% in patients with a 90-minute CTFC of 0 to 13 frames to 2.7% in patients with a CTFC of 14 to 40 (CTFC of 40 had previously been identified as the cutpoint for TIMI grade 3 flow) to 6.4% in patients with a CTFC > 40 ($p = 0.003$) (17). The coronary flow corresponding to CTFC <14, which is faster than the 95th percentile for normal flow, has been considered as expression of hyperemia and termed "TIMI 4 flow." The clinical significance of hyperemic epicardial flow has been recently evaluated in patients included in the Clopidogrel as Adjunctive Reperfusion Therapy–TIMI 28 (CLARITY-TIMI 28) (18). In patients who underwent fibrinolytic therapy, hyperemic flow on initial diagnostic coronary angiography two to eight days following drug administration was associated with improved outcomes. On the contrary, in patients who underwent PCI at this time point, hyperemic flow following intervention was associated with an increased incidence of adverse outcomes, including death and myocardial infarction. This adverse association appeared to occur exclusively in patients with suboptimal myocardial perfusion, whereas hyperemic flow with normal myocardial perfusion was associated with a low incidence of 30-day mortality. Although the pathophysiological mechanism is not well understood, it has been suggested that hyperemic flow with associated impaired myocardial perfusion may be a marker of more extensive microembolization.

Myocardial Perfusion Grade

While TIMI flow grade and CTFC are indicative of the quality of epicardial coronary flow, myocardial reperfusion is better evaluated using myocardial blush grade (MBG), on the basis of visually assessed contrast density in the infarcted myocardium after reperfusion therapy (Table 14.3). In a study by van't Hof et al. (19) including 777 patients who had undergone primary PCI, the decrease in MBG from 3 (normal myocardial blush) to 0 (no myocardial blush) was associated in a stepwise fashion with an increase in enzymatic infarct size ($p < 0.0001$) and in LV dysfunction ($p < 0.0001$). Mortality rates of patients with MBG 3, 2, and 0/1 were 3%, 6%, and 23% ($p < 0.0001$), respectively. Multivariate analysis showed that the MBG was a predictor of long-term mortality, independent of Killip class, TIMI grade flow, and left ventricular ejection fraction (LVEF). In a more recent study of the same group, MBG was shown to be a strong predictor of mortality beyond TIMI grade 3 flow (20). In 924 consecutive patients with TIMI grade 3 flow after primary PCI, mortality was significantly higher in patients with MBG 0/1 compared to patients with MBG 2/3 (relative risk 4.7; 95% CI, 2.3–9.5; $p < 0.001$). Enzymatic infarct size was larger and residual LVEF was lower in patients with MBG 0/1 compared to patients with MBG 2/3 (20). Similar results have been reported in the 1301 patients with AMI randomized to balloon angioplasty versus stenting, each with or without abciximab, who had been enrolled in the Controlled Abciximab and Device Investigation to Lower Late Angioplasty Complications (CADILLAC) trial (21). Despite TIMI grade 3

Table 14.3 Myocardial Blush Grade

Grade 0–No myocardial blush or contrast density.
Grade 1–Minimal contrast blush or contrast density.
Grade 2–Moderate myocardial blush or contrast density but less than that observed in a contralateral or ipsilateral non-infarct-related coronary artery.
Grade 3–Normal myocardial blush or contrast density, comparable with that observed in a contralateral or ipsilateral non-infarct-related coronary artery.

The persistence of myocardial blush suggests leakage of contrast medium into the endovascular space and is classified as grade 0.
Source: From Ref. 19.

flow restoration in 96.1% of patients, MBG 3 was found in only 17.4%, while MBG 2 occurred in 33.9% and MBG 0/1 in 48.7%. Myocardial perfusion status post-PCI stratified patients into three distinct categories with one-year mortality rates of 1.4 (MBG 3), 4.1% (MBG 2), and 6.2% (MBG 0/1), respectively ($p = 0.01$).

While MBG uses static densitometric evaluation of the intensity of myocardial blush, a different method—on the basis of the dynamic evaluation of entrance and exit of contrast medium in the myocardium supplied by the infarct vessel—was developed by the TIMI study group (22). The TIMI myocardial perfusion grade (TMPG) evaluates the duration of the myocardial blush, rather than its brightness or density (Table 14.4). In a study including 762 patients of the TIMI 10B trial (22), there was a mortality gradient across the TMPGs, with mortality lowest in patients with TMPG 3 (2.0%), intermediate in TMPG 2 (4.4%), and highest in TMPG 0/1 (6%; 3-way $p = 0.05$). The use of the TMPG allowed additional risk stratification even in patients with TIMI grade 3 flow in the epicardial artery. Mortality at 30 days was 0.7% for TMPG 3, 2.9% for TMPG 2, and 5.0% for TMPG 0/1. TMPG 3 was a correlate of 30-day mortality (OR 0.35, $p = 0.054$) in a multivariate model adjusted for the presence of TIMI grade 3 flow, CTFC, AMI location, and age. Thus, the TMPG appears to add prognostic information to the conventional epicardial TIMI flow grade and CTFC, which evaluate the quality of blood

Table 14.4 TIMI Myocardial Perfusion Grade

Grade 0–Failure of contrast material to enter the microvasculature. Either minimal or no ground-glass appearance ("blush") or opacification of the myocardium in the distribution of the culprit artery.
Grade 1–Contrast material slowly enters but fails to exit the microvasculature. There is the ground-glass appearance (blush) or opacification of the myocardium in the distribution of the culprit lesion that fails to clear from the microvasculature, and dye staining is present on the next injection (~30 seconds between injections).
Grade 2–Delayed entry and exit of contrast material from the microvasculature. There is the ground-glass appearance (blush) or opacification of the myocardium in the distribution of the culprit lesion that is strongly persistent at the end of the washout phase (contrast material is strongly persistent after three cardiac cycles of the washout phase and either does not or only minimally diminishes in intensity during washout).
Grade 3–Normal entry and exit of contrast material from the microvasculature. There is the ground-glass appearance (blush) or opacification of the myocardium in the distribution of the culprit lesion that clears normally and is either gone or only mildly/moderately persistent at the end of the washout phase, similar to that in an uninvolved artery.

Source: From Ref. 19.

flow in the epicardial coronary artery. Similar results have recently been obtained in patients with AMI treated with primary PCI. In the subset of 1018 patients included in the Assessment of Pexelizumab in AMI (APEX-AMI) trial, TMPG 2/3 occurred in 91%. After adjustment for baseline characteristics, TMPG 2/3 after PCI was associated with younger age, pre-PCI TIMI grade 2/3 flow, and ischemic time. TMPG 2/3 after PCI, in combination with TIMI grade 3 flow, identified a group of patients with a nearly 50% lower incidence of death, or heart failure, or shock at 90 days compared with patients with neither one of these indexes of successful reperfusion (23).

Myocardial Contrast Echocardiography

While in the past the only way to obtain myocardial contrast echocardiography (MCE) was intracoronary injection of sonicated microbubbles, the development of new contrast agents, which can opacify the myocardium after intravenous infusion, has given rise to the hope of a diffusion of this method to evaluate microvascular perfusion. Ultrasound contrast agents consist of high density and high molecular weight gas encased by an outer shell. They are able to pass through an intact microvasculature and cannot diffuse out of the intravascular space. Therefore, microbubbles behave as pure tracers of myocardial flow and allow an accurate assessment of microvascular perfusion. During constant intravenous infusion of microbubbles, the contrast intensity seen within the myocardium reflects the concentration of bubbles, which is proportionate to the capillary blood volume. During high-power imaging, microbubbles are destroyed, and the rate of increase in signal intensity can be measured. Decrease in myocardial blood flow is associated with a reduced rate of increase of signal intensity, which depends on microbubble entry into the microvasculature. Microvascular status evaluation is based on both the change in myocardial signal intensity throughout the replenishment curve and the degree of opacification at the peak contrast effect (24). Unfortunately, severe adverse events, which have been observed during the i.v. infusion of ultrasound contrast agents, have prevented until now a more extensive use of such agents to study patients with AMI or other unstable conditions.

The main goals of MCE in the setting of AMI are the evaluation of the area at risk and the assessment of reperfusion in terms of microvascular flow restoration.

The accurate evaluation of the risk area size by MCE requires that the microbubbles enter both coronary arteries to identify the contribution of collateral supply. Collateral blood flow may limit the infarct size and preserve LV function during acute coronary occlusion. Experimental data have confirmed that the infarct size is smaller and the recovery of LV function faster when collateral flow is present (25).

After the infarct artery is fully reopened, microvascular flow in the reperfused area is spatially heterogeneous (Fig. 14.2) (26,27). In the salvaged myocardium, microvasculature is maintained structurally intact, and flow may be normal or hyperemic, while contractile function is often transiently impaired (stunned myocardium). In the infarcted area, a mixture of intact and structurally damaged microvasculature is present, conditioning the coexistence of hyperemia, normal flow (both with impaired flow reserve), low flow, or no-reflow. Because microbubbles cannot enter an area with damaged microvasculature, a persistent MCE defect after recanalization of the infarct artery indicates low flow or no-reflow and is associated with the presence of necrotic myocardium. On the other hand, the demonstration by MCE of perfusion recovery in the risk area does not exclude necrosis, since MCE performed immediately after recanalization of the infarct artery may underestimate the infarct size, due to the presence of hyperemia or normal flow. Therefore, infarct size is more accurately evaluated at a time distance from the acute phase, although the optimal time is not precisely defined. Alternatively, infarct size shortly after infarct artery recanalization may be better quantified using a vasodilator stimulus. Necrotic regions, which initially maintain a relatively preserved resting flow, have an impaired flow reserve and, consequently, MCE perfusion defects during vasodilatation may more closely indicate infarct extent (27).

Numerous studies using MCE have shown that despite epicardial coronary artery patency, a large number of patients have perfusion defects, indicating low flow or no-reflow. In a study including 86 patients with first anterior AMI who underwent MCE before and immediately after revascularization by PCI or thrombolysis, epicardial coronary flow was graded according to the TIMI grade system (28). All 18 patients with TIMI grade 2 flow had no-reflow at MCE; no-reflow was present also in 11 of the 68 patients with TIMI grade 3 flow (16%). Among patients with TIMI grade 3 flow, only those with reflow showed a significant improvement in systolic function at one-month follow-up. In other studies (29–33), which used MCE shortly after reopening of the infarct artery, absence of microvascular reperfusion despite epicardial coronary artery patency was observed in 27% to 33% of the patients. Patients with no-reflow in the risk area immediately after reperfusion did not show late improvement in LV regional wall motion, while patients with reflow in the risk area showed late improvement in regional wall motion (Fig. 14.3). Therefore, no-reflow is indicative of failure of myocardial salvage and predicts poor LV functional recovery. Nevertheless, functional recovery cannot be demonstrated in all patients with reflow and in all reperfused segments. In a study (31) in 30 patients with AMI treated with PCI, of 72 reperfused

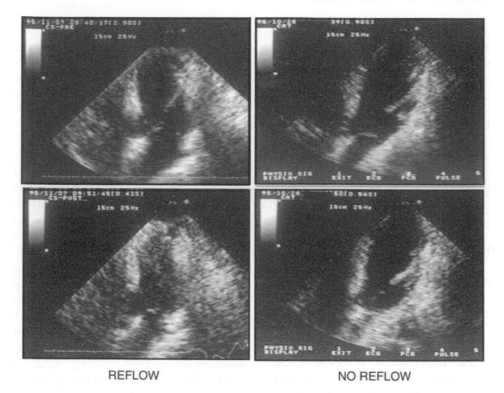

REFLOW   NO REFLOW

Figure 14.2 MCE before (*upper*) and after (*lower*) successful coronary angioplasty of the mid left anterior descending artery in two different patients with anterior AMI, one with reflow (*right*) and the other with no-reflow (*left*). (*Left*) Pre-PCI MCE identifies the risk area including the distal septum and the apex of the left ventricle (*upper*); post-PCI MCE shows reperfusion of the distal septum, although a perfusion defect persists at the apex (*lower*). (*Right*) Pre-PCI MCE identifies the risk area including the distal septum and the apex of the left ventricle (*upper*); post-PCI MCE shows the persistence of a large perfusion defect, suggesting no-reflow (*lower*). *Abbreviations*: MCE, myocardial contrast echocardiography; PCI, percutaneous coronary intervention; AMI, acute myocardial infarction.

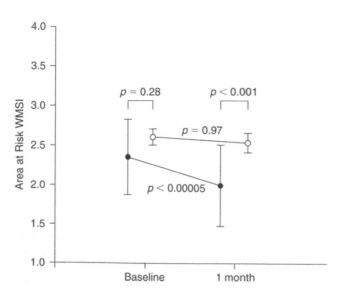

Figure 14.3 Plots of WMSI in the area at risk in the acute and chronic stages of myocardial infarction in patients with no-reflow (*open circles*) and with reflow (*solid circles*). *Abbreviation*: WMSI, wall motion score index. *Source*: From Ref. 31.

segments, only 27 (37%) showed an improvement in wall motion score after one month while 45 did not. This result confirms that contrast enhancement shortly after reperfusion does not necessarily imply myocardial salvage and LV functional recovery. It is possible that the execution of MCE at a time outside the temporal range of the dynamic changes of flow occurring immediately after reperfusion may estimate myocardial viability more accurately (32,33). A better indicator of viability may be dobutamine stimulation, especially in the absence of flow-limiting lesions. In patients with AMI successfully treated with primary PCI, we compared the ability of MCE performed immediately after reflow and low-dose dobutamine echocardiography performed three days after AMI to predict late functional recovery (31). Only half of the segments with homogeneous contrast enhancement had preserved contractile reserve and demonstrated improvement at follow-up. The sensitivities of the two methods were similar but specificity, positive predictive value, and global accuracy of dobutamine echocardiography were significantly better (Fig. 14.4).

The long-term prognostic value of microvascular dysfunction by MCE after successful reopening of the infarct

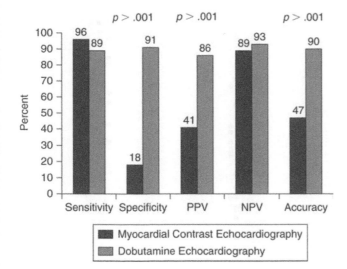

Figure 14.4 Comparison on segment basis of the results of MCE and of those of dobutamine echocardiography in predicting late functional recovery. *Abbreviation*: MCE, myocardial contrast echocardiography. *Source*: From Ref. 31.

artery was investigated in a study by Bolognese et al. (34). The incidence of LV remodeling was significantly greater among patients with microvascular dysfunction than among those without (63% vs. 11%, $p < 0.0001$). During a mean follow-up of 46 ± 32 months, patients with microvascular dysfunction had a higher rate of death and cumulative adverse events than those without. By multivariate analysis, microvascular dysfunction was identified as an independent predictor of cardiac death (OR 0.26; 95% CI, 0.09–0.72; $p = 0.014$). Similar data have been reported in patients with anterior AMI and LV dysfunction (35). Recently the value of microvascular dysfunction in the prediction of LV remodeling was compared with established parameters of reperfusion, such as peak creatine kinase (CK), ST segment resolution, TIMI flow grade, and MBG (36). At multivariate analysis, only the endocardial length of contrast defect on MCE and TIMI flow <3 were independent predictors of LV remodeling. In the subset of patients with a TIMI grade 3 flow, only the endocardial length of MCE perfusion defect predicted LV remodeling.

Nuclear Imaging

In humans, the first demonstration of no-reflow after AMI was obtained by Shofer et al. in 1985 using dual myocardial scintigraphy with thallium-201 (Tl-201) and technetium-99m (Tc-99m) microalbumin aggregates performed before and immediately after intracoronary thrombolysis (37). Since then, nuclear imaging has been extensively used to evaluate the results of reperfusion therapy, as it has the

potential to assess both myocardial perfusion and viability.

Myocardial perfusion scintigraphy with Tl-201 was initially used to evaluate the efficacy of coronary reperfusion in AMI (38,39). However, the use of Tl-201 in this setting has important limitations, which were overcome by the introduction of Tc-99m sestamibi. The absence of significant redistribution and the independence from postreperfusion hyperemia allow to inject Tc-99m sestamibi before starting reperfusion therapy and to collect images even several hours later, without delaying therapy and when the patient's condition is relatively stabilized. Therefore, patients can be injected with the tracer before the application of treatment; the perfusion defect, seen in the images acquired in the subsequent hours, is assumed to demonstrate the area at risk. Myocardial scintigraphy after a second injection of Tc-99m sestamibi can be repeated hours or days after the first examination; the perfusion defect on the second study is assumed to indicate the final infarct size. The decrease in the perfusion defect size between the first and the second study is considered to represent the extent of myocardial salvage, that is, the extent of reperfused viable myocardium (Fig. 14.5). In a study (40) from our group all patients who showed a remarkable decrease in the perfusion defect size had a late reduction in wall motion abnormalities; in contrast, patients who showed a limited or negligible reduction in the perfusion defect size did not have changes in regional LV wall motion. The modification of the perfusion defect size between the first and the second scintigraphic study was highly correlated with the reduction in the asynergic area extent score between admission and follow-up echo examinations (40,41). The demonstrated ability of serial Tc-99m sestamibi scintigraphy to detect myocardium salvage induced Gibbons et al. (42) to use this method to compare the results of intravenous thrombolysis and direct PCI. Myocardial salvage was 27% of the left ventricle for patients treated with fibrinolytic therapy versus 31% of the left ventricle for patients undergoing primary PCI and the difference was not significant.

While the functional outcome of salvaged myocardium is easily predicted by its preserved perfusion and viability, the fate of the myocardium included in the posttreatment perfusion defect is more uncertain. Several studies have demonstrated that in a consistent part of patients the defect size continued to decrease late after fibrinolytic therapy (43–45). The reduction in the perfusion defect size was associated with an improvement in LVEF and regional wall motion and a reduction in end-systolic and end-diastolic volumes (45). Therefore, while the MCE perfusion defect extent may overestimate the extent of myocardial salvage early after reperfusion treatment, the scintigraphic perfusion defect may underestimate the presence of viable myocardium. A more reliable marker of viability may be

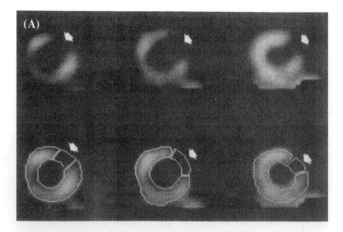

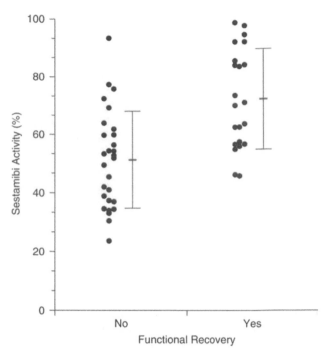

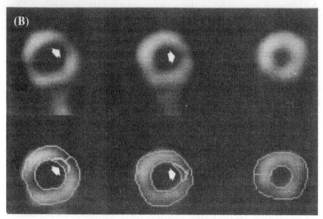

Figure 14.5 Short-axis images (from *left to right*: basal, midventricular, and subapical slices). (**A**) The prethrombolytic treatment images; a clear-cut anterolateral perfusion defect is shown (*top row, arrows*). (**B**) The five-day images; a noteworthy reduction in the defect can be appreciated (*top row, arrows*). In the respective bottom rows, the computer-assisted, manually drawn perfused and nonperfused areas (*arrows*) are shown. The difference in perfusion defect size between the first and the second study represents the extent of myocardial salvage. *Source*: From Ref. 40.

Figure 14.6 Scatterplot of sestamibi activity in perfusion risk area segments divided according to the presence or absence of functional recovery in follow-up echocardiography. Individual data points and mean ± SD are shown. *Source*: From Ref. 46.

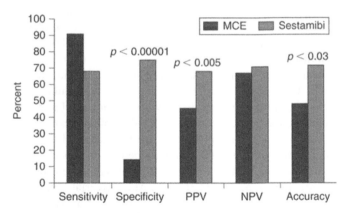

Figure 14.7 Comparison on segment basis of the results of MCE and of those of Tc-99m sestamibi SPECT in the identification of myocardial salvage. *Abbreviation*: MCE, myocardial contrast echocardiography. *Source*: From Ref. 46.

the demonstration of preserved tracer activity (>60% of peak activity) within the perfusion defect using delayed Tc-99m sestamibi perfusion imaging (Fig. 14.6). In a study (46) including 26 patients with AMI treated with successful primary PCI, MCE showed a higher sensitivity in detecting viable myocardium, whereas Tc-99m sestamibi SPECT showed significantly higher specificity and positive predictive value (Fig. 14.7). The demonstration of a concordant improvement in perfusion and function suggests the possibility that hypoperfused but viable myocardium (i.e., hibernating myocardium) is present in a relevant proportion of patients with persistent perfusion defect after reperfusion therapy. Lomboy et al. (47), using rest-redistribution Tl-201 scintigraphy, demonstrated viable myocardium early after AMI in 48% of patients; on follow-up these patients

showed improved LV function. In patients with AMI and TIMI grade 3 flow in the infarct vessel after fibrinolytic therapy, Maes et al. (48), using positron emission tomography (PET) to study myocardial blood flow and metabolism, observed that patients with high flow values had preserved regional contractile function at three months, while patients with reduced flow despite successful thrombolysis showed recovery of LV function only if PCI succeeded in treating the residual stenosis of the infarct vessel corresponding to regions with flow-metabolism mismatch, suggesting hibernation. In a more recent study (49) including 18 patients with TIMI grade 3 flow after successful reperfusion, the same group observed that in infarct-related regions, myocardial blood flow, glucose uptake, and oxygen consumption were decreased, compared with remote regions; however, a significant linear correlation was observed between LVEF at three months and oxidative metabolism in the infarct area ($p < 0.0001$). The evaluation of the contractile reserve of the infarct zone using dobutamine echocardiography and the assessment of the tracer activity of the infarct zone or infarct severity using Tc-99m sestamibi SPECT early after AMI were shown to be able to identify patients who had late LVEF improvement (50). In 51 patients with AMI who underwent primary PCI with TIMI grade 3 flow restoration, the late outcome of the LVEF was established after a six-month follow-up. In the early phase after AMI, dobutamine echocardiography achieved a receiver-operating curve (ROC) area of 0.75 ± 0.07 with 74% sensitivity, 71% specificity, and 73% overall accuracy. Of the Tc-99m sestamibi SPECT parameters, the extent of the infarct had no diagnostic value according to ROC analysis; on the other hand, the mean activity of the infarct zone had an ROC area of 0.64 ± 0.09 with 82% sensitivity, 50% specificity, and 73% overall accuracy, and the infarct severity had an ROC area of 0.76 ± 0.08 (not significant vs. mean activity and vs. contractile reserve) with 77% sensitivity, 71% specificity, and 75% overall accuracy (Fig. 14.8).

Magnetic Resonance Imaging

Contrast-enhanced magnetic resonance imaging (MRI) with gadolinium chelates is becoming one of the most interesting techniques to assess myocardial perfusion and viability following AMI (51–54). Although gadolinium is an extracellular contrast agent that diffuses into the interstitial space, on early first-pass imaging (i.e., the first minute after intravenous bolus), gadolinium behaves as an intravascular agent. Therefore, the hypoenhanced region (low signal intensity) subtended by the infarct artery represents an area of no-reflow or slow flow compared to the normal adjacent myocardium. In addition to the assessment of perfusion status, contrast-enhanced MRI can also evaluate the infarcted tissue. After intravenous injection, gadolinium extravasates into the interstitium. While the contrast medium is rapidly washed out of normal myocardium, it remains entrapped in infarcted myocardium because of the slow washout from poor blood flow and increased volume of distribution in this abnormal tissue. When contrast-enhanced images are obtained late (approximately 10–15 minutes after gadolinium injection), infarcted myocardium appears as a hyperenhanced region

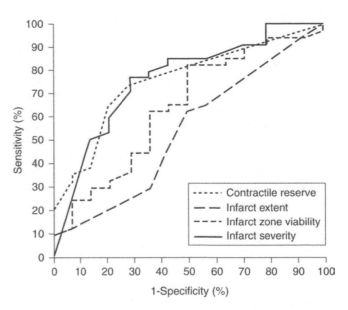

Figure 14.8 ROCs constructed using contractile reserve assessed by dobutamine echocardiography, and three different parameters derived from Tc-99m sestamibi SPECT for detection of significant late LVEF improvement after primary PCI. *Abbreviations*: ROC, receiver-operating curve; LVEF, left ventricular ejection fraction. *Source*: From Ref. 50.

with high signal intensity, which is easily distinguishable from the dark-gray appearance of surrounding normal myocardium. In 30% to 40% of patients, a hypoenhanced core region can be seen within gadolinium late hyperenhanced area, which is smaller than the perfusion defect on first-pass imaging. This area is usually located in the subendocardium and shows a variable degree of transmurality. It has been suggested that the perfusion defect on first-pass imaging represents an area with microvascular dysfunction, which may reduce, but not completely abolish, blood flow in the microvessels. The hypoenhanced core inside the hyperenhanced infarct region on delayed imaging may indicate a higher degree of damage, with profound microvascular alterations or obstruction, which prevent gadolinium to diffuse into the interstitium even after prolonged time period. Using a canine model of AMI, Wu et al. (55) compared MCE versus contrast-enhanced delayed MRI and S-thioflavin staining in the quantification of microvascular obstruction. MRI detected infarcted regions of <40% blood flow when compared with remote nonischemic regions, whereas MCE detected regions of <60% blood flow. Although both methods correctly identify regions of microvascular damage, MCE demarcates a larger region. When present, the size of hypoenhanced core peaks at approximately 48 hours and then diminishes as the area with severely damaged microvasculature turns into scar tissue. Although the hypoenhanced core may be still present one month after AMI, it is no longer present at six months (56).

Despite successful reopening of the infarct artery, patients with microvascular dysfunction detected by contrast-enhanced MRI have larger infarcts, more ventricular remodeling, less myocardial functional recovery, and worse clinical outcome.

Perfusion defects on first-pass imaging are present in 84% to 95% of patients with reperfused AMI. Taylor et al. (57) in 20 AMI patients treated with successful PCI showed that delay of contrast wash-in by more than two seconds compared to remote segments and infarct transmurality were both independent predictors of reduced systolic thickening at three months. Yan et al. (58) in 25 AMI patients studied within 72 hours of successful reperfusion demonstrated that the size of the perfusion defect had a strong correlation with TIMI frame count and infarct size.

The hypoenhanced core region within gadolinium late enhancement, when present, portends a worse prognosis in comparison with the perfusion defect seen in first-pass imaging. In a study (56) including 44 patients who underwent MRI 10 ± 6 days after AMI, patients with microvascular dysfunction, as demonstrated by the presence of a hypoenhanced core region, had more cardiovascular events than those without (45% vs. 9%). The risk of adverse events increased with infarct extent (30%, 43%, and 71% for small, mid-sized, and large infarcts, respectively). Even at multivariate analysis, the presence of microvascular dysfunction remained a prognostic marker of post-infarction complications. Hombach et al. (59) in 110 AMI patients imaged at six days, and again at six to nine months, found that the combination of severe microvascular damage demonstrated by the presence of the hypoenhanced core region, infarct size, and transmurality were predictors for the occurrence of adverse remodeling. The presence of microvascular damage also identified patients with a higher incidence of major adverse cardiac events including death, reinfarction, rehospitalization for cardiac failure, unstable angina, and revascularization procedures (21% vs. 8%). Bogaert et al. (60) in 52 patients with a successfully reperfused AMI observed that the hypoenhanced core area in the context of an hyperenhanced infarct area was associated with larger infarct area, worse systolic wall thickening in the infarct and peri-infarct area, and lower LVEF. At four months, infarcts with severe microvascular damage showed more adverse remodeling and lack of functional improvement in comparison with infarcts without the hypoenhanced core area.

Multidetector Computed Tomography

Multidetector computed tomography (MDCT) is mainly used to study coronary arteries, while evaluation of the myocardium is performed less often. Therefore, limited data are available about the diagnostic value of MDCT to assess myocardial perfusion and viability. MDCT has shown strong similarities with contrast-enhanced MRI in animals and humans (61–63). After recanalization of the infarct artery, on initial scan performed during the first pass of an iodinated contrast agent, the risk area with a preserved microvasculature becomes normally enhanced, while infarcted myocardium with microvascular dysfunction appears as a perfusion defect. On delayed imaging, performed five to six minutes after contrast injection, infarcted myocardium appears as a hyperenhanced area. The pharmacokinetic of iodinated contrast agents is similar to that of gadolinium chelates. Cell death together with microvascular damage results in accumulation of the contrast agent in the expanded extracellular space of the infarct area, which remains hyperenhanced because of the slow washout (64,65). In an experimental model of reperfused AMI, the infarct size measured on MDCT on the basis of delayed hyperenhancement correlated well with the infarct size measured on histochemical imaging (66). In humans, a strong association has been demonstrated between the presence and size of myocardial hyperenhancement on late scans and the likelihood of persistent mechanical dysfunction after AMI. In 52 consecutive patients with a first AMI, 64-slice MDCT was performed immediately after primary PCI. In patients with transmural delayed hyperenhancement, the recovery in global LV function was significantly poorer and LV remodeling was more frequently observed than in patients with only subendocardial hyperenhancement or patients with no hyperenhancement. On the other hand, the absence of myocardial hyperenhancement predicted myocardial functional recovery (67,68). Similar to MRI, the presence of a hypoenhanced core in the hyperenhanced region is thought to represent severe microvascular damage at the infarct center. The presence of hypoenhancement was associated with the lack of functional recovery of the myocardial segments involved (68).

Doppler Imaging

The use of intracoronary Doppler flow-wire has been proposed to demonstrate microvascular damage. In humans the no-reflow phenomenon determines a pattern of coronary blood flow velocity, which is characterized by three main elements: early systolic flow reversal (SFR), reduced anterograde systolic flow, and forward diastolic flow with a rapid deceleration slope (69,70). In 42 patients with AMI treated with PCI (70), coronary flow velocity measured by Doppler flow-wire was related to the results of MCE performed before and after PCI. Peak velocity and duration of systolic coronary flow were significantly

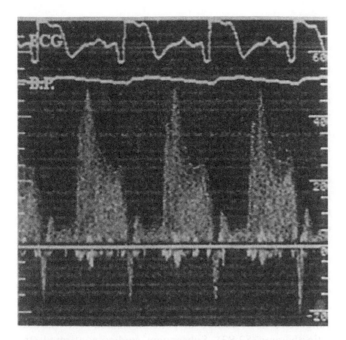

Figure 14.9 Coronary flow velocity spectrum in a patient with no-reflow on MCE. Note early systolic retrograde flow and rapid diastolic deceleration rate. *Abbreviation*: MCE, myocardial contrast echocardiography. *Source*: From Ref. 70.

less in patients with MCE no-reflow than in those with MCE reflow (8 ± 4 vs. 17 ± 10 cm/sec and 207 ± 79 vs. 289 ± 55 milliseconds, respectively; $p < 0.01$). Patients with MCE no-reflow showed early SFR more frequently than those with MCE reflow (91% vs. 3%; $p < 0.001$). Although peak diastolic flow velocity was similar in the two subsets of patients, diastolic deceleration rate was significantly higher in patients with MCE no-reflow than in those with MCE reflow (107 ± 76 vs. 56 ± 31 cm/sec²; $p < 0.01$) (Fig. 14.9). The changes observed in the coronary flow velocity pattern in patients with no-reflow have been explained as the consequence of extensive microvascular damage, resulting in decrease in intramyocardial blood pool and increase in microvascular impedance. In patients with no-reflow, the blood pool would be rapidly filled in the early phase of diastole, with the consequence of a rapid deceleration in diastolic anterograde flow. The increase in myocardial stress during systole usually squeezes the intramyocardial blood, which is pooled during diastole, into the coronary venous circulation, but in patients with no-reflow the pooled blood cannot easily cross the microvasculature due to the high microvascular impedance and will be pushed back to the epicardial coronary artery, producing the early SFR (70). A second blood flow velocity pattern has been described as associated with TIMI grade 2 flow, characterized by slow anterograde systolic and diastolic flow velocity

waveforms. This pattern has been related to an increase in arterial resistance, possibly associated with a large thrombus burden with high probability of microvascular obstruction by microemboli (71).

The evaluation of coronary flow velocity after successful epicardial reperfusion appears to predict recovery of LV function. In 68 consecutive patients (72) who underwent successful primary PCI, resting average peak velocity ≤10 cm/sec, average systolic peak velocity ≤5 cm/sec, rapid diastolic deceleration time <600 milliseconds, and early SFR significantly predicted a composite end point combining cardiac death, recurrent MI, and congestive heart failure. At multivariate analysis, the only Doppler-derived parameter independently associated with a worse outcome was rapid diastolic deceleration time (OR 5.4; 95% CI, 1.5–19.3; $p = 0.01$).

While coronary blood flow velocity patterns have been extensively studied in the setting of reperfused AMI, less data exist regarding the clinical value of coronary flow reserve (CFR) measured immediately after reperfusion. In the experimental model (73), viable reperfused myocardium had normal basal flow, while CFR, which was intact at the start of reperfusion, decreased in the first few hours, and recovered completely within one week. In irreversibly damaged myocardium, both basal flow and CFR were severely and permanently impaired. In 67 consecutive patients (74) who had a first anterior AMI and were treated with primary PCI, CFR significantly correlated with the change of wall motion score at three weeks; the optimal cutoff value for CFR for predicting wall motion recovery was 1.4 (sensitivity 85%, specificity 94%).

Recent studies suggest the possibility of evaluating the occurrence of no-reflow using noninvasive transthoracic Doppler echocardiography in patients with anterior AMI. Short deceleration time of early diastolic flow velocity has been described to identify the no-reflow after anterior AMI. In 15 patients with anterior AMI who were successfully reperfused by primary PCI, diastolic deceleration time correlated well with myocardial viability predicted by myocardial fluorodeoxyglucose uptake (75). In this study, diastolic deceleration time <190 milliseconds was always associated with nonviable myocardium. However, whether flow velocity profile assessed by transthoracic Doppler echocardiography predicts myocardial viability remains uncertain (76).

Cardiac Biomarkers

Successful reperfusion is associated with a rapid release of many myocardial proteins into the blood stream, which is considered to be the result of the washout after perfusion restoration at the cellular level. Therefore, the analysis of the rate of release of markers such as myoglobin, troponin, and CK during the first minutes after the application of reperfusion treatment might allow identification of patients with myocardial tissue reperfusion. Obviously, the study of the kinetics of cardiac biomarker release to derive information about the result of reperfusion treatment is limited to patients treated with i.v. fibrinolytic therapy, since in patients treated with PCI, a direct evaluation of the result in terms of recanalization of the infarct artery and restoration of TIMI grade 3 flow may be directly performed at the end of the invasive procedure. Characteristics of a cardiac biomarker as an ideal marker of reperfusion would be early release after reperfusion, rapid clearance from blood, high myocardial specificity, and availability of a rapid quantitative assay. Myoglobin has been considered a suitable marker, due to its cytosolic location, small size, early peak, and rapid clearance after successful reperfusion (77), but troponins and CK have also been proved useful to predict early reperfusion success. In a study (78) including 105 patients with AMI who underwent early angiography after streptokinase, serial blood samples were collected to assay CK-MB mass, troponin T, and myoglobin concentrations. The ratios of the 60- and 90-minute concentrations to prefibrinolytic values were used to determine an index that could identify failure to achieve TIMI grade 3 flow in the infarct artery at 90 minutes. Ratios ≤ 5 at 60 minutes after thrombolysis detected failure to achieve 90-minutes TIMI grade 3 flow with 92% to 97% sensitivity, 43% to 60% specificity, 63% to 76% positive, and 86% to 94% negative predictive values. Ratios ≤ 10 at 90 minutes showed 88% to 95% sensitivity, 49% to 65% specificity, 61% to 69% positive, and 86% to 94% negative predictive values for TIMI flow grade <3. The overall predictive values were similar for all three markers. In another study from the same group (79), blood levels of troponin T, CK-MB, and myoglobin were measured before and 60 minutes after starting streptokinase infused for 30 to 60 minutes in 107 patients, who presented within 12 hours of symptom onset and underwent angiography at 90 minutes. On multivariate analysis, the factors associated with failure to achieve TIMI grade 3 flow were ST resolution <70% ($p = 0.009$), 60-min/baseline troponin T ratio of ≤ 5 ($p = 0.0004$), baseline CK-MB level of >4 μg/L ($p = 0.039$), or baseline myoglobin level of >85 μg/L ($p = 0.048$). On the basis of results of this study, a risk score, including clinical variables, ST resolution, and 60-min/baseline ratios of troponin T, CK-MB, and/or myoglobin, was developed, which allowed the prediction of failure to achieve TIMI grade 3 flow with 90% accuracy. The evaluation of this score might facilitate triage of patients at 60 minutes after fibrinolysis to additional reperfusion treatment.

ST-Segment Resolution

The ST-segment elevation observed on the electrocardiogram during acute ischemia is related to the functional damage of the involved myocytes, which, deprived of oxygen, lose adenosine triphosphate–dependent transmembrane ion gradients (80). After the application of reperfusion treatment, ST-segment recovery identifies the reversal of this condition due to myocardial reperfusion in the presence of maintained myocardial viability. In the experimental model of coronary occlusion reperfusion, the restoration of myocardial perfusion was associated with rapid normalization of ST-segment elevation (81). In the clinical setting the relevance of ST-segment evaluation was first defined by Schröder et al. (82,83), who proposed a classification based on the degree of ST-segment resolution: complete ($\geq 70\%$), partial (31–69%), or none ($\leq 30\%$). They found that the degree of ST-segment resolution could predict accurately the risk of death and congestive heart failure in patients treated with fibrinolytic therapy (82,83). Subsequent studies confirmed statistically significant differences between the three groups of ST-segment resolution evaluated at 90 to 180 minutes after thrombolysis. One-month mortality increased from 1.0% to 2.8% in patients with complete ST-segment resolution to 4.2% to 6.0% in patients with partial resolution to 5.9% to 17.5% in patients with no resolution (84). These results confirm that ST-segment resolution is a reliable predictor of mortality.

The better outcome of patients with rapid ST-segment resolution may be related to a more complete restoration of myocardial perfusion. In the TIMI-14 substudy (85,86), where tPA and a combination of abciximab plus reduced-dose tPA were used, patients with complete ST-segment resolution at 90 minutes had a 94% likelihood of infarct artery patency and a 79% probability of TIMI grade 3 flow. In the HIT-4 study (87), where streptokinase was used, the likelihood of infarct artery patency in patients with complete ST-segment resolution was 92%, and the probability of TIMI grade 3 flow was 69%. While complete ST-segment resolution is a highly accurate predictor of infarct artery patency, the absence of ST-segment resolution does not accurately predict an occluded infarct artery. In the TIMI-14 substudy (85), patients with no ST-segment resolution had a persistent occlusion of the infarct artery in only 32% of cases while 68% still had a patent infarct artery, 44% with TIMI grade 3 flow. In the HIT-4 study (87), the likelihood of infarct artery occlusion in patients with no ST-segment resolution was 59%; however, 41% of patients with no ST-segment resolution had a patent infarct artery, 16% with TIMI grade 3 flow. The absence of ST-segment resolution despite a patent infarct artery may be an indicator of irreversible myocardial damage or may reflect an incomplete restoration of perfusion within the jeopardized

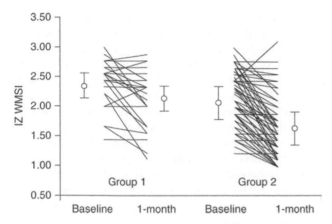

Figure 14.10 Plot of IZ WMSI at baseline and at follow-up in the 35 patients with no reduction in ST elevation (*group 1*) and in the 67 patients with ≥ 50% reduction in ST-segment elevation (*group 2*). Infarct zone wall motion score index decreased by 0.22 in 12 group 1 patients (34%) and in 52 group 2 patients (78%) (*p* < 0.001). *Abbreviation*: IZ WMSI, infarct zone wall motion score index. *Source*: From Ref. 88.

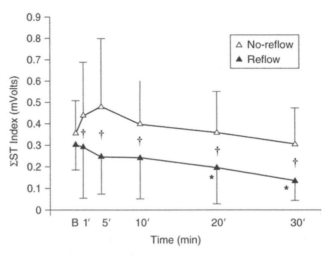

Figure 14.11 Time course of the ΣST index (in mV) in patients with myocardial reflow (*solid triangles*) and in patients with no-reflow phenomenon (*open triangles*). Data are reported as mean values ± SD. B = baseline. Analysis of variance for repeated measures: *p* < 0.005 versus baseline (within groups); †*p* < 0.005 (between groups). *Abbreviations*: ΣST index, ST-segment elevation sum index. *Source*: From Ref. 91.

myocardium due to microvascular damage. Since the demonstration of a TIMI grade 3 flow does not ensure restoration of myocardial tissue perfusion, rapid ST-segment resolution might be a more reliable marker of successful myocardial reperfusion. In patients treated with successful primary PCI, rapid ST-segment resolution was shown to predict greater improvement in LVEF, smaller infarct size, and more favorable prognosis as compared with delayed ST-segment resolution (88–90). In a study from our group (88) patients with ST-segment reduction ≥50% observed in a single selected lead 30 minutes after the end of the procedure had lower peak CK release and better LV functional recovery than those with persistent ST-segment elevation (Fig. 14.10). At one-month follow-up, LVEF was significantly higher in patients with rapid ST-segment resolution. At multivariate analysis, rapid ST-segment resolution was the only independent predictor of functional recovery (*p* < 0.001).

The relation between ST-segment changes and microvascular perfusion was evaluated in a study (91) including patients with AMI who had got the infarct artery recanalized by primary PCI with restoration of a TIMI grade 3 flow. Myocardial perfusion in the infarct area was assessed by MCE, performed before PCI to evaluate the risk area, and shortly after the end of the procedure to evaluate microvascular reperfusion. ST-segment changes were evaluated before PCI and, afterward, for a period of 30 minutes after TIMI grade 3 flow restoration. MCE showed recovery of perfusion in 26 patients and no-reflow in 11 patients. In patients with myocardial reperfusion, the ST-segment elevation progressively declined, while in patients with no-reflow, no significant change was observed (Fig. 14.11). Reduction ≥50% in ST-segment elevation occurred in 20 of the 26 patients with reflow and in 1 of the 11 with no-reflow (*p* = 0.0002). An additional increase ≥30% in ST-segment elevation occurred in three patients with reflow and in seven with no-reflow (Fig. 14.12). The increase in ST-segment elevation was transient in all the three patients with myocardial reflow because they had a ≥50% reduction on the 30-minute electrocardiogram. The increase in ST-segment elevation also showed a reduction in the seven patients with no-reflow, but this reduction was <50% compared with the baseline value. The additional increase in ST-segment elevation, occurring immediately after the restoration of a TIMI grade 3 flow, might be related to the myocardial cell injury induced by reperfusion. The different speed and magnitude of the subsequent ST-segment resolution might reflect different degrees of myocyte injury, light and reversible in patients with reflow, severe and irreversible in patients with no-reflow. However, the significance of the additional ST-segment elevation observed in patients with no reflow remains uncertain. In 26 patients with no reflow identified on the basis of MCE performed immediately after successful PCI, 13 patients showed >30% additional increase in ST-segment elevation, whereas 13 did not. The additional increase in ST-segment elevation was not associated with more severe microvascular damage on MCE, higher peak CK, higher incidence of LV remodeling, or worse outcome at follow-up (92). It has been hypothesized that, with similar extension of microvascular damage, the additional increase in ST-segment

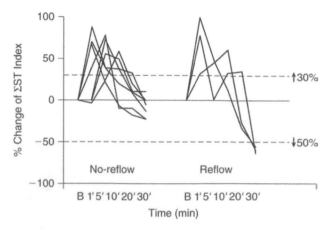

Figure 14.12 Percent changes in ΣST Index (in mV) on the electrocardiograms recorded before coronary angioplasty and at 1, 5, 10, 20, and 30 minutes after the first restoration of a TIMI grade 3 flow in patients with myocardial reflow (*right*) and in patients with no-reflow phenomenon (*left*) who had a ≥ 30% additional increase in ΣST index. The increase in ΣST index was transient in all three patients with myocardial reflow because they had a ≥ 50% reduction on the 30-minute electrocardiogram. The increase in ΣST index showed a reduction also in the seven patients with no-reflow, but this reduction was <50% compared with the baseline value. *Abbreviations*: TIMI, Thrombolysis in Myocardial Infarction; SST index, ST-segment elevation sum index. *Source*: From Ref. 91.

elevation represents a response of residual viable cells to reperfusion in the jeopardized myocardium.

On the basis of these studies, the analysis of ST-segment resolution, using both static serial electrocardiograms and continuous ST-monitoring, may be considered a valid method to evaluate myocardial reperfusion and viability. Complete ST-segment resolution at 30 to 180 minutes after reperfusion treatment indicates high probability of successful reperfusion at both epicardial and microvascular level; in this condition the prognosis of patients is excellent, and the probability of LV functional recovery is high. On the other hand, no ST-segment resolution suggests either an occluded artery or a patent artery with failure of microvascular or myocardial reperfusion; in this case the short-term and long-term mortality is higher than that observed in patients with complete or partial ST-segment resolution (93). However, which is the optimal cutoff temporal value to distinguish patients with and without optimal reperfusion remains undetermined. It is possible that different parameters have to be considered for fibrinolytic therapy and primary PCI. Since the achievement of reperfusion after initiation of fibrinolysis occurs generally after 45 to 60 minutes, the traditional cutoff of 90 minutes to evaluate ST-segment resolution may be the best option. On the other hand, in patients treated with primary PCI, the optimal time window for evaluating ST-segment resolution is probably

shorter, since patients with normal versus impaired myocardial tissue perfusion after primary PCI have been demonstrated to differ in 30-minute ST-segment resolution but not in 60- or 90-minute ST-segment resolutions (94). Similarly, which is the optimal entity of ST-segment resolution (50% or 70%) in comparison with the ST-segment level recorded before the application of reperfusion therapy to predict the outcome of patients is unclear. In a study by our group in patients with AMI treated with primary PCI and adjunctive abciximab therapy, ST-segment elevation resolution was showed to require a high threshold to maximize the classification of patients. In this study, the optimal ST-resolution cutoff was > 60% with 77% sensitivity and 51% specificity for predicting a favorable outcome (95).

CONCLUSIONS

The first step in the optimal management of AMI is to obtain the early and complete restoration of anterograde flow. However, epicardial coronary artery recanalization may not be sufficient to ensure a benefit in terms of myocardial salvage because this requires restoration of myocardial tissue perfusion and preserved myocardial viability. It has been demonstrated that a large part of patients with patent epicardial coronary artery and TIMI grade 3 flow have a severe microvascular damage conditioning the occurrence of no-reflow. Patients with no-reflow have poor LV functional recovery and are at high risk of early and late congestive heart failure and death. Despite its prognostic relevance, the accurate assessment of microvascular reperfusion in AMI and its effects on myocardial tissue is difficult. The ideal modality would combine information on microvascular perfusion and myocardial viability. The development of new angiographic indexes has improved the ability of coronary angiography to provide a more accurate evaluation of microvascular reperfusion. However, no information on myocardial viability can be obtained. The extensive use of MCE, which is a potentially interesting method to explore myocardial perfusion, has been prevented by the report of severe side effects related to the use of ultrasound contrast agents in unstable patients. Intracoronary Doppler flow-wire is an invasive tool, which may offer some information about microvascular status but not on myocardial viability. Other imaging methods, including nuclear scintigraphy, MRI, and MDCT, have the advantage of evaluating both myocardial perfusion and viability. Cardiac MRI has the potential to assess myocardial perfusion, characterize myocardial tissue (viable or scar), and evaluate contractile function and reserve. Nuclear scintigraphy has similar diagnostic capabilities but a suboptimal spatial resolution. Concerns about MDCT are the use of iodinated contrast agents and high radiation exposure to the patient.

However, all these techniques require a complex organization and are inadequate to provide early and rapid information about myocardial reperfusion and viability. Serum cardiac markers have been evaluated in their ability to identify the success or failure of epicardial reperfusion, but their utility is limited to an indirect assessment of the result in patients treated with fibrinolytics. The electrocardiographic evaluation of ST-segment resolution allows a rapid, simple, inexpensive, and readily available assessment of myocardial tissue reperfusion, but remains a qualitative method, which does not quantify the extent of damage.

EDITOR'S COMMENT

A plethora of markers of myocardial perfusion is available. Most markers, but ST-segment elevation changes, have the major limitation that can provide only a snapshot of the microcirculation function at a defined time. An abnormal microvasculature function immediately after PCI may improve during hours or days after reperfusion. Conversely, a normal microvasculature function after PCI cannot exclude a **progressive** subsequent deterioration due to reperfusion injury. As a consequence, for practical purpose, in the setting of emergency PCI for AMI, ST-segment monitoring remains the more reliable marker of the effectiveness of reperfusion in AMI.

REFERENCES

1. Kloner RA, Ganote CE, Jennings RB. The "no-reflow" phenomenon after temporary coronary occlusion in the dog. J Clin Invest 1974; 54:1496–1508.
2. Rezkalla SH, Kloner RA. No-reflow phenomenon. Circulation 2002; 105:656–662.
3. Engler RL, Schmid-Scoenbein GW, Pavelec RS. Leukocyte capillary plugging in myocardial ischemia and reperfusion in the dog. Am J Pathol 1983; 111:98–111.
4. Murohara T, Buerke M, Lefer AM. Polymorphonuclear leukocyte-induced vasocontraction and endothelial dysfunction. Role of selectins. Arterioscler Thromb 1994; 14:1509–1519.
5. Minamino T, Kitakaze M, Asanuma H, et al. Endogenous adenosine inhibits P-selectin-dependent format of coronary microemboli during hypoperfusion in dogs. J Clin Invest 1998; 101:1643–1653.
6. Gavin JB, Maxwell L, Edgar SG. Microvascular involvement in cardiac pathology. J Mol Cell Cardiol 1998; 30:2531–2540.
7. Kiyak JH, Zerbino DD. Pathogenesis and morphogenesis of microcirculatory disorders in myocardial infarction: clinical and ultrastructural examination. Pol J Pathol 1996; 47:27–32.
8. Gregorini L, Marco J, Kozakova M, et al. α-Adrenergic blockade improves recovery of myocardial perfusion and function after coronary stenting in patients with acute myocardial infarction. Circulation 1999; 99:482–490.
9. Lefroy DC, Wharton J, Crake T. Regional changes in angiotensin II receptor density after experimental myocardial infarction. J Mol Cell Cardiol 1996; 28:429–440.
10. Lerman A, Holmes DR, Herrmann J, et al. Microcirculatory dysfunction in ST-elevation myocardial infarction: cause, consequence, or both? Eur Heart J 2007; 28:788–797.
11. TIMI Study Group. The Thrombolysis in Myocardial Infarction (TIMI) trial: phase I findings. N Engl J Med 1993; 329:673–682.
12. Anderson JL, Karagounis LA, Califf RM. Meta analysis of five reported studies on the relation of early coronary patency grades with mortality and outcomes after acute myocardial infarction. Am J Cardiol 1996; 78:1–8.
13. Grines CL, Cox DA, Stone GW, et al. Coronary angioplasty with or without stent implantation for acute myocardial infarction: Stent Primary Angioplasty in Myocardial Infarction Study Group. N Engl J Med 1999; 341:1949–1956.
14. The Global Use of Strategies to Open Occluded Coronary Arteries in Acute Coronary Syndromes (GUSTO IIb) Angioplasty Substudy Investigators: a clinical trial comparing primary coronary angioplasty with tissue plasminogen activator for acute myocardial infarction. N Engl J Med 1997; 336:1621–1628.
15. Stone GW, Brodie BR, Griffin JJ, et al. Clinical and angiographic follow-up after primary stenting in acute myocardial infarction: the Primary Angioplasty in Myocardial Infarction (PAMI) stent pilot trial. Circulation 1999; 99:1548–1554.
16. Gibson CM, Cannon CP, Daley WL, et al. The TIMI frame count: a quantitative method of assessing coronary artery flow. Circulation 1996; 93:879–888.
17. Gibson CM, Murphy SA, Rizzo MJ, et al. Relationship between TIMI frame count and clinical outcomes after thrombolytic administration. Circulation 1999; 99:1945–1950.
18. Gibson CM, Pride YB, Buros JL, et al. Relation of hyperemic epicardial flow to outcomes among patients with ST-segment elevation myocardial infarction receiving fibrinolytic therapy. Am J Cardiol 2008; 1001:1232–1238.
19. van't Hof AWJ, Liem A, Suryapranata H, et al. Angiographic assessment of myocardial reperfusion in patients treated with primary angioplasty for acute myocardial infarction. Myocardial blush grade. Circulation 1998; 97:2302–2306.
20. Henriques JPS, Zijlstra F, van 't Hof AWJ, et al. Angiographic assessment of reperfusion in acute myocardial infarction by myocardial blush grade. Circulation 2003; 107:2115–2119.
21. Costantini CO, Stone GW, Mehran R, et al. Frequency, correlates, and clinical implications of myocardial perfusion after primary angioplasty and stenting, with and without glycoprotein IIb/III inhibition, in acute myocardil infarction. J Am Coll Cardiol 2004; 21:44:305–312.
22. Gibson CM, Cannon CP, Murphy SA, et al., for the TIMI Study Group. Relationship of TIMI myocardial perfusion

grade to mortality after administration of thrombolytic drugs. Circulation 2000; 101:125–130.

23. Brener SJ, Moliterno DJ, Aylward PE, et al. Reperfusion after primary angioplasty for ST-elevation myocardial infarction: predictors of success and relationship to clinical outcomes in the APEX-AMI Angiographic Study. Eur Heart J 2008; 29:1127–1135.

24. Agati L, Tonti G, Pedrizzetti G, et al. Clinical application of quantitative analysis in real-time MCE. Eur J Echocardiogr 2004; 45(suppl 2):S9–S15.

25. Cheirif JB, Narkiewicz-Jodko JB, Hawkins HK, et al. Myocardial contrast echocardiography: relation of collateral perfusion to extent of injury and severity of contractile dysfunction in a canine model of coronary thrombosis and reperfusion. J Am Coll Cardiol 1995; 26:537–546.

26. Cobb FR, Bache RJ, Rivas F, et al. Local effects of acute cellular injury on regional myocardial blood flow. J Clin Invest 1976; 57:1359–1368.

27. Villanueva FS, Galsheen WP, Sklenar J, et al. Characterization of spatial patterns of flow within the reperfused myocardium by myocardial contrast echocardiography. Implications in determining extent of myocardial salvage. Circulation 1993; 88:2596–2606.

28. Ito H, Tomooka T, Sakai N, et al. Lack of myocardial perfusion immediately after successful thrombolysis. A predictor of poor recovery of left ventricular function in anterior myocardial infarction. Circulation 1992; 85:1699–1705.

29. Lim YJ, Nanto S, Masuyama T, et al. Myocardial salvage: its assessment and prediction by the analysis of serial myocardial contrast echocardiograms in patients with acute myocardial infarction. Am Heart J 1994; 128:649–656.

30. Kenner MD, Zajac EJ, Kondos GT, et al. Ability of the no-reflow phenomenon during an acute myocardial infarction to predict left ventricular dysfunction at one-month follow-up. Am J Cardiol 1995; 76:861–868.

31. Bolognese L, Antoniucci D, Rovai D, et al. Myocardial contrast echocardiography versus dobutamine echocardiography for predicting functional recovery after acute myocardial infarction treated with primary coronary angioplasty. J Am Coll Cardiol 1996; 28:1677–1683.

32. Ragosta M, Camarano G, Kaul S, et al. Microvascular integrity indicates myocellular viability in patients with recent myocardial infarction. New insights using myocardial contrast echocardiography. Circulation 1994; 89:2562–2569.

33. Camarano G, Ragosta M, Gimple LW, et al. Identification of viable myocardium with contrast echocardiography in patients with poor left ventricular systolic function caused by recent or remote myocardial infarction. Am J Cardiol 1995; 75:215–219.

34. Bolognese L, Carrabba N, Parod G, et al. Impact of microvascular dysfunction on left ventricular remodeling and long-term clinical outcome after primary coronary angioplasty for acute myocardial infarction. Circulation 2004; 109:1121–1126.

35. Khumri TM, Nayyar S, Idupulapati M, et al. Usefulness of myocardial contrast echocardiography in predicting late mortality in patients with anterior wall acute myocardial infarction. Am J Cardiol 2006; 98:1150–1155.

36. Galiuto L, Garramone B, Scarà A, et al. The extent of microvascular damage during myocardial contrast echocardiography is superior to other known indexes of post-infarct reperfusion in predicting left ventricular remodeling. J Am Coll Cardiol 2008; 51:552–559.

37. Schofer J, Montz R, Mathey DG. Scintigraphic evidence of the "no reflow" phenomenon in human beings after coronary thrombolysis. J Am Coll Cardiol 1985; 5:593–598.

38. Reduto LA, Freund GC, Gaeta JM, et al. Coronary artery reperfusion in acute myocardial infarction: beneficial effects of intracoronary streptokinase on left ventricular salvage and performance. Am Heart J 1981; 102:1168–1177.

39. De Coster PM, Melin JA, Detry JMR, et al. Coronary artery reperfusion in acute myocardial infarction: assessment by pre- and post-intervention thallium-201 myocardial perfusion imaging. Am J Cardiol 1985; 55:889–895.

40. Santoro GM, Bisi G, Sciagrà R, et al. Single photon emission computed tomography with technetium-99m-hexakis-2-methoxy-isobutyl isonitrile in acute myocardial infarction before and after thrombolytic treatment: assessment of salvaged myocardium and prediction of late functional recovery. J Am Coll Cardiol 1990; 15:301–314.

41. Bisi G, Sciagrà R, Santoro GM, et al. Comparison of tomographic and planar imaging for the evaluation of thrombolytic therapy in acute myocardial infarction using pre- and post-treatment myocardial scintigraphy- with technetium-99m sestamibi. Am Heart J 1991; 122:13–22.

42. Gibbons RJ, Holmes DR, Reeder GS, et al. Immediate angioplasty compared with the administration of a thrombolytic agent followed by conservative treatment for myocardial infarction. N Engl J Med 1993; 328:685–691.

43. Wackers FJ, Gibbons RJ, Verani MS, et al. Serial quantitative planar technetium-99m isonitrile imaging in acute myocardial infarction: efficacy for non-invasive assessment of thrombolytic therapy. J Am Coll Cardiol 1989; 14:861–873.

44. Pellikka PA, Behrenbeck T, Verani MS, et al. Serial changes in myocardial perfusion using tomographic technetium-99m-hexakis-2methoxy-2-methylpropyl-isonitrile imaging following reperfusion therapy of myocardial infarction. J Nucl Med 1990; 31:1269–1275.

45. Galli M, Marcassa C, Boili R, et al. Spontaneous delayed recovery of perfusion and contraction after the first five weeks after anterior infarction. Circulation 1994; 90:1386–1397.

46. Sciagrà R, Bolognese L, Rovai D, et al. Detecting myocardial salvage after primary PTCA: early myocardial contrast echocardiography versus delayed sestamibi perfusion imaging. J Nucl Med 1999; 40:363–370.

47. Lomboy CT, Schulman DS, Grill HP, et al. Rest-redistribution thallium-201 scintigraphy to determine myocardial viability early after myocardial infarction. J Am Coll Cardiol 1995; 25:210–217.

48. Maes A, Van de Werf F, Nuyts J, et al. Impaired myocardial tissue perfusion early after successful thrombolysis. Impact on myocardial flow, metabolism, and function at late follow-up. Circulation 1995; 92:2072–2078.

49. Maes AF, Van de Werf F, Mesotten LV, et al. Early assessment of regional myocardial blood flow metabolism in thrombolysis in myocardial infarction flow grade 3 reperfused myocardial infarction using carbon-11acetate. J Am Coll Cardiol 2001; 37:30–36.

50. Sciagrà R, Sestini S, Bolognese L, et al. Comparison of dobutamine echocardiography and 99mTc-sestamibi tomography for prediction of left ventricular ejection fraction outcome after acute myocardial infarction treated with successful primary coronary angioplasty. J Nucl Med 2002; 43:8–14.

51. Lima JA, Judd RM, Bazille A, et al. Regional heterogeneity of human myocardial infarcts demonstrated by contrast-enhanced MRI. Potential mechanisms. Circulation 1995; 92:1117–1125.

52. Judd RM, Lugo-Olivieri CH, Arai MKT, et al. Physiologic basis of myocardial contrast enhancement in fast magnetic resonance images of 2-day-old reperfused canine infarcts. Circulation 1995; 92:1092–1010.

53. Kim RJ, Chen EL, Lima JA, et al. Myocardial Gd-DTPA kinetics determine MRI contrast enhancement and reflect the extent and severity of myocardial injury after acute reperfused infarction. Circulation 1996; 94:3318–3326.

54. Duffy KJ, Ferrari VA. Prognosis following acute myocardial infarction: insights from cardiovascular magnetic resonance. Curr Cardiol Rep 2007; 9:57–62.

55. Wu KC, Kim RJ, Bluemke DA, et al. Quantification and time course of microvascular obstruction by contrast-enhanced echocardiography and magnetic resonance imaging following acute myocardial infarction and reperfusion. J Am Coll Cardiol 1998; 32:1756–1764.

56. Wu KC, Zerhouni EA, Judd RM, et al. Prognostic significance of microvascular obstruction by magnetic resonance imaging in patients with acute myocardial infarction. Circulation 1998; 97:765–772.

57. Taylor AJ, Al-Saadi N, Abdel-Aty H, et al. Detection of acutely impaired microvascular reperfusion after infarct angioplasty with magnetic resonance imaging. Circulation 2004; 109:2080–2085.

58. Yan AT, Gibson CM, Larose E, et al. Characterization of microvascular dysfunction after acute myocardial infarction by cardiovascular magnetic resonance first-pass perfusion and late gadolinium enhancement imaging. J Cardiovasc Magn Reson 2006; 8:831–837.

59. Hombach V, Grebe O, Merkle N, et al. Sequelae of acute myocardial infarction regarding cardiac structure and function and their prognostic significance as assessed by magnetic resonance imaging. Eur Heart J 2005; 26:549–557.

60. Bogaert J, Kalantzi M, Rademakers FE, et al. Determinants and impact of microvascular obstruction in successfully reperfused ST-segment elevation myocardial infarction. Assessment by magnetic resonance imaging. Eur Radiol 2007; 17:2572–2580.

61. Mahnken AH, Koos R, Katoh M, et al. Assessment of myocardial viability in reperfused acute myocardial infarction using 16-slice computed tomography in comparison to magnetic resonance imaging. J Am Coll Cardiol 2005; 45:2042–2047.

62. Lardo AC, Corderiro MA, Silva C, et al. Contrast-enhanced multidetector computed tomography viability imaging after myocardial infarction: characterization of myocyte death, microvascilar obstruction, and chronic scar. Circulation 2006; 113:394–404.

63. Gerber BL, Belge B, Legros GJ, et al. Characterization of acute and chronic myocardial infarcts by multidetector computed tomography: comparison with contrast-enhanced magnetic resonance. Circulation 2006; 113:823–833.

64. Hoffmann U, Millea R, Enzweiler C, et al. Acute myocardial infarction: contrast-enhanced multidetector row CT in a porcine model. Radiology 2004; 231:607–701.

65. Gosalia A, Haramati LB, Sheth MP, et al. CT detection of acute myocardial infarction. AJR Am J Roentgenol 2004; 182:1563–1566.

66. Baks T, Cademartiri F, Moelker AD, et al. Assessment of acute reperfused myocardial infarction with delayed enhancement 64-MDCT. AJR Am J Roentgenol 2007; 188:W135–W137.

67. Sato A, Hiroe M, Nozato T, et al. Early validation study of 64-slice multidetector computed tomography for the assessment of myocardial viability and the prediction of left ventricular remodelling after acute myocardial infarction. Eur Heart J 2008; 29:490–498.

68. Lessick J, Dragu R, Mutlak D, et al. Is functional improvement after myocardial infarction predicted with myocardial enhancement patterns at multidetector CT? Radiology 2007; 244:736–744.

69. Nakamura M, Tsunoda T, Wakatsuki T, et al. Distal coronary flow velocity immediately after direct angioplasty for acute myocardial infarction. Am Heart J 1996; 132:251–257.

70. Iwakura K, Ito H, Takiuchi S, et al. Alternation in the coronary blood flow velocity pattern in patients with no reflow and reperfused acute myocardial infarction. Circulation 1996; 94:1269–1275.

71. Yamamoto K, Ito H, Iwakura K, et al. Two different coronary blood flow velocity patterns in Thrombolysis in Myocardial Infarction flow grade 2 in acute myocardial infarction. Insight into mechanisms of microvascular dysfunction. J Am Coll Cardiol 2002; 40:1755–1760.

72. Furber AP, Prunier F, Nguyen HCP, et al. Coronary blood flow assessment after successful angioplasty for acute myocardial infarction predicts the risk of long-term cardiac events. Circulation 2004; 110:3527–3533.

73. Vanhaecke J, Flameng W, Borgers M, et al. Evidence for decreased coronary flow reserve in viable postischemic myocardium. Circ Res 1990; 67:1201–1210.

74. Takahashi T, Hiasa Y, Ohara Y, et al. Usefulness of coronary flow reserve immediately after primary coronary stenting in predicting wall motion recovery in patients with anterior wall acute myocardial infarction. Am J Cardiol 2004; 94:1033–1037.

75. Saraste A, Koskenvuo JW, Saraste M, et al. Coronary artery flow velocity profile measured by transthoracic Doppler echocardiography predicts myocardial viability after acute myocardial infarction. Heart 2007; 93:456–457.

76. Voci P, Mariano E, Pizzuto F, et al. Coronary recanalization in anterior myocardial infarction. The open perforator hypothesis. J Am Coll Cardiol 2002; 40:1205–1213.

77. Jurlander B, Clemmensen P, Ohman E, et al. Serum myoglobin for the early non-invasive detection of coronary reperfusion in patients with acute myocardial infarction. Eur Heart J 1996; 17:399–406.

78. Stewart JT, French JK, Theroux P, et al. Early noninvasive identification of failed reperfusion after intravenous thrombolytic therapy in acute myocardial infarction. J Am Coll Cardiol 1998; 31:1499–1505.

79. French JK, Ramanathan K, Stewart JT, et al. A score predicts failure of reperfusion after fibrinolytic therapy for acute myocardial infarction. Am Heart J 2003; 145:508–514.

80. Maroko PR, Libby P, Ginks WR, et al. Coronary artery reperfusion. I. Early effects on local myocardial function and the extent of myocardial necrosis. J Clin Invest 1972; 51:2710–2716.

81. Kleber AG. ST-segment elevation in the electrocardiogram: a sign of myocardial ischemia. Cardiovasc Res 2000; 45:111–118.

82. Schröder R, Dissmann R, Bruggemann T, et al. Extent of early ST segment elevation resolution: a simple but strong predictor of outcome in patients with acute myocardial infarction. J Am Coll Cardiol 1994; 24:384–391.

83. Schröder R, Wegscheider K, Schroder K, et al., for the INJECT Trial Group. Extent of early ST segment elevation resolution: a strong predictor of outcome in patients with acute myocardial infarction and a sensitive measure to compare thrombolytic regimens. A substudy of the International Joint Efficacy Comparison of Thrombolytics (INJECT) trial. J Am Coll Cardiol 1995; 26:1657–1664.

84. Neuhaus KL, Tebbe U, Schröder R. Resolution of ST segment elevation is an early predictor of mortality in patients with acute myocardial infarction: meta-analysis of three thrombolysis trials. Circulation 1998; 98(suppl I):I–632 (abstr).

85. de Lemos JA, Antman EM, Gibson CM, et al. Abciximab improves both epicardial flow and myocardial reperfusion in ST elevation myocardial infarction: observations from the TIMI 14 trial. Circulation 2000; 101:239–243.

86. de Lemos JA, Antman EM, McCabe CH, et al. ST-segment resolution and infarct related artery patency and flow after thrombolytic therapy. Am J Cardiol 2000; 85:299–304.

87. Zeymer U, Schröder R, Neuhaus KL. Noninvasive detection of early infarct vessel patency by resolution of ST-segment elevation in patients with thrombolysis for acute myocardial infarction: results of the angiographic substudy of the Hirudin for Improvement of Thrombolysis (HIT)-4 trial. Eur Heart J 2001; 22:769–775.

88. Santoro GM, Antoniucci D, Valenti R, et al. Rapid reduction of ST-segment elevation after successful direct angioplasty in acute myocardial infarction. Am J Cardiol 1997; 80:685–689.

89. van't Hof A, Liem A, de Boer M, et al. Clinical value of 12-lead electrocardiogram after successful reperfusion therapy for acute myocardial infarction. Lancet 1997; 350:615–619.

90. Matetzky S, Novikov M, Gruberg L, et al. The significance of persistent ST elevation versus early resolution of ST segment elevation after primary PTCA. J Am Coll Cardiol 1999; 34:1932–1938.

91. Santoro GM, Valenti R, Buonamici P, et al. Relation between ST-segment changes and myocardial perfusion evaluated by myocardial contrast echocardiography in patients with acute myocardial infarction treated with direct angioplasty. Am J Cardiol 1998; 82:932–937.

92. Carrabba N, Parodi G, Valenti R, et al. Significance of additional ST segment elevation in patients with no reflow after angioplasty for acute myocardial infarction. J Am Soc Echocardiogr 2007; 20:262–269.

93. de Lemos JA, Braunwald E. ST segment resolution as a tool for assessing the efficacy of reperfusion therapy. J Am Coll Cardiol 2001; 38:1283–1294.

94. Terkelsen CJ, Norgaard BL, Lassen JF, et al. Potential significance of spontaneous and interventional ST-changes in patients transferred for primary percutaneous coronary intervention: observations from the ST-monitoring in acute myocardial infarction study (the MONAMI study). Eur Heart J 2006; 27:267–275.

95. Sciagrà R, Parodi G, Migliorini A, et al. ST-segment analysis to predict infarct size and functional outcome in acute myocardial infarction treated with primary coronary intervention and adjunctive abciximab therapy. Am J Cardiol 2006; 97:48–54.

Index

Printed and bound by CPI Group (UK) Ltd, Croydon, CR0 4YY

18/10/2024

01776250-0019